NEW CONCEPTS IN MEDICINE
Volume II

New Concepts in Disease Spread
&
Control of Disease Spread
Part I
1ˢᵗ Edition

Disease Spread during Late Decades in Brief
Helicobacter pylori and Disease Spread; Misconception& Facts
Functional Dyspepsia
Misconception and Misbehavior towards *H. pylori* is Leading to Major Spread of Illness
Stop Fighting the Stomach Bacterium; Acid Reflux was not as Such before the Anti-*H. pylori* Antibiotics
The Real Fact in Spastic Colitis& Irritable Bowel Syndrome; *Spastic Colitis is a Big Scientific Lie*
The Dramatic Spread of Diabetes Mellitus Worldwide and Influence of Helicobacter pylori. *The World's Burden of DM during Late Decades is not on the Account of Type II Diabetes but on Stress Diabetes due to a Biological Colonic Toxic Stress; Stress Diabetes could be Corrected*
The Truth in the Challenge of Childhood Diabetes during Late Decades
How Should the World Manage the Challenge of Diabetes Mellitus!!
An Alternative Approach for the Rising Challenge of Hypertensive Illness via *H. pylori* Eradication; *Most Patients Could Quit Medications and Maintain Normal BP Values after Colon Clear*
Improvement of Idiopathic Cardiomyopathy After Colon Clear; *Not All Cardiomyopathy in Late Decades is Related to Viral Myocarditis but Mostly Toxic Myocarditis*
Influence of *Helicobacter pylori* on Thrombocytopenia in Children
Male Pelvic Congestion and Erectile Dysfunction; Obscure Reasons for an Obvious Phenomenon among the Young
Why Do Physicians Diagnose Gout in Young Adults with Perfect Kidney Function!!
Endometriosis and Ovarian Cystic Disease; Why so Linked as if Born Simultaneous!!
The Secret of the Silence of the Silent Maxillary Sinus Syndrome
Autism; An Approach for Definite Etiology and Definitive Etiologic Management; *Autism Might Not be a Disease of Definitive Cure but it is a Typical Disease of Definite Prevention*
Alzheimer and Helicobacter Pylori, Should We Fight and Kill or Save *H. Pylori*!! We Should Save H. Pylori; *Alzheimer Could be Readily Delayed until End of Life of a Person*
Autism and Alzheimer; the Etiopathologic Twins
Frequency of Leukemia during Late Decades May Indicate that the Anti-*Helicobacter Pylori* Antibiotic Strategy was a Therapeutic Mistake; *Does Leukemia in Late Decades Constitute an Influenza*
A Pathologic Etiology for the Rising World Challenge of Obesity and Dyslipidemia during Latest Three Decades; *Dyslipidemia was the Fake of Last Century*
The Hidden Truth behind Osteoporosis and Vitamin D Deficiency; *Why Osteoporosis and Vitamin D Deficiency are Lately Running among People like Common Cold!!*
A Simple Sustained Solution for Dissolution of the Cellulite

ABDULLAH M NASRAT
2019

Printed in the United States of America

Library of Congress Control Number: 2020900597
ISBN:Softcover   978-1-64376-791-8
eBook   978-1-64376-790-1

Republished by: PageTurner Press and Media LLC
Publication Date: 04/21/2020

To order copies of this book, contact:

PageTurner Press and Media
Phone: 1-888-447-9651
order@pageturner.us
www.pageturner.us

NEW CONCEPTS IN MEDICINE

Volume II

New Concepts in Disease Spread
&
Control of Disease Spread

Part I
1st Edition

BY
Abdullah M Nasrat
MBBS, MS

Revised by
Randa M Nasrat, MD   *Mohammad M Nasrat, MBBS*

Proof-Reviewed by
Salwa A Nasrat, BSPT, MSc
2019

<u>Preface Notice</u>

All venturesome scientists are aware of the many chances of going astray as they enter a new field. Michael Faraday, a prince of experimenters, testified that "I may be largely wrong, I am free to admit who can be right altogether in physical science which is essentially progressive and corrective". If Faraday could have such feeling towards experimentation in the territory of physics, how much readier to acknowledge the possibility of error should be an investigator who leads into the more complex and difficult field of biology.

Medicine is an ever-changing science; hence, was the name of this book "*New Concepts in Disease Spread and Control of Disease Spread*" under a main title of "*New Concepts in Medicine*". Disease spread was lately major and beyond control in spite of the many advances in medicine; therefore, introduction of new concepts in control of disease spread that could be truly of benefit to patients and practitioners was the motive and interest of the authors to provide this issue.

The "*New Concepts in Control of Disease Spread*" in this book depend mainly on three elements of a "*New Concept of Natural Drug-Free Therapy*" which is constituted of colon care, colon clear mediated by vinegar therapy and the potent natural senna purge and sero-clearanc done via blood-let out cupping therapy. In this book, the elements which are majorly used for control of disease spread are colon care and colon clear which are vinegar therapy and the senna purge while cupping therapy has been saved for a separate book which is volume IV the "*New Concepts in Blood-let Out Cupping Therapy*".

Here arise the question; could three elements only of a natural therapy, whatever its nature, control or share in the control of the current disease spread aggressively invading the whole world!! The answer is very simple; the clue in disease control is recognition of pathology as fundamental cure is withdrawal of pathology not introduction of pills and definitive cure is treatment of pathology but not merely treatment of symptoms. The main first hidden reason behind chronic and major illness is accumulation of toxins and inflammatory mediators in the circulation; the author of this fact is Morishita who is the Nobel Prize holder in 1968, while the second hidden reason is accumulation of potential toxins in the colon. These two reasons could account for the pathogenesis of more than 90% of diseases that require treatment; according to this clinical sense, three elements of an effective natural therapy could help to control most of the challenging current disease spread. The natural therapy and drug-free therapies are known and available in the East, Far East and many elsewhere but they lead the same mistake as the modern medicine which is introduction of herbs instead of pills but not taking the pathology out. The "New Concept of Drug-Free Therapy" in this book works on withdrawal of pathology or dealing with the real pathology if it includes introduction of therapeutic material; therefore, it is decisive.
October, 2019.

<u>Overview of the Book:</u>

This issue *"New Concepts in Disease Spread& Control of Disease Spread"* demonstrates that chronic illness has been flaring up worldwide beyond the traditional rules of spread of these diseases. The rising figures of disease spread are not scientifically logic and do not coincide with any medical statistics. This means that traditional measures employed to control these diseases could never be decisive or successful.

The *"New Concepts in Disease Spread& Control of Disease Spread"* also emphasizes that the current chronic diseases are mostly inadequately controlled in spite of extreme scientific efforts; this could further indicate the possibility of existence of a missed underlying common pathologic environmental error behind the world's burden of this disease spread. Therefore, most patients with chronic illness are inadequately controlled in spite of regular follow up of their medications and extreme carefulness about style of life.

The value of the *"New Concepts in Disease Spread& Control of Disease Spread"* lies in the true promising opportunity it gives for many patients of an adequate and permanent cure as fundamental cure is treatment of pathology but not of the symptoms and definitive cure is withdrawal of pathology not merely introduction of pills. It also lies in the real chance it gives for many people of adequate protection from major, chronic illness and cancer.

All the literature included in the *"New Concepts in Disease Spread& Control of Disease Spread"* has been peer-reviewed by International reviewers, accepted and already published in American and Canadian medical journals with digital object identification (DOI) which means that it is NCBI-indexed in addition of being available on Google as an open access except for an article concerning thrombocytopenia (ITP) in children which has been included because of its importance to patients, families and practitioners but it is still Google-indexed as an open access.

Word of the Author

Any patient with chronic illness would have a continued dream of fundamental cure; nobody can blame a patient for this dream even he seeks a treatment which is based upon controversial or new ideas. Controversy is always there and nobody can prevent that; from controversy new ideas arise and that is how knowledge and science move forwards. It is worthy to mention that the new ideas and new concepts of this book stand over solid scientific grounds as being peer-reviewed, accepted and published in International medical journals.

The rising figures of disease spread all over the world do not coincide with the traditional risk rules of spread of these diseases. Furthermore; the world literature demonstrates that most diseases are inadequately controlled despite the great advances in medicine. These facts were striking enough to attract the scientific enthusiasm of the authors together with their concern about patient's welfare in order to produce this issue of "_New Concepts in Disease Spread& Control of Disease Spread_".

<u>*The Author: Biography of the Author:*</u>

Egyptian, born in May 1950, General surgeon, graduated from Faculty of Medicine/Cairo University in June 1975, qualified in surgery from Faculty of Medicine/Cairo University in May 1979, he was research investigator since 1985, working as drug-free therapy consultant and chronic-illness control advisor in the Middle East since 2004, international speaker and international author having more than 36 international speaker presentations in East/West/Middle East and the Gulf, having 3 abstract publications in the American Medical Association journal, he is having 36 original article publications in American and Canadian International medical journals and 3 original articles published in Indian medical journals.

October, 2019

The Scientific Research Activity of the Author Published with Digital Object Identification (DOI) in International Medical Journals is listed at End of the Book

Introduction to the 1ˢᵗ Edition

"*New Concepts in Disease Spread& Control of Disease Spread*" is the second volume of a series of "*New Concepts in Medicine*" which are:

1. *New Concepts in Diabetes.*

2. *New Concepts in Disease Spread& Control of Disease Spread.*

3. *New Concepts on **Helicobacter pylori.***

4. *New Concepts in Blood-Let out Cupping Therapy.*

5. *New Concepts in Fundamental Therapy& Definitive Cure.*

6. *New Concepts in Natural Nutritional Drug-Free Therapy.*

7. *New Concepts in Physio-Benefits of Human Body Balance.*

The authors are wishing that patients, readers and medical practitioners would keep expecting these issues and evaluate the knowledge included in them as application of any new knowledge to the practice is the best valid proof that confirms its credibility and value reality. The first volume of this series which is "*New Concepts in Diabetes*" could be considered a revolution in diabetes knowledge of the last three decades as it is sufficient to prove that the world's burden of diabetes during late decades is not on the account of type II but on stress diabetes; type II diabetes is not curable but stress diabetes could be corrected.

"*New Concepts in Disease Spread& Control of Disease Spread*" will concentrate mainly on the new information of a disease with reference in brief to the established knowledge of the current disease spread and chronic illness in order to allow proper attention to what is new.

The authors are wishing that patients, readers and medical practitioners would benefit the *new concepts of knowledge in this issue of "Disease Spread& Control of Disease Spread"*.

October, 2019.

Dedication

I would like to dedicate this work to the family; all members of the family I owe them great favors.

This work is specially presented to whom I owe the motives, the emotions and even the troubles that accompanied every success in my life and the sweet taste of success to introduce this bookl, I owe her different love to the life since she is there in my way; she is my *"Salwa"*.

Abdullah M Nasrat

Acknowledgment

"*ACCEPT OUR THOUGHTS OF THANKS,*
WE HAVE NO WORDS, WORDS CAN NEVER SAY"
Gratitude Is Extended To All Who Helped To Make This Work Possible

A Message to Patients

We, the authors, would like to confirm to our patients and readers that the material in this book is all original material; moreover, the knowledge and results included in this book have been repeatedly and continuously justified over the past 15 years. We were approaching patients in their own places even treating them freely to observe progress and improvement of their conditions as we believe that the patient himself is the sole constantly open book for a medical knowledge; it is in turn the best way for re-assessment of any new concept in medicine. Our patients were followed up for at least 18 months but many of them were followed for 7-9 years.

All the knowledge of the *"New Concepts in Disease Spread& Control of Disease Spread"* contained within this book have been sufficiently accepted and presented in more than thirty international conferences. In addition, it is all reviewed, accepted and published in international peer-reviewed medical journals.

We would like also to re-assure our patients that most disease spread diagnosed during the last three decades (around 90%) were found typical cases of ***Helicobacter pylori***-related chronic illness; meaning that these diseases could be just potential conditions that could readily improve or completely recover if properly managed via an effective ***H. pylori*** eradication employing natural measures.

We have also made great concern to describe the characteristic manifestations of ***H. pylori***-induced dyspepsia in adequate detailed explanation in the first book of this series which is *"New Concepts in Diabetes"* and also in this book in order to be of good benefit for those targeted individuals to help discover the relation of their illness to the associated dyspeptic symptoms.

The advantage of following the instructions and advices of the *"New Concepts in Disease Spread& Control of Disease Spread"* will be summarized and confirmed in a separate section at the end of this book.

The future Part II of the *"New Concepts in Disease Spread& Control of Disease Spread"* is expected to include also new definitive strategic concepts for the control of spread of further many diseases. Until then, people can consult for any query concerning a current illness on the phone or e-mail as shown in the questionnaires and queries chapter at end of the book.

Table of Contents

DISEASE SPREAD DURING LATE DECADES IN BRIEF

Disease spread worldwide is lately leading a flare up plateau that has been described in some diseases as the fire while spreading in hay giving the term "chronic illness epidemics" an actual credibility,[1] or the term "disease industry"; as if a hidden cunning factor or an evil offensive party is manufacturing, producing or breeding diseases.

Chronic illness has been flaring up worldwide beyond the traditional rules of disease spread; which means that traditional measures employed to control these diseases can never be decisive or successful.[2] Vitamin D deficiency for example is spreading worldwide like common cold, whenever a person is investigated for vitamin D, he is deficient although not every person you meet would have common cold, vitamin D deficiency is then more than the common cold in its spread or it is uncommon cold which is medically non-sense.

The current chronic diseases are mostly inadequately controlled in spite of extreme scientific efforts; this could further indicate the possibility of existence of a missed underlying common pathologic environmental error behind the world's burden of this disease spread. Unless withdrawal of the underlying pathology is successful or treatment of the etiologic pathology is definitive, adequate and fundamental cure can mot be achieved.[3,4]

REFERENCES:

1. Al-Nozha MM, Al-Maatouq MA, Al-Mazrou YY, et al. Diabetes mellitus in Saudi Arabia. Saudi Med J 2004 Nov; 25 (11): 1603-10.

2. **Nasrat AM. The world misconception and misbehavior towards Helicobacter pylori is leading to major spread of illness. The 7th Anti-Aging Medicine World Congress, Monte-Carlo, Monaco, 2009 Mar. Available from URL, www.euromedicom.com**

3. **Nasrat SAM, Nasrat RM, Nasrat MM, et al. The dramatic spread of diabetes mellitus worldwide and influence of Helicobacter t**

HELICOBACTER PYLORI AND DISEASE SPREAD; MISCONCEPTIONS AND FACTS

The latest reports in literature confirm the prevalence of abnormal *Helicobacter pylori* strains with flare up of a lot of medical challenges related to it through immune, inflammatory, toxic or different unknown reasons; *H. pylori*-related dysglycemia or diabetes is one of these challenges. *H. pylori*-associated autoimmune pancreatitis is not behind the development of DM as autoimmune pancreatitis affects mainly the exocrine function of the pancreas but not the endocrine one. *H. pylori*-related dysglycemia or diabetes is a potential condition developing due to toxic biological stress due to accumulation of potential toxins in the colon.[1-4] In the same way, accumulation of toxins in the colon secondary to excessive migration of *H. pylori* strains to the colon could have been an integral hidden reason behind disease spread during late decades.

H. pylori colonized the stomach since an immemorial time as if both the stomach wall and the bacterium used to live together in peace harmless to each other. *H. pylori* could migrate or get forced to migrate to the colon under the influence of the antibiotic violence; *H. pylori* in the colon will continue producing ammonia for a reason or no reason, unopposed or buffered by any acidity unlike in the stomach, leading to accumulation of profuse toxic amounts of ammonia. Accumulation of toxic amounts of ammonia in the colon could lead to different adverse effects or a biological toxic stress to the body with its various sequels among predisposed or susceptible individuals.[2,4]

Scientific reports refer to *H. pylori* as being a natural bacterium due to its existence since an immemorial time, its huge biological defense talents of survival, its recurrence in the stomach is un-avoidable and its high biological protective functions.[2,4] The highly biologic protective functions of *H. pylori* is an integral subject which will be issued in details in the future book of "*New Concepts in Helicobacter pylori*". These scientific reports also refer to the frank possibility that *H. pylori* is not essentially pathologic by its own but it is forced to all pathologic attitudes related to it due to misbehavior in food habits or the antibiotic violence towards it. This concept is supported by the facts that *H. pylori* has got a mostly harmless long history inside the stomach, its existence in the stomach is major while gastric complications were minor, its complications due to misbehavior in food habits were limited to the stomach in minor incidence and more apparently, the complications related to *H. pylori* did not exceed the limits of the stomach except after the antibiotic violence towards it. The last three decades demonstrated flare up of abnormal-behavior *H. pylori* strains, development of the *H. pylori* antibiotic eradication strategies and extensive spread of diseases related to these abnormal-behavior *H. pylori* strains; any medical which does not correlate between these three facts, is definitely not implementing a clinical sense or even a common sense.[2-5]

REFERENCES:

1. **Andreoli TE.** Cecil Essentials of Medicine. *WB Saunders Company. 2001; 5th Ed: 334.*

2. **Farinha P, Gascoyne RD. Helicobacter pylori and MALT Lymphoma. Gastroenterology 2005 May; 128 (6): 1579-605.**

3. **Nasrat SAM, Nasrat RM, Nasrat MM, et al. The dramatic spread of diabetes mellitus worldwide and influence of Helicobacter pylori.** *General Med J 2015; 3 (1): 159-62.*

4. **Nasrat AM. The world misconception and misbehavior towards Helicobacter pylori is leading to major spread of illness.** *The 7th Anti-Aging Medicine World Congress, Monte-Carlo, Monaco, 2009 Mar.* **Available from URL,** *www.euromedicom.com*

5. **Nasrat AM, Nasrat SAM, Nasrat RM, et al. Misconception and misbehavior towards Helicobacter pylori is leading to major spread of illness.** *General Med 2015; S1: 002.*

FUNCTIONAL DYSPEPSIA

Functional Dyspepsia: Published in Journal of General Medicine 2015; 3 (3): 192. (Open Access). Nasrat AM. Functional dyspepsia. *General Med 2015; 3 (3): 192. [doi: 10.4172/2327-5146.1000192]*

Functional dyspepsia is a clinical syndrome defined by chronic or recurrent pain or discomfort in the upper abdomen of a variable origin. A general agreement exists on the irrelevant role played by *Helicobacter pylori* in the pathophysiology of most cases of functional dyspepsia worldwide.[1]

Diagnosis is based on the clinical picture and detection of *H. pylori* serum antibodies. The following clinical symptoms are considered; upper gastrointestinal pain, burping, gastric distension, halitosis, and hyperacidity. Specific sensitive diagnostic tests such as urea breath and *H. pylori* fecal antigen tests are available; *H. pylori* serum antibodies, though non-specific, is suggested because of being cost effective as the matter of *H. pylori* dyspepsia is a typical subject of cost-effectiveness.[2,3]

It is necessary to effectively deal with *H. pylori* dyspepsia due to its associated risk with many reasons of chronic illness like diabetes, hypertension, thyroiditis, carditis, dermatitis and nephritis through inflammatory, toxic, immune or other different reasons.[2]

The efficacy of antibiotic treatment for non-ulcer dyspepsia is controversial, different trails have given conflicting results. Overall, antibiotic eradication treatment for non-ulcer dyspepsia symptoms had no significant effect on quality of life compared with placebo and was found more costly if compared to antacid treatment.[4,5] Bio-organic acids; lactic, formic and acetic, have been proved effective in symptomatic and clinical cure of dyspepsia.[6,7]

Eradication of clinical symptoms *H. pylori* dyspepsia should be considered a clinical cure; patients who are rendered asymptomatic after treatment do not need further investigation or treatment, they can just return for re-assessment if they develop further symptoms. Evaluation of eradication after *H. pylori* treatment markedly increases cost with no clear improvement in results.[8]

H. pylori is not just a bad bug in all instances; the juxta-mucosal ammonia produced by *H. pylori* protects the gastric wall from its acid if it goes in excess. The residual ammonia inside the lumen of the stomach resulting from the buffering process between the ammonia and the gastric acid is not toxic, it is even beneficial; as it functions as smooth muscle tonic maintaining the integrity of the gastro-esophageal sphincter and hence preventing reflux.[2,7]

It was amazing to the team working with the author of this study to get the news of a nine years old Saudi girl living with her family in Switzerland to have a diagnosis of reflux disease. The symptoms of this kid just all disappeared after stopping un-necessary antibiotics for every throat infection, restriction of outside-home meals and fast food in addition to intake of natural probiotics. Normal behavior **_H. pylori_** strains are supposed to be protective; it should not be kicked out from the stomach but should be saved.

REFERENCES:

1. **Stanghellini V, De Ponti F, De Giorgio R, et al.** New developments in the treatment of functional dyspepsia. *Drugs 2003; 63 (9): 869-92.*

2. **Farinha P, Gascoyne RD. Helicobacter pylori and MALT Lymphoma.** *Gastroenterology 2005 May; 128(6): 1579-605.*

3. **Garcia-Altes A, Jovell AJ, Serra-Part M, et al. Management of Helicobacter pylori in duodenal ulcer: a cost-effectiveness analysis.** *Aliment Pharmacol Ther 2000 Dec; 14 (12): 1631-8.*

4. **McColl K, Murray L, el-Omar E, et al. Symptomatic benefit from eradicating Helicobacter pylori infection in patients with nonulcer dyspepsia.** *N Eng J Med 1998; 339: 1869-74.*

5. **Moayyedi P, Soo S, Deeks J, et al. Systemic review and economic evaluation of Helicobacter pylori eradication treatment for non-ulcer dyspepsia.** *Dyspepsia Review Goup. BMJ 2000 Sep 16; 321 (7262): 659-64.*

6. **Midolo PD, Lambert JR, Hull R, et al. In vitro inhibition of Helicobacter pylori NCTC 11637 by organic acids and lactic acid bacteria.** *J Appl Bacteriol. 1995 Oct; 79 (4); 475-9.*

7. **Nasrat AM. The world misconception and misbehavior towards Helicobacter pylori is leading to major spread of illness.** *The 7th Anti-Aging Medicine World Congress, Monte-Carlo, Monaco, 2009 Mar.* **Available from URL,** *www.euromedicom.com*

8. **Phull PS, Halliday D, Price AB, et al. Absence of dyspeptic symptoms as a test for Helicobacter pylori eradication.** *BMJ 1996 Feb 10; 312 (7027): 349-50.*

MISCONCEPTION AND MISBEHAVIOR TOWARDS HELICOBACTER PYLORI IS LEADING TO MAJOR SPREAD OF ILLNESS

Introduction: The widespread prevalence and the challenges constituted by ***Helicobacter pylori***; namely its close relation to acid peptic disease, gastric carcinoma and lymphoma have led to the widely-established medical concept that ***H. pylori*** eradication should be a necessary attempt. The annual cost associated with peptic ulcer disease in the United States is estimated to be 6 billion dollars and gastric cancer kills over 700,000 people every year in the world.[1,2]

H. pylori is an extremely common bacterium which is considered by quite many investigators upon statistical basis or relative association with some diseases to be pathogenic bacterium that is able to alter the host physiology; subverting its immune response and allowing it to persist for the life of the host. The prevalence of ***H. pylori*** remains high; over 50% in most of the world, although existence rates are dropping in some developed countries. The drop in ***H. pylori*** prevalence could be a double-sided matter; reducing the incidence of gastric diseases while increasing the risk of allergies, auto-immunity and esophageal diseases.[2,3]

The latest reports in literature demonstrate a definite flare up of many medical challenges related to ***H. pylori*** through immune or different unknown reasons. Thyroiditis, autoimmune pancreatitis, immune thrombocytopenic purpura and acute inflammatory demyelinating polyradiculoneuropathy are examples of these challenges.[3-6] These autoimmune medical challenges related to ***H. pylori*** are sufficient to render the matter that ***H. pylori*** can reside hidden somewhere in the body be taken seriously.

The list of diseases potentially related to ***H. pylori*** continues to grow, however, explanations of how ***H. pylori*** could contribute to extra-gastric diseases lag far behind clinical studies. A number of host factors and ***H. pylori*** virulence factors act together to determine which individuals are most predisposed and susceptible or are at the highest risk of illness. These factors include bacterial cytotoxins and polymorphisms in host genes responsible for manipulating the immune response.[2,7,8]

H. pylori could migrate or get forced or migrate to the colon under the influence of antibiotic violence where it will continue producing ammonia for a reason or no reason, unopposed or buffered by any acidity unlike in the stomach leading to accumulation of profuse amounts of ammonia as gastric juxta-mucosal ammonia of ***H. pylori*** is strictly liberated in response to any acidity approaching the gastric mucosa. Accumulation of excess ammonia in the body is toxic that could lead to adverse biological effects in the body among predisposed disadvantaged population. Ammonia is smooth muscle tonic and therefore; excess ammonia in the colon could be spastic causing multiple colonic spasms.[9-12]

REFERENCES:

1. **Ge Z.** Potential of fumarate reductase as a novel therapeutic target in Helicobacter pylori infection. *Expert Opin Ther Targets 2002 Apr; 6(2): 135-46.*

2. **Testerman TL, Morris J. Beyond the stomach: An updated view of Helicobacter pylori pathogenesis, diagnosis, and treatment.** *World J Gastroenterol 2014 Sep 28; 20 (36): 12781-12808.*

3. **Segni M, Borrelli O, Pucarelli I, et al. Early manifestations of gastric autoimmunity in patients with juvenile autoimmune thyroid disease.** *J Clin Endocrinol Metab 2004Oct; 89 (10):4944-8.*

4. **Kountouras J, Zavos C, Chatzopoulos D. A concept on the role of Helicobacter pylori infection in autoimmune pancreatitis.** *J Cell Mol Med 2005Jan-Mar; 9 (1): 196-207.*

5. **Kountouras J, Deretzi G, Zavos C, et al. Association between Helicobacter pylori infection and acute inflammatory demyelinating polyradiculoneuropathy.** *Eur J Neurol 2005 Feb; 12 (2):139-43.*

6. **Veneri D, Krampera M, Franchini M. High prevalence of sustained remission of idiopathic thrombocytopenic purpura after Helicobacter pylori eradication: a long-term follow-up study.** *Platelets 2005 Mar; 16 (2):117-9.*

7. **Farinha P, Gascoyne RD. Helicobacter pylori and MALT Lymphoma.** *Gastroenterology 2005 May; 128 (6): 1579-605.*

8. **Cirak MY, Ozdek A, Yilmaz D, et al. Detection of Helicobacter pylori and its CagA gene in tonsil and adenoid tissues by PCR.** *Arch Otolaryngol Head Neck Surg. 2003 Nov; 129 (11): 1225-9.*

9. **Nasrat AM. The world misconception and misbehavior towards Helicobacter pylori is leading to major spread of illness.** *The 7th Anti-Aging Medicine World Congress, Monte-Carlo, Monaco, 2009 Mar.* **Available from URL,** *www.euromedicom.com*

10. **Nasrat SAM, Nasrat RM, Nasrat MM, et al. The dramatic spread of diabetes mellitus worldwide and influence of Helicobacter pylori.** *General Med J 2015; 3 (1): 159-62.*

11. **Nasrat SAM, Nasrat AM. An alternative approach for the rising challenge of hypertensive illness via Helicobacter pylori eradication.** *J Cardiol Res 2015; 6 (1): 221-225.*

12. **Nsarat RM, Nasrat MM, Nasrat AM, et al. Improvement of idiopatic cardiomyopathy after colon clear.** *J Cardiol Res 2015 Apr; 6 (2): 249-254.*

SCIENTIFIC EVIDENCES ON THE FINDING THAT MISCONCEPTION AND MISBEHAVIOR TOWARDS HELICOBACTER PYLORI IS LEADING TO MAJOR SPREAD OF ILLNESS

Misconception and Misbehavior towards Helicobacter pylori is leading to Major Spread of Illness: Published in the Journal of General Medicine 2015; S1: 002. (Open Access). Nasrat et al. Misconception and misbehavior towards Helicobacter pylori is leading to major spread of illness. *General Med 2015; S 1: 002.* *[doi: 10.4172/2327-5146.1000S1-002]*

Background: The widespread prevalence and the challenges constituted by **Helicobacter pylori**; namely its close relation to acid peptic disease, gastric carcinoma and lymphoma have led to the widely-established medical concept that **H. pylori** eradication should be a necessary attempt.[1-6] The flare up of these medical problems indicates that the current combined antibiotic therapy is not an effective measure to control all the challenges related to the stomach bug. **H. pylori** colonized the stomach since an immemorial time, the antibiotics could force **H. pylori** to migrate to another shelter which would oblige it to become a source of illness.[7-9]

Objective: This study aimed to demonstrate that the antibiotic violence has rendered a domestic bug (**H. pylori**) to become wild in attitude instead of getting rid of it.

Design & Setting: Prospective study done in Balghsoon Cinics in Jeddah/ Saudi Arabia during 2012/2013.

Patients & Methods: The scientific interest of this study was focused on three groups of clinical conditions associated with **H. pylori** dyspepsia; chronic and recurrent colitis, uncontrolled hypertension under medication and newly discovered diabetes mellitus in adults. The patients were randomly included in the study without selection. The rectal spasm was detected by proctoscopy or sigmoidoscopy, while the multiple colonic spasms were demonstrated by colonoscopy. The management of cases constituted eradication of **H. pylori** by natural measures employing the senna purge and vinegar therapy.

Results: All patients became free of any dyspeptic symptoms. The integral colonic function has been easily rectified in 33 patients. 15 hypertensive patients were able to quit their antihypertensive pills and maintain normal blood pressure values although they were inadequately controlled in spite of regular follow up of medications and extreme carefulness about their life style. The diabetic condition has been successfully and permanently corrected in 10 newly discovered cases.

Ethical Considerations: An informed signed consent was taken from all patients, they were made aware about safety of the natural colon clear remedy; they were free to quit the study whenever they like. The research proposal was approved and the study followed the rules of the Research Ethics Committee of Balghsoon Clinics in Jeddah, Saudi Arabia.

Discussion: Most of the diabetic and hypertensive patients in the world are inadequately controlled in spite of regular follow up of medications and strict carefulness about their style of life; this could further indicate the presence of a missed underlying pathology.[9-11]

A general impression has developed that the antibiotic violence has forced ***H. pylori*** to migrate in panic to the colon and/or the rectum. Migration of ***H. pylori*** will be accompanied by accumulation of profuse toxic amounts of ammonia in the colon which will lead to multiple colonic and a high rectal spasm. This matter is manifested by marked constipation and passage of small pieces of dried stool which have been observed as integral entity of ***H. pylori***-related dyspepsia. These spasms are so resistant to ordinary laxative measures leading to loss of the integral colonic function and set up of a state of irritable or spastic colitis.[9]

The development of multiple colonic spasms with subsequent severe constipation and interference with the integral colonic function will establish a colonic re-absorption error with retention of fluids, salts and toxins inside the body. This could lead to hypertension which is expected to remain inadequately controlled without correction of the underlying colonic re-absorptive error. Hypertension, a disease of rich, is now flaring up as a challenge among poor population. Some reports consider hypertension in developing countries a consequence of progress and life style changes. In spite of that, traditional risk factors do not appear fully sufficient to explain the rising figures of hypertensive illness.[11-14]

Accumulation of profuse toxic amounts of ammonia in the colon constitutes a biological toxic stress to the body that could lead to stress diabetes among disadvantaged susceptible people. Administration of oral hypoglycemic drugs to a stressed pancreas means an insistence to flog a tired horse turning a potential condition into an established chronic illness with consequent flare up of the diabetic phenomena all over the world. Traditional risk rules are not sufficient to explain the dramatic spread of diabetes all over the world; this indicates that traditional measures employed to control the problem can never be adequate or decisive.[9,10]

Misconception of most investigators about the nature of ***H. pylori*** and their misbehavior towards it is possibly leading in great part to the major spread of pathologic conditions associated with ***H. pylori*** existence. ***H. pylori*** colonized the stomach since an immemorial time;[7] as if both the stomach and the bug used to live together in peace, harmless to each other. This also indicates that the commonest natural habitat of ***H. pylori*** is the stomach; if ***H. pylori*** is kicked outside the stomach by antibiotics, it will become a foreign structure the tissues and is rendered a poison itself by causing local tissue pathology or becomes a source of poison by encoding autoimmunity or by leading to accumulation of profuse toxic amounts of ammonia somewhere in the body.[7,9] Recurrence of ***H. pylori*** existence is un-avoidable or hardly avoidable;[7,8] as if it is a matter of natural existence of a bacterium. Existence of abnormal-behavior ***H. pylori*** strains is essentially a sanitary conflict before it is a medical challenge,[7] sanitary problems are treated with antiseptic measures but not antibiotics. If investigators and therapists keep these findings in consideration, most of the challenges associated with ***H. pylori*** would disappear. Moreover, the continued flare up of the medical problems associated with ***H. pylori*** indicates that the current combined antibiotic therapy is not an effective measure to control all the challenges related to the stomach bacterium.

The senna leaves extract purge effectively and readily kills and expels all migrated colonic ***H. pylori*** strains. Vinegar therapy maintains colon clear by interference with re-set up of abnormal-behavior ***H. pylori*** strains due to interference with the energy metabolism and respiratory chain metabolism of ***H. pylori*** via inhibition of the pyruvate dehydrogenase complex according to the rules of feedback regulation and product inhibition with consequent inhibition of pyruvate metabolism which is the main source of energy production by for ***H. pylori***.[7,9-12]

The dramatic response achieved in this study confirms the concept that the etiologic pathology associated with *H. pylori* was simply the colon-spastic and toxic effect of ammonia produced by *H. pylori* in the colon. The integral colonic function was resumed by rectifying the multiple colonic spasms, blood pressure values were maintained with quit of antihypertensive medications by correction of the colonic re-absorptive error and recovery of the newly discovered diabetic condition was achieved by elimination of the biological toxic stress situation via mere natural eradication of *H. pylori* from the colon.

Conclusion: It seems that most of the budget of searching and researching after *H. pylori* should be redirected towards raising the standard of life and ensuring sanitary water supply for poor population, patient and family education as regards misbehavior in food habits and antibiotic abuse, and orientation in primary health care units as concerns natural measures towards *H. pylori* dyspepsia.

REFERENCES:

1. Ge Z. Potential of fumarate reductase as a novel therapeutic target in Helicobacter pylori infection. *Expert Opin Ther Targets 2002 Apr; 6 (2): 135-46.*

2. **Testerman TL, Morris J. Beyond the stomach: An updated view of Helicobacter pylori pathogenesis, diagnosis, and treatment.** *World J Gastroenterol 2014 Sep 28; 20 (36): 12781-12808.*

3. **Segni M, Borrelli O, Pucarelli I, et al. Early manifestations of gastric autoimmunity in patients with juvenile autoimmune thyroid disease.** *J Clin Endocrinol Metab 2004 Oct; 89 (10):4944-8.*

4. **Kountouras J, Zavos C, Chatzopoulos D. A concept on the role of Helicobacter pylori infection in autoimmune pancreatitis.** *J Cell Mol Med 2005 Jan-Mar; 9 (1): 196-207.*

5. **Kountouras J, Deretzi G, Zavos C, et al. Association between Helicobacter pylori infection and acute inflammatory demyelinating polyradiculoneuropathy.** *Eur J Neurol 2005 Feb; 12 (2): 139-43.*

6. **Veneri D, Krampera M, Franchini M. High prevalence of sustained remission of idiopathic thrombocytopenic purpura after Helicobacter pylori eradication: a long-term follow-up study.** *Platelets 2005 Mar; 16 (2): 117-9.*

7. **Farinha P, Gascoyne RD. Helicobacter pylori and MALT Lymphoma.** *Gastroenterology 2005 May; 128 (6): 1579-605.*

8. **Cirak MY, Ozdek A, Yilmaz D, et al. Detection of Helicobacter pylori and its CagA gene in tonsil and adenoid tissues by PCR.** *Arch Otolaryngol Head Neck Surg. 2003 Nov; 129 (11): 1225-9.*

9. **Nasrat AM. The world misconception and misbehavior towards Helicobacter pylori is leading to major spread of illness.** *The 7th Anti-Aging Medicine World Congress, Monte-Carlo, Monaco, 2009 Mar.* **Available from URL,** *www.euromedicom.com*

10. **Nasrat SAM, Nasrat RM, Nasrat MM, et al. The dramatic spread of diabetes mellitus worldwide and influence of Helicobacter pylori.** *General Med J 2015; 3 (1): 159-62.*

11. **Nasrat SAM, Nasrat AM. An alternative approach for the rising challenge of hypertensive illness via Helicobacter pylori eradication.** *J Cardiol Res 2015; 6 (1): 221-225.*

12. **Nsarat RM, Nasrat MM, Nasrat AM, et al. Improvement of idiopatic cardiomyopathy after colon clear.** *J Cardiol Res 2015 Apr; 6 (2): 249-254.*

13. **Bakris G, Hill M, Mancia G, et al. Achieving blood pressures goals globally: five core actions for health-care professionals. A worldwide call to action.** *J Hum Hypertens 2008 Jan; 22 (1): 63-70.*

14. **Reddy KS, Naik N, Prabhakaran D. Hypertension in developing world: a consequence of progress.** *Curr Cardiol Rep 2006 Nov; 8 (6); 399-404.*

STOP FIGHTING THE STOMACH BACTERIUM HELICOBACTER PYLORI;ESOPHAGEAL REFLUX WAS NOT AS SUCH BEFORE THE ANTI-H. PYLORI ANTIBIOTICS

Introduction: Functional dyspepsia is a clinical syndrome defined by chronic or recurrent pain or discomfort in the upper abdomen of a variable origin. A general agreement exists on the irrelevant role played by ***Helicobacter pylori*** in the pathophysiology of most cases of functional dyspepsia worldwide.[1]

Diagnosis of functional dyspepsia is based on the clinical picture and detection of ***H. pylori*** serum antibodies. The following clinical symptoms are considered; upper gastrointestinal pain, burping, gastric distension, halitosis, hyperacidity and acid reflux. Specific sensitive diagnostic tests such as urea breath and ***H. pylori*** fecal antigen tests are available; ***H. pylori*** serum antibodies, though non-specific, is suggested as screening test because of being cost effective as the matter of ***H. pylori*** dyspepsia is a typical subject of cost-effectiveness.[2,3]

Esophageal acid reflux disease has been demonstrated lately to widely spread beyond medical limits and rules in both sexes among different age groups and social classes to the extent that it was found prevalent even among children.[2,4,5]

It is necessary to effectively deal with ***H. pylori*** dyspepsia due to its associated risk with many reasons of chronic illness like diabetes, hypertension, thyroiditis, carditis, dermatitis and nephritis through inflammatory, toxic, immune or other different reasons.[2]

The efficacy of antibiotic treatment for non-ulcer dyspepsia is controversial, different trails have given conflicting results. Overall, antibiotic eradication treatment for non-ulcer dyspepsia symptoms had no significant effect on quality of life compared with placebo and was found more costly if compared to antacid treatment.[6,7] Bio-organic acids; lactic, formic and acetic, have been proved effective in symptomatic and clinical cure of dyspepsia.[4,8]

Eradication of clinical symptoms ***H. pylori*** dyspepsia should be considered a clinical cure; patients who are rendered asymptomatic after treatment do not need further investigation or treatment, they can just return for re-assessment if they develop further symptoms. Evaluation of eradication after ***H. pylori*** treatment markedly increases cost with no clear improvement in results.[9]

REFERENCES:

1. **Stanghellini V, De Ponti F, De Giorgio R, et al.** New developments in the treatment of functional dyspepsia. *Drugs 2003; 63 (9): 869-92.*

2. **Farinha P, Gascoyne RD. Helicobacter pylori and MALT Lymphoma.** *Gastroenterology 2005 May; 128 (6): 1579-605.*

3. Garcia-Altes A, Jovell AJ, Serra-Part M, et al. Management of Helicobacter pylori in duodenal ulcer: a cost-effectiveness analysis. *Aliment Pharmacol Ther 2000 Dec; 14 (12): 1631-8.*

4. Nasrat AM. The world misconception and misbehavior towards Helicobacter pylori is leading to major spread of illness. *The 7th Anti-Aging Medicine World Congress, Monte-Carlo, Monaco, 2009 Mar.* Available from URL, *www.euromedicom.com*

5. Nasrat AM, Nasrat SAM, Nasrat RM, et al. Misconception and misbehavior towards Helicobacter pylori is leading to major spread of illness. *Gen Med 2015; S1: 002.* [Open Access]

6. McColl K, Murray L, el-Omar E, et al. Symptomatic benefit from eradicating Helicobacter pylori infection in patients with nonulcer dyspepsia. *N Eng J Med 1998; 339: 1869-74.*

7. Moayyedi P, Soo S, Deeks J, et al. Systemic review and economic evaluation of Helicobacter pylori eradication treatment for non-ulcer dyspepsia. *Dyspepsia Review Goup. BMJ 2000 Sep 16; 321 (7262): 659-64.*

8. Midolo PD, Lambert JR, Hull R, et al. In vitro inhibition of Helicobacter pylori NCTC 11637 by organic acids and lactic acid bacteria. *J Appl Bacteriol. 1995 Oct; 79(4); 475-9.*

9. Phull PS, Halliday D, Price AB, et al. Absence of dyspeptic symptoms as a test for Helicobacter pylori eradication. *BMJ 1996 Feb 10; 312 (7027): 349-50.*

SCIENTIFIC EVIDENCES ON THE FLARE UP OF ACID REFLUX DISEASE AFTER HELICOBACTER PYLORI ERADICATION FROM THE STOMACH

Stop Fighting the Stomach Bacterium Helicobacter pylori; Acid Reflux was not as Such before the Anti-H. pylori Antibiotics: Published in the American Journal of Medicine and Medical Sciences; 2017; 7 (4): 196-201. Nasrat et al. Stop Fighting the Stomach Bacterium Helicobacter pylori; Acid Reflux was not as Such before the Anti-H. pylori Antibiotics. Am J Med Med Sci 2017; 7 (4): 196-201. *[doi: 10.5923/j.ajmms.20170704.07]*

Background: Esophageal acid reflux disease has been demonstrated lately to widely spread beyond medical limits and rules in both sexes among different age groups and social classes to the extent that it was found prevalent even among children. *Helicobacter pylori* colonized the stomach since an immemorial time; as if both the gastric wall and the bacterium used to live together in peace harmless to each other. *H. pylori* has been shown to be protective against low acidity-related problems. It was suggested that *H. pylori* is protective against development of esophageal reflux disease and eradication treatment may increase the incidence of reflux symptoms.[1-6]

The efficacy of antibiotic treatment for non-ulcer dyspepsia is controversial, different trails have given conflicting results. Overall, antibiotic eradication treatment for non-ulcer dyspepsia symptoms had no significant effect on quality of life compared with placebo and was found more costly if compared to antacid treatment. Bio-organic acids; lactic, formic and acetic, have been proved effective in symptomatic and clinical cure of dyspepsia.[5-9]

Objective: Demonstration of recent etiologic reasons behind the apparent phenomena of increasing figures of gastro-esophageal reflux during latest decades.

Design&Setting: A Prospective study done in Balghsoon Clinics in Jeddah/Saudi Arabia between October 2014 and October 2015.

Patients& Methods: It was amazing to the research team of this study to receive the news of a nine years old Saudi girl living with her family in Switzerland to have a diagnosis of reflux disease; the family was actually seeking a medical advice. All the symptoms of this kid just totally disappeared after stopping unnecessary antibiotic use for every throat infection, complete restriction of outside-home meals and fast food in addition to intake of natural probiotic supplements. That was the real motive of this study to investigate for an underlying pathologic reason for the flare up of the esophageal acid reflux disease.

Two equal groups of patients with dyspepsia and acid reflux symptoms, 20 children between 9 and 15 years of age and 20 adults between 30-45 years old, were randomly included in the study, both groups were equally distributed between males and females. The following clinical symptoms of *H. pylori* dyspepsia; heart burn, abdominal distension, constipation, were considered. *H. pylori* existence was confirmed by specific tests; urea breath test and *H. pylori* fecal antigen.[2] All patients underwent upper endoscopy to confirm the diagnosis of acid reflux disease. All patients were given a natural remedy of colon care and colon clear for eradication of the abnormal-behavior *H. pylori* strains from the stomach and colon by vinegar therapy and senna leaves extract purge for eradication of colonic *H. pylori* strains. The vinegar therapy consists of vinegar-mixed salad to be taken with principal meals once or twice per day, 3-5 days every week.[10] Patients were requested to avoid antibiotics unless strictly indicated and to restrict out-side home meals during the period of the study. They were given natural probiotic supplements in the form of acid butter milk; one third of a glass, once or twice per day and a whole glass at bedtime for ten days.

Results: More than 95% of the screened sample for the purpose of their inclusion in the study were demonstrated to have an element of dyspepsia or colonic upsets. *H. pylori* fecal antigen test was proved positive in 90% of patients; 19 children and 17 adults. Urea breath test was positive in 25% of patients; 3 children and 7 adults. A total of 28 patients (70%); 17 children and 11 adults were confirmed positive for acid reflux by endoscopy. 7 adults were having endoscopic signs of mild esophagitis. Eradication of the abnormal *H. pylori* strains from the colon was confirmed *H. pylori* fecal antigen test. Urea breath test was rendered negative in all patients after three days of vinegar therapy. Dyspeptic and acid reflux symptoms disappeared in all patients before completing seven days of commencing the probiotic supplementation.

Ethical Considerations: An informed signed consent was taken from all patients, they were made aware about safety of the natural colon clear; they were free to quit the study whenever they like. The research proposal was approved and the study followed the rules of the Research Ethics Committee of Balghsoon Clinics in Jeddah, Saudi Arabia.

Discussion: It was not surprising while screening patients for symptoms of dyspepsia before their inclusion in the study to have a finding indicating the possibility that almost all the population living in a developing country lifestyle are suffering from dyspeptic symptoms and colonic troubles; this finding actually conforms with the current social and health standards in these countries.[2,10]

Migration of *H. pylori* to the colon is a fact that has been reported in literature; *H. pylori* could migrate or could get forced to migrate to the colon under the influence of antibiotic violence.[2,4,5,11] Antibiotics are seldom effective against extra-gastric *H. pylori* strains;[12] It was suggested that the antibiotic violence could have forced the stomach bug to migrate to the colon rather than eradicating it from the stomach.[4,5,13] This suggestion is supported by the finding that pseudo-membranous toxic colitis and toxic megacolon have developed after eradication of *H. pylori* by antibiotic therapy.[14,15] It seems that antibiotics do not have any influence towards *H. pylori* except forcing it to migrate from the stomach which is actually the reason of initiating risks and complications.[4,5] *H. pylori* in the colon will continue producing ammonia for a reason or no reason leading to accumulation of profuse toxic amounts of ammonia, unopposed or buffered by any acidity, carrying the risk of various biologic toxic effects in the body and leading to multiple colonic spasms interfering with the integral colonic function and causing recurrent colonic upsets.[10,16]

Survival of *H. pylori* inside the stomach is achieved through various defense mechanisms. The bacterium resides and colonizes under the layer of mucus overlying gastric mucosa, although gastric acid plays an important role in the protection against many enteric organisms, and *H. pylori* can be readily killed by a brief exposure to diluted hydrochloric acid solutions; the organism's intense urease activity produces ammonia from organic urea in gastric juice in such amounts that can buffer the pH of gastric acid. The gastric mucus layer is relatively thick and viscous allowing for *H. pylori* pH gradients from approximately pH 2 close to the gastric lumen until pH 7.4 immediately adjacent to the mucosa. The high motility of *H. pylori* via its flagellae even in very viscous mucus allows the organism to swim and migrate freely to reach the most favorable pH gradient. Furthermore, elaboration of ammonia from endogenous urea that buffers gastric acid in the immediate vicinity of the bacterium constitutes an essential mechanism for survival of *H. pylori* in its gastric habitat.[17-21]

Existence of ammonia in the stomach was described as early as 1852, in 1930s it was reported that ammonia in the stomach is due to a urease activity, and it was further reported in 1960s that gastric urease activity is not a property of the stomach but is of a bacterial origin. Early in 1980s it was emphasized that ammonia of the stomach does not exist in toxic concentrations but in residual amounts and it is even useful. Amazingly; *H. pylori* may not be just a bad bug in all instances, as complete eradication of the bacterium might introduce new problems due to the low gastric acidity. *H. pylori* has been shown to be a protective against low pH-related carcinomas involving the cardia of the stomach.[2] Data from observational studies have proposed a protective role of *H. pylori* against the development of gastro-esophageal reflux disease, and suggested that *H. pylori* eradication treatment may increase the incidence of reflux symptoms. It was observed that prevalence of *H. pylori* has been decreasing in developed countries, while the prevalence of gastro-esophageal reflux disease and esophageal adenocarcinoma have been increasing since 1930s.[22-25]

A normal-behavior *H. pylori* never exists inside the gastric lumen during presence of food, it remains under the gastric mucus layer until travel of food from the stomach and drop of gastric acid to a residual level where the bacterium picks up its nutrition from remnants of food within gastric lumen in a blink like momentum protected with a shield of ammonia around its immediate vicinity before it returns back to its natural secure habitat under the gastric mucus layer leaving behind it a residual ammonia scattered in the gastric lumen. This scattered residual ammonia excites the gastric wall to secrete the acid preventing in this way absence of the protective role of the gastric acid during absence of food and serving in turn to guard against low acidity-related complications at the cardiac end of the stomach. Ammonia is smooth muscle tonic; therefore, residual gastric ammonia resulting from flash moves of *H. pylori* to seek its nutrition helps to maintain the integrity of the gastro-esophageal tone and to protect accordingly from incidents of acid reflux.[2,4,5,10]

As the use of antibiotics in children is more than in adults due to the frequent incidence of throat and upper respiratory troubles, migration of *H. pylori* to the colon was manifested in children more than the adults of this study as demonstrated by a lesser incidence of positive urea breath test, higher incidence of acid reflux confirmed by endoscopy and higher incidence of positive *H. pylori* fecal antigen test.

Colon clear employing the senna leaves extract purge was done in this study to eradicate the *H. pylori* strains migrated to the colon in order to correct the resulting colonic troubles. Migration of colonic *H. pylori* strains remains lifelong unless eradicated as antibiotics are seldom effective against extra-gastric *H. pylori* strains,[2,12] and there is no effective measure to eradicate *H. pylori* from the colon except the senna purge. The senna purge kills and expels all colonic *H. pylori* strains as it was found that three-times dilution of the standard senna extract has got a direct lethal effect on *H. pylori* culture media.[10,13,26,27]

Colon care which consists of vinegar-mixed salad to be taken with principal meals was meant to get rid of the abnormal-behavior gastric *H. pylori* strains that exists in gastric lumen during presence of food leading to a lot of gastric upsets. It was also aimed to eradicate these strains before migrating to the colon.[5,10] The complex nutritional requirements of *H. pylori* are achieved via its unique energy metabolism which exhibits characteristic dislocation sites. These sites can be considered as targets that should attract any attempts to fight the organism.[28,29] As acetate is demonstrated as an end product among the metabolic pathway of *H. pylori*;[30,31] therefore, addition of acetic acid in the atmosphere around *H. pylori* could compromise the energy metabolism of *H. pylori* or interfere with its respiratory chain metabolism. This suggestion is supported by the fact that the major routes of generation of energy for *H. pylori* are via pyruvate and the activity of the pyruvate dehydrogenase complex is controlled by the rules of product inhibition and feedback regulation.[32,33] For the same reason, addition of pyruvate to different solid culture media was found to inhibit bacterial growth, and this inhibition was attributed to accumulation of acetate and formate;[34] As the matter includes interference with the energy metabolism and the respiratory chain metabolism of **H. pylori**; an immediate paralysis of the bacterium could be considered leading to immediate eradication of the abnormal-behavior gastric **H. pylori** strains. Twenty-times dilution of dietary white vinegar 6% was demonstrated to have an immediate lethal effect on **H. pylori**.[10,13]

Natural probiotics play an important role in human health by promoting nutrient supply, preventing pathogen colonization, shaping and maintaining normal mucosal immunity. Natural gut bacteria have been recently appreciated as having a true symbiotic relationship with the host; within this large pool of bacteria, probiotic supplements containing lactic acid-producing bacteria (LAPB) like *Lactobacilli* have been claimed to have a variety of beneficial effects on human health. LAPB are facultative anaerobic organisms that grow in abundance in the digestive tract of vertebrate animals. LAPB also represent some of the most commonly used probiotic bacteria and are extensively used in food products. LAPB generate large amounts of the healthy bio-organic lactic acid that helps to improve dyspeptic symptoms.[35-37] Natural Probiotic supplements were used in this study in the form of acid butter milk in order to improve symptoms of dyspepsia until the natural **H. pylori** strains are replaced to take over the function of maintaining the integrity of gastro-esophageal tone and protecting from acid reflux.

Disappearance of symptoms of dyspepsia and acid reflux was considered in this study clinical cure with no need for further confirmation by endoscopy as **H. pylori** is a typical subject of cost-effectiveness and evaluation of eradication after **H. pylori** treatment markedly increases cost with no clear improvement in results.[9]

H. pylori colonized the stomach since an immemorial time;[2] as if both the gastric wall and the bacterium used to live together in peace harmless to each other. Existence of **H. pylori** in the stomach is lifelong unless eradicated but recurrence of **H. pylori** in the stomach is unavoidable.[16,38,39] In children, existence of **H. pylori** starts trans-familial early during childhood, and the **H. pylori** strain is often identical with that of parents. Interestingly, children maintain the same strain genotype even after moving to a different environment.[6] In children, elimination of **H. pylori** is probably common due to the frequent antibiotic use for other different reasons; yet, trans-familial recurrence in children is still hardly avoidable.[6,39] It seems that **H. pylori** is a natural bacterium habitat of the stomach as evidenced by the scientific facts of its existence since an immemorial time, having huge biological talents for survival inside the strongly acidic gastric lumen, its recurrence in the stomach is unavoidable and its biological benefits of protection towards low acidity-related complications at the cardia of the stomach and guard against acid reflux disease.

Conclusion: The bacterium **H. pylori** is leading the behavior of natural useful bacteria of the gut and its function might be properly assessed, saved and not offended before adequate justification of the sequels of offensive attitudes towards it. Experimental and observational findings support the scientific fact that the antibiotic violence towards **H. pylori** could have been the reason for the rising figures of acid reflux disease during latest decades.

Conflict of Interest: There is no conflict of interest existing.

REFERENCES:

1. **Stanghellini V, De Ponti F, De Giorgio R, et al.** New developments in the treatment of functional dyspepsia. *Drugs 2003; 63 (9): 869-92.*

2. **Farinha P, Gascoyne RD. Helicobacter pylori and MALT Lymphoma.** *Gastroenterology 2005 May; 128 (6): 1579-605.*

3. **Garcia-Altes A, Jovell AJ, Serra-Part M, et al. Management of Helicobacter pylori in duodenal ulcer: a cost-effectiveness analysis.** *Aliment Pharmacol Ther 2000 Dec; 14 (12): 1631-8.*

4. **Nasrat AM. The world misconception and misbehavior towards Helicobacter pylori is leading to major spread of illness.** *The 7th Anti-Aging Medicine World Congress, Monte-Carlo, Monaco, 2009 Mar.* **Available from URL,** *www.euromedicom.com*

5. **Nasrat AM, Nasrat SAM, Nasrat RM, et al. Misconception and misbehavior towards Helicobacter pylori is leading to major spread of illness.** *Gen Med 2015; S1: 002.* **[Open Access]**

6. **McColl K, Murray L, el-Omar E, et al. Symptomatic benefit from eradicating Helicobacter pylori infection in patients with nonulcer dyspepsia.** *N Eng J Med 1998; 339: 1869-74.*

7. **Moayyedi P, Soo S, Deeks J, et al. Systemic review and economic evaluation of Helicobacter pylori eradication treatment for non-ulcer dyspepsia.** *Dyspepsia Review Goup. BMJ 2000 Sep 16; 321 (7262): 659-64.*

8. **Midolo PD, Lambert JR, Hull R, et al. In vitro inhibition of Helicobacter pylori NCTC 11637 by organic acids and lactic acid bacteria.** *J Appl Bacteriol. 1995 Oct; 79 (4); 475-9.*

9. **Phull PS, Halliday D, Price AB, et al. Absence of dyspeptic symptoms as a test for Helicobacter pylori eradication.** *BMJ 1996 Feb 10; 312 (7027): 349-50.*

10. **Nasrat AM, Nasrat SAM, Nasrat RM, et al. An alternate natural remedy for symptomatic relief of Helicobacter pylori dyspepsia. Gen Med 2015**; *3 (4).* **[Open Access]**

11. **Matsuo S, Mizuta Y, Hayashi T, et al. Mucosa-associated lymphoid tissue lymphoma of the transverse colon: a case report. World** *J Gastroenterol 2006 Sep 14; 12 (34): 5573-6.*

12. **Grünberger B, Wöhrer S, Streubel B, et al. Antibiotic treatment is not effective in patients infected with Helicobacter pylori suffering from extragastric MALT lymphoma.** *J Clin Oncol 2006 Mar 20; 24 (9):1370-5.*

13. **Nasrat RM, Nasrat MM, Nasrat AM, et al. Improvement of idiopathic cardiomyopathy after colon clear.** *J Cardiol Res 2015 Apr; 6 (2): 249-254***. [Open Access]**

14. **Kubo N, Kochi S, Ariyama I, et al. Pseudomembranous colitis after Helicobacter pylori eradication therapy.** *Kansenshogaku Zasshi 2006 Jan; 80 (1): 51-5.*

15. **Schweigart U, Franck H, Schepp W, et al. Toxic megacolon after Helicobacter pylori eradication therapy.** *Internist (Berl) 1997 Apr; 38 (4): 352-4.*

16. **Andreoli TE. Cecil Essentials of Medicine.** *WB Saunders Company. 2001; 5th Ed: 334.*

17. **Baron S. Baron's medical microbiology.** *Churchill Livingstone. 2000; 4th Ed: 346.*

18. **Zentilin P, Iiritano E, Vingale C, et al. Helicobacter pylori infection is not involved in the Pathogenesis of either erosive or non-erosive gastro-oesophageal reflux disease.** *Aliment Pharmacol Ther 2003 Apr; 17(8): 1057-64.*

19. **Volk WA, Gebhardt BM, Hammarskjold M-L, et al. Essential of Medical Microbiology. Lippincott-Raven. 1996; 5th Ed: 377.**

20. **Cotran RS, Kumar V, Collins T. Robins Pathologic Basis of Disease.** *WB Saunders Company. 1999; 6th Ed: 790.*

21. **Sleigh JD, Timbury MC. Notes on Medical Microbiology**. *Churchill Livingstone. 1998; 5th Ed: 232.*

22. **Issing WJ. Gastroesophageal reflux - a common illness.** *Laryngorhinootologie 2003 Feb; 82 (2): 118-22.*

23. **Labenz J, Blum AL, Bayerdorffer E, et al. Curing Helicobacter pylori infection in patients with duodenal ulcer may provoke reflux esophagitis.** *Gastroenterology 1997; 112: 1442-47.*

24. **Sharma P, Vakil N. Review article: Helicobacter pylori and reflux disease.** *Aliment Pharmacol Ther 2003 Feb; 17 (3): 297-305.*

25. **Vakil N. Gastroesophageal reflux disease and Helicobacter pylori infection.** *Rev Gastroenterol Disord 2003 winter; 3 (1):1-7*

26. **Keskin D, Toroglu S. Studies on antimicrobial activities of solvent extracts of different species.** *J Environ Biol 2011 Mar; 32 (2): 251-6.*

27. **Guarizel L, Costa JC, Dutra LB, et al. Anti-inflammatory, laxative and intestinal motility effects of Senna macranthera leaves.** *Nat Prod Res 2012; 26 (4): 331-43.*

28. **Ge Z. Potential of fumarate reductase as a novel therapeutic target in Helicobacter pylori infection.** *Expert Opin Ther Targets 2002 Apr; 6 (2): 135-46.*

29. **Mendz GL, Hazell SL, Burns BP. Glucose utilization and lactate production by Helicobacter pylori.** *J Gen Microbiol 1993 Dec; 139 (Pt 12): 3023-8.*

30. **Mendz GL, Hazell SL. Fumarate catabolism in Helicobacter pylori.** *Biochem Mol Biol Int. 1993 Oct; 31 (2):325-32*

31. **Mendz GL, Hazell SL, van Gorkom L. Pyruvate metabolism in Helicobacter pylori.** *Arch Microbiol. 1994; 162 (3):187-92.*

32. **Hughes NJ, Clayton CL, Chalk PA, et al. Helicobacter pylori porCDAB oorDABC genes encode distinct pyruvate: flavodoxin and 2-oxoglutarate: acceptor oxidoreductases which mediate electron transport to NADP.** *J Bacteriol 1998 Mar; 180 (5): 1119-28.*

33. **Berg JM, Tymoczko JL, Stryer L. Biochemistry.** *WH Freeman and Company. 2002; 5th Ed: 480.*

34. **Mendz GL, Ball GE, Meek DJ, Pyruvate metabolism in Campylobacter spp.** *Biochim Biophys Acta 1997 Mar 15; 1334 (2-3): 291-302.*

35. **Sears CL. A dynamic partnership: Celebrating our gut flora.** *Anaerobe 2005 Oct; 11 (5): 247-51.*

36. **O'Hara AM, Shanahan F. The gut flora as a forgotten organ.** *EMBO Rep 2006 Jul; 7 (7): 688-93.*

37. **Flint HJ, O'Toole PW, Walker AW. The human intestinal microbiota.** *Microbilogy 2010 Nov; 156 (11): 3203-4.*

38. **Asaka M. Epidemiology of Helicobacter pylori infection in Japan.** *Nippon Rinsho 2003 Jan; 61 (1): 19-24.*

39. **Cirak MY, Ozdek A, Yilmaz D, et al. Detection of Helicobacter pylori and its CagA gene in tonsil and adenoid tissues by PCR.** *Arch Otolaryngol Head Neck Surg. 2003 Nov; 129 (11): 1225-9.*

THE REAL FACT IN SPASTIC COLITIS AND IRRITABLE BOWEL SYNDROME
Spastic Colitis is a Big Scientific Lie

Introduction: Irritable bowel syndrome (IBS) is a common condition that can have significant impact on a person's quality of life. It is a chronic relapsing gastrointestinal disorder characterized by recurring abdominal pain or discomfort associated with disturbed bowel habit or both in the absence of structural abnormalities likely to account for these symptoms. It is a common disorder that affects 5–11% of the population in most countries. The cause of IBS is unknown but several mechanisms have been proposed including visceral hypersensitivity, central sensitization, abnormal gut motility and altered gut micro-flora. IBS is challenging to manage and many patients report insufficient symptomatic relief from treatment. It is one of the most common bowel diseases which seriously affects the quality of patient's life and consumes a considerable amount of medical resources. To date, there is no universally accepted method to effectively cure this disease. Most popular medicines, including antispasmodics, anti-diarrhea measures and laxatives only treat the symptoms of IBS and are therefore not ideal.[1-3]

IBS is a disabling gastrointestinal problem that affects psychosocial function of a person as well as the quality of his life. IBS has been considered as a bio-psychosocial disorder that could results from the interaction of multiple systems including central nervous system, increased sensitivity of the intestine and psychological factors such as stressful life events. IBS patients often have more psychological disorders than healthy people. A substantial number of studies indicated that IBS patients have abnormal personality with higher anxiety-depression scores. Hence, several studies were conducted to evaluate the effectiveness of antidepressants on IBS.[2-5]

Approximately 60% of patients identify food as a trigger for their symptoms and there has been interest in exclusion diets for managing IBS. Dietary adaptation is a common self-management strategy for patients with IBS, with many self-diagnosing intolerance to specific foods. This may lead to patients adopting over-restrictive or inappropriate diets. In recent years, a diet low in poorly absorbed short-chain carbohydrates, known collectively as FODMAPs (fermentable oligosaccharides, disaccharides, monosaccharides and polyols) has been advocated for the treatment of IBS.[6]

As all theories of irritable bowel disease are not definite and most therapeutic attempts are inadequate while most dyspeptic and colonic symptoms are readily cured after ***Helicobacter pylori*** eradication from the colon, ***H. pylori*** should be rendered into consideration in the etiologic pathology in most cases of IBS and natural eradication of colonic ***H. pylori*** strains should be an integral element in the management of IBS.[7-11]

REFERENCES:

1. **Everhart JE, Ruhl CE.** Burden of digestive disease in the United States part I: overall and upper gastrointestinal diseases. *Gastroenterology 2009; 136 (2): 376-86.*

2. **Xie C, Tang Y, Wang Y. Efficacy and safety of antidepressants for the treatment of irritable bowel syndrome: A meta-analysis.** *Plos One 2015; 10(8): e0127815. .*

3. **Tripathi R, Mehrotra S. Irritable bowel syndrome and its psychological management.** *Ind Psychiatry J 2015 Jan-Jun; 24 (1): 91-3.*

4. **Porcelli P. Psychological abnormalities in patients with irritable bowel syndrome.** *Indian J Gastroenterol 2004; 23: 63-9.*

5. **Hayee B, Forgacs I. Psychological approach to managing irritable bowel syndrome.** *BMJ 2007; 334: 1105-9. Gastroenterology. 2015 Aug 5; pii: S0016-5085 (15) 01086-0.* **doi: 10.1053/j.gastro.2015.07.054.**

6. **Bohn L, Storsrud S, Liliebo T, et al. Diet low in FODMAPs reduces symptoms of irritable bowel syndrome as well as traditional dietary advice: A randomized controlled trial.** *Gastroenterol 2015 Aug 5.* **[Epub ahead of print]**

7. **Farinha P, Gascoyne RD. Helicobacter pylori and MALT Lymphoma.** *Gastroenterology 2005 May; 128 (6): 1579-605.*

8. **Nasrat SAM, Nasrat AM. An alternative approach for the rising challenge of hypertensive illness via Helicobacter pylori eradication.** *J Cardiol Res 2015; 6 (1): 221-225.*

9. **Nasrat AM. The world misconception and misbehavior towards Helicobacter pylori is leading to major spread of illness.** *The 7th Anti-Aging Medicine World Congress, Monte-Carlo, Monaco, 2009 Mar.* **Available from URL,** *www.euromedicom.com*

10. **Nasrat AM, Nasrat SAM, Nasrat RM, et al. Misconception and misbehavior towards Helicobacter pylori is leading to major spread of illness.** *Gen Med 2015; S1: 002.* **[Open Access]**

11. **Nasrat AM, Nasrat SAM, Nasrat RM, et al. The definitive eradication of Helicobacter pylori from the colon.** *General Med 2015; S1: 5.*

SCIENTIFIC EVIDENCES ON THE REAL FACT IN IRRITABLE BOWEL SYNDROME

Scientific Evidences on the Fallacy of Spastic Colitis

The Real Fact in Irritable Bowel Syndrome: Published in Journal of General Medicine 2015; 3(6): 213. (Open Access). Nasrat et al. The real fact in irritable bowel syndrome. *General Med 2015; 3(6): 213. [doi: 10.4172/2327-5146.1000213]*

Background: Irritable bowel syndrome (IBS) is a common condition that can have a significant impact on a person's psychology and quality of life. It is a chronic relapsing gastrointestinal disorder characterized by recurring abdominal pain or discomfort associated with disturbed bowel habit. The cause of IBS is still unclear and most patients report insufficient symptomatic relief in spite of treatment.[1-6]

Helicobacter pylori should be rendered into consideration in the etiologic pathology in most cases of IBS and natural eradication of colonic ***H. pylori*** strains should be an integral element in the management of IBS.[7-10]

Objective: Demonstration of a missing fact about the major role of abnormal-behavior colonic ***H. pylori*** strains in IBS.

Design & Setting: Prospective study done in Balghsoon Clinics in Jeddah, Saudi Arabia between October 2012 and May 2014.

Patients & Methods: Twenty patients were consecutively selected and included in the study so that they are suffering the worst symptoms of spastic colitis or IBS regardless of their age, body built or food habits and life style except those following regular medications for any other chronic illness. One patient was 70 years old who used to fast every other day because of his bowel disorders, but he was craving for a single meal of frayed eggs. Another patient was a private pilot; he was generally fit and free of any disease except his irritable bowel condition that was so severe to the extent that he was not able to sleep at night unless he is having an ice pack under his left flank which is very drastic. Another patient expressed that he is having long history of IBS as if himself and the bowel syndrome were born together. Another patient used to sleep at night on his right side with a warm water bag under him; he mentioned that he feels that his body is divided into two halves; a clear left side and abnormal sensation of the right side even for the hand touch, hearing and vision. He used also to have migraine headache on the right side only. Existence of colonic ***H. pylori*** strains was confirmed by ***H. pylori*** fecal antigen test.[7] Natural eradication of colonic ***H. pylori*** strains was employed for all patients using the natural senna leaves pure, while colon care/colon clear was maintained by vinegar therapy.[8,9] Confirmation of ***H. pylori*** eradication from the colon was done using ***H. pylori*** fecal antigen test.[7]

Results: All patients were positive for colonic ***H. pylori*** strains and they turned negative after employing the senna purge. All patients without exception became within 3-5 days free of any dyspeptic symptoms, abdominal cramps or distension regardless of the quality of their food. The patient's expressions were interesting and indicative; one patient said "spastic colitis, was it a big lie of whole my life!!": that was the patient's own words. Another patient said "I can not believe that I am able to have all frayed vegetables like frayed green pepper or frayed onion even frayed eggplant and everything frayed not only frayed eggs without developing distension and cramps". It is interesting to know that the patient who had different sensation of his two halves of the body has gained equal normal sensation of both sides, his right-sided migraine headache almost disappeared as he had only two mild attacks in 12 months follow up.

Ethical Considerations: An informed signed consent was taken from all patients; they were made aware about safety of the natural remedies employed for them. Although they were ready to try any new measure that could offer them comfortable solution for their problem; they were free to quit the study whenever they like. They were requested to gradually withdraw their colonic medications and they were allowed to lead their routine style of life except restriction of outside-home meals.

Discussion: In spite of the extensive scientific efforts and adequate therapeutic trials, the etiologic pathology of IBS is still unclear and patients remain in agony;[2,3] which could further indicate existence of a missing fact or a missed underlying pathology in this matter.

Food should be essentially innocent; it is the abuse of antibiotics or the antibiotic violence towards ***H. pylori*** which render the stomach bacterium panic in attitude escaping from the stomach to the colon upon every delicious meal which raises the appetite and increases the gastric acid secretion that terrifies the bacterium.[10] If the patient's comments in this study indicated that their symptoms of IBS had been eliminated; it means that it is the stomach bacterium which undergoes irritability not the colon as the senna purge eliminates the panic colonic ***H. pylori*** strains but not the colon. In turn, it is irritability of the bacterium which reflects its effect on the colon.

H. pylori could migrate or get forced to migrate to the colon; ***H. pylori*** in the colon will continue producing ammonia for a reason or no reason leading to accumulation of profuse amounts of ammonia, unopposed or buffered by any acidity. Ammonia is smooth muscle tonic; therefore, accumulation of profuse amounts of ammonia in the colon will interfere with the colonic function by causing multiple colonic spasms leading to cramps, distension and digestive upsets. These spasms are known to be so solid and resistant to all symptomatic measures.[10] In the current study, a high rectal spasm was detected by proctoscopy or sigmoidoscopy, while a high sigmoid and multiple colonic spasms were demonstrated by colonoscopy.

In this study and other studies, the effect of three times dilution of the natural senna leaves extract and twenty times dilution of dietary white vinegar (acetic acid 6%) were found directly lethal to ***H. pylori*** culture media.[8,9]

The senna purge kills and expels all migrated colonic ***H. pylori*** strains.[10] Dietary vinegar (acetic acid 6%) has been recently demonstrated as dramatic, effective and decisive solution for all the challenges and medical problems related to ***H. pylori*** including eradication and recurrence. The vinegar therapy is simply based on a definite pathophysiologic principle offering in this way wonderful promises for many patients.[11] The complex nutritional requirements of ***H. pylori*** are achieved through its unique energy metabolism, which exhibits characteristic dislocation sites. These sites can be considered as targets that should attract any attempts to fight the organism.[12] As acetate is demonstrated as an end product among the metabolic pathway of ***H. pylori***; this means that addition of acetic acid in the atmosphere around ***H. pylori*** could compromise the energy metabolism of ***H. pylori***, or interfere with the organism's respiratory chain metabolism. This suggestion is supported by the fact that the major routes of generation of energy for ***H. pylori*** are via pyruvate and the activity of the pyruvate dehydrogenase complex is controlled by the rules of product inhibition and feedback regulation. It is further supported by the observation that addition of pyruvate to different solid culture media was found to inhibit bacterial growth, and this inhibition was attributed to accumulation of acetate and formate.[11-13] As the matter includes interference with the energy metabolism and the respiratory chain of ***H. pylori***; an immediate paralysis of the bacterium can be considered with dramatic relief of patient's symptoms. The fast immediate influence of acetic acid on *H. pylori* gives no chance for the bacterium to resist the treatment with vinegar or to mutate and develop resistant strains.

As concerns the patient with different sensations of his two sides of the body, his condition was explained to him by the fact that he used to lie mainly over one side because of the warm water bag under him, owing to the colonic re-absorptive error because of the multiple colonic spasms; there should be retention of fluids from the colon into the body with hypostatic gravitation of these fluids towards the dependant side; these accumulated fluids in one side more than the other could account for that different sensation in his both sides of the body. Definitely that heterogeneous sensation should disappear after his colon got cleared.

Conclusion: H. pylori may be behind the real pathology in most cases of IBS as it is the stomach bacterium which undergoes irritability but not the colon or it is irritability of the bacterium which reflects its effect on the colon. Revision of the guidelines of IBS treatment may be needed and accurate redetermination of natural measures of *H. pylori* management for their wider practical employment is becoming mandatory and urgent in order to stop the chronic agony of IBS patients.

Acknowledgment: The study appreciates the facilities and time allowed by Balghsoon Clinics in Jeddah/ Saudi Arabia. The continuous support offered by Abdul-Aziz Al-Sorayai Investment Company (ASIC) in Jeddah/Saudi Arabia, the scientific and emotional support of Dr Ahmed S. Balghsoon are extremely valued and appreciated.

Conflict of Interest: No conflict of interest is existing.

REFERENCES:

1. **Everhart JE, Ruhl CE.** Burden of digestive disease in the United States part I: overall and upper gastrointestinal diseases. *Gastroenterology 2009; 136 (2): 376-86.*

2. **Xie C, Tang Y, Wang Y. Efficacy and safety of antidepressants for the treatment of irritable bowel syndrome: A meta-analysis.** *Plos One 2015; 10 (8): e0127815. .*

3. **Tripathi R, Mehrotra S. Irritable bowel syndrome and its psychological management.** *Ind Psychiatry J 2015 Jan-Jun; 24 (1): 91-3.*

4. **Porcelli P. Psychological abnormalities in patients with irritable bowel syndrome.** *Indian J Gastroenterol 2004; 23: 63-9.*

5. **Hayee B, Forgacs I. Psychological approach to managing irritable bowel syndrome.** *BMJ 2007; 334: 1105-9.* **Gastroenterology. 2015 Aug 5. pii: S0016-5085 (15) 01086-0. doi: 10.1053/j.gastro.2015.07.054.**

6. **Bohn L, Storsrud S, Liliebo T, et al. Diet low in FODMAPs reduces symptoms of irritable bowel syndrome as well as traditional dietary advice: A randomized controlled trial.** *Gastroenterol 2015 Aug 5.* **[Epub ahead of print]**.

7. **Farinha P, Gascoyne RD. Helicobacter pylori and MALT Lymphoma.** *Gastroenterology 2005 May; 128 (6): 1579-605.*

8. **Nasrat SAM, Nasrat AM. An alternative approach for the rising challenge of hypertensive illness via Helicobacter pylori eradication.** *J Cardiol Res 2015; 6 (1): 221-225.*

9. **Nsarat RM, Nasrat MM, Nasrat AM, et al. Improvement of idiopatic cardiomyopathy after colon clear.** *J Cardiol Res 2015 Apr; 6 (2): 249-254.*

10. Nasrat AM. The world misconception and misbehavior towards Helicobacter pylori is leading to major spread of illness. *The 7th Anti-Aging Medicine World Congress, Monte-Carlo, Monaco, 2009 Mar.* Available from URL, *www.euromedicom.com*

11. Nasrat AM. A new approach for the hematologic challenges of Helicobacter pylori infection in children. The *International Symposium of the Egyptian Society of Pediatric Hematology/Oncology, 2006 Mar. Available from URL, www. espho.org*

12. Ge Z. Potential of fumarate reductase as a novel therapeutic target in Helicobacter pylori infection. *Expert Opin Ther Targets 2002 Apr; 6(2): 135-46.*

13. Nasrat SAM, Nasrat RM, Nasrat MM, et al. The dramatic spread of diabetes mellitus worldwide and influence of Helicobacter pylori. *General Med 2015; 3 (1): 159-62.*

HELICOBACTER PYLORI-INDUCED DIABETES THE DRAMATIC SPREAD OF DIABETES MELLITUS WORLDWIDE AND INFLUENCE OF HELICOBACTER PYLORIC

The World's Burden of DM during Late Decades is not on the Account of Type II Diabetes but on Stress Diabetes due to a Biological Colonic Toxic Stress; Stress Diabetes Could be Corrected

Introduction: The widespread prevalence and the challenges constituted by *Helicobacter pylori*; namely its close relation to acid peptic disease, gastric carcinoma and lymphoma have led to the widely-established medical concept that *H. pylori* eradication should be a necessary attempt. Although eradication regimens do eradicate *H. pylori* from the stomach; the emergence of antibiotic-resistant *H. pylori* strains, the severe side effects and the high costs are major drawbacks of these treatments.[1-3] More efficient, economic and friendly drugs need to be developed.

The latest reports in literature demonstrate a definite flare up of many medical challenges strictly related to *H. pylori* existence through immune or many different unknown reasons. Autoimmune thyroiditis, autoimmune pancreatitis, idiopathic or immune thrombocytopenic purpura and acute inflammatory demyelinating polyradiculoneuropathy (Guillian-Barre Syndrome) are examples of these challenges.[2] The flare up of these *H. pylori*-related medical challenges is sufficient to denote that the current combined antibiotic eradication strategies are inadequate to control all the problems associated with the stomach bug.

H. pylori colonized the stomach since an immemorial time;[2] as if both the stomach and the bug used to live together in peace, harmless to each other which could further suggest that *H. pylori* is essentially a natural bacterium.

DM in developing countries has been lately described as the fire when spreads in hay; giving the title "diabetic epidemic" an actual credibility.[4,5] Traditional risk factors do not appear fully sufficient to explain this dramatic spread of diabetes in these countries; in a way that further indicates that traditional measures employed to control the spread of the disease would never be adequate or successful.

A general impression has developed that the ill-decisiveness and the obvious length of the current *H. pylori* eradication treatment courses allowed the chance to the stomach bug to mutate and develop drastic or resistant strains. In addition, the aggression made by antibiotics towards *H. pylori* could have forced it to hide or migrate where it could influence or compromise the immune system. This concept is being supported by the fact that tonsils and adenoids have been lately discovered as secondary reservoirs for *H. pylori*.[2,6]

DM which was once considered a disease of the developed world has become a worldwide pandemic, resembling an ocean wave flooding the whole world with two thirds of the diabetic population living in the developing side of the globe. As much as the precise statistical revision strongly correlates between the prevalence of **H. pylori** and the flare up of DM in developing countries, it also reveals that the diabetic challenge was not as such in these countries before attacking **H. pylori** with antibiotics.[7-12]

A lot of controversy has been encountered as concerns the current strategies of **H. pylori** eradication. The efficacy of **H. pylori** eradication strategies, the appropriate length of treatment and the cost effectiveness, all appear controversial.[13-16] Further reports in literature have devaluated the triple therapy and suggested a quadruple one.[17] **H. pylori** recurrence; whether it is gastric recurrence from dental plaques, fecal-oral recurrence or recurrence via oral intake, is hardly avoidable.[18]

The current antibiotic therapies appear to be successful only in forcing **H. pylori** to migrate outside the stomach to recur later or migrate and hide elsewhere mostly in the colon. The migrated **H. pylori** strains in the colon would continue producing ammonia for a reason or no reason leading to accumulation of profuse toxic amounts of ammonia, un-opposed or buffered by any acidity. Accumulation of profuse amounts of ammonia in the colon is toxic and constitutes a biological toxic stress to the body that could lead to stress diabetes. Administration of traditional oral hypoglycemic pills to a stressed pancreas means an insistence to flog a tired horse leading to turn a potential condition into an established chronic illness with consequent dramatic flare up of the diabetic phenomena.[4,19]

Dietary vinegar (acetic acid 5%) has been recently shown to be an effective and decisive measure for the clinical cure of **H. pylori** dyspepsia with an immediate dramatic relief of patient's symptoms.[4] **H. pylori** is essentially a sanitary conflict before it is a medical challenge,[20] sanitary problems should be treated by hygienic and antiseptic measures but not antibiotics; vinegar could be an answer. Accordingly, colon clear followed by a vinegar-mixed food for few days could constitute an effective decisive natural measure that could help to correct most diabetic conditions developing in relation to **H. pylori**.

REFERENCES:

1. **Volk WA, Gebhardt BM, Hammarskjold M-L, et al.** *Essential of Medical Microbiology. Lippincott-Raven. 1996; 5th Ed: 377.*

2. **Farinha P, Gascoyne RD. Helicobacter pylori and MALT Lymphoma.** *Gastroenterology 2005 May; 128 (6): 1579-605.*

3. **3. Garcia-Altes a, Jovell AJ, Serra-Part M, et al. Management of Helicobacter pylori in duodenal ulcer: a cost-effectiveness analysis.** *Aliment Pharmacol Ther 2000 Dec; 14 (12): 1631-8.*

4. **Nasrat AM. The world misconception and misbehavior towards Helicobacter pylori is leading to major spread of illness.** *The 7th Anti-Aging Medicine World Congress, Monte-Carlo, Monaco, 2009 Mar.* **Available from URL,** *www.euromedicom.com*

5. **Al-Nozha MM, Al-Maatouq MA, Al-Mazrou YY, et al. Diabetes mellitus in Saudi Arabia.** *Saudi Med J 2004 Nov; 25 (11): 1603-10.*

6. **Cirak MY, Ozdek A, Yilmaz D, et al. Detection of Helicobacter pylori and its CagA gene in tonsil and adenoid tissues by PCR.** *Arch Otolaryngol Head Neck Surg. 2003 Nov; 129 (11): 1225-9.*

7. **Katulanda P, Sheriff MH, Matthews DR. The diabetes epidemic in Sri Lanka-a growing problem.** *Ceylon Med J 2006 Mar; 51 (1): 26-8.*

8. Wissow LS. Diabetes, poverty and Latin America. *Patient Educ Couns 2006 May; 61 (2): 169-70. Epub 2006 Apr 18.*

9. Hossain P, Kawar B, El Nahas M. Obesity and diabetes in developing world-a growing challenge. *N Engl J Med 2007 Jan 18; 356 (3): 213-5.*

10. Einecke D. Like a tsunami: diabetes wave floods the whole world. *MMC 2006 Apr 6; 148 (14): 4-6.*

11. Yach D, Stuckler D, Brownell KD. Epidemiologic and economic consequences of the global epidemics of obesity and diabetes. *N Med 2006 Jan; 12 (1): 62-6.*

12. Narayan K, Zhang P, Williams D, et al. How should developing countries manage diabetes? *CMAJ 2006 Sep 26; 175 (7): 733.*

13. McColl K, Murray L, el-Omar E, et al. Symptomatic benefit from eradicating Helicobacter pylori infection in patients with nonulcer dyspepsia. *N Eng J Med 1998; 339: 1869-74.*

14. Laheij RJ, Van Rossum LG, Verbeek AL, et al. Helicobacter pylori infection treatment for nonulcer dyspepsia: An analysis of meta-analysis . *J Clin Gastroenterol 2003 Apr; 36 (4): 315-20.*

15. Ikeda S, Tamamuro T, Hamashima C, et al. Evaluation of the cost-effectiveness of Helicobacter pylori eradication triple therapy vs. conventional therapy for ulcers in Japan. *Aliment Pharmacol Ther 2001 Nov: 15 (11): 1777-85.*

16. 16. Mason J, Axon AT, Forman D, et al. The cost-effectiveness of population Helicobacter pylori screening and treatment: a Markov model using economic data from a randomized controlled trial. *Aliment Pharmacol Ther 2002 Mar; 16 (3): 559-68.*

17. Songür Y, Senol A, Balkarl A, et al. Triple or quadruple tetracycline-based therapies versus standard triple treatment for Helicobacter pylori treatment. *Am J Med Sci 2009 May 26.* [Epub ahead of print]

18. McPhee SJ, Lingappa VR, Ganong WF. Pathophysiology of Disease, An introduction to Clinical Medicine. *Lange Medical Books/McGraw-Hill. 1996; 4th Ed: 361.*

19. Nasrat AM. The dramatic spread of diabetes mellitus and influence of Helicobacter pylori. *The 1st American Diabetes Association Congress in the Middle East, Dubai, 2012 Dec.* Available from URL, *www.ADA-me.org*

20. Zaterka S, Eisig JN, Chinzon D, Rothstein W. Factors related to Helicobacter pylori prevalence in an adult population in Brazil. *Helicobacter 2007 Feb; 12 (1):82-8.*

SCIENTIFIC EVIDENCES ON THE INFLUENCE OF HELICOBACTER PYLORIC ON THE DRAMATIC SPREAD OF DIABETES MELLITUS

***T**he Dramatic Spread of Diabetes Mellitus Worldwide and Influence of Helicobacter pylori:* Published in Journal of General Medicine 2015; 3 (1): 159. (Open Access): Nasrat et al. The dramatic spread of diabetes mellitus worldwide and influence of Helicobacter pylori. *General Med 2015; 3 (1): 159.* *[doi: 10.4172/2327-5146.1000159]*

Background: The flare up of a lot of medical challenges related to ***Helicobacter pylori*** through immune or different unknown reasons made the medical world believe that ***H. pylori*** eradication should be a necessary attempt.[1] These ***H. pylori***-related medical problems are sufficient to render the matter that ***H. pylori*** can reside hidden somewhere in the body be taken seriously and is sufficient to denote that the current combined antibiotic eradication strategies are inadequate to control all the problems associated with the stomach bug.

The spread of diabetes mellitus (DM) is rising in a dramatic way as the fire spreading in hey especially in developing countries giving the term "diabetic epidemic" an actual credibility.[2] ***H. pylori*** could migrate or get forced to migrate to the colon leading to accumulation of profuse toxic amounts of ammonia unopposed or buffered by any acidity leading to biological stress to the body that could predispose to stress diabetes among disadvantaged susceptible people.[3,4]

H. pylori colonized the stomach since an immemorial time;[2] as if both the stomach and the bug used to live together in peace, harmless to each other.

Objective: Demonstration of an influence of the bacterium ***H. pylori*** on the dramatic spread of DM among many patients during latest decades.

Design: Prospective study.

Patients& Methods: The scientific interest of this study was focused on the pathologic effect of ***H. pylori*** in leading to an onset of diabetes. The study was held in Balghsoon Clinics in Jeddah, Saudi Arabia, during the period between May, 2011 and October, 2013. 18 cases of newly discovered DM associated with frank history of ***H. pylori*** dyspepsia were randomly included in the study once the onset of diabetes was recognized without any selection. The protocol of the study has been approved by the institutional review board of King Abdul-Aziz University Hospital in Jeddah, Saudi Arabia. An informed signed consent has been obtained from all patients.

Screening of patients for existence of ***H. pylori*** was based on clinical symptoms and detection of ***H. pylori*** serum antibodies. A brief history suggestive of ***H. pylori*** dyspepsia was taken, the following dyspeptic symptoms; epigastric discomfort, heart burn, abdominal distension and constipation were considered. Detection of ***H.***

pylori serum antibodies, though non-specific, was used for screening as being cost-effective.[3] Existence of **H. pylori** was confirmed by reliable specific and sensitive tests; **H. pylori** fecal antigen and urea breath tests.[4]

The **H. pylori** serum antibodies test was available from Semen Co., USA with Batch No. 104132 while the urea breath test was available from Helicap Co., Sweden with Batch No. HCO1150108-E10. The **H. pylori** fecal antigen test was obtained from Acon Laboratory, USA, Batch No. HP8040008.

Detection of raised random blood sugar samples in three successive days was the criterion to include cases in the study, while recovery from diabetes after eradication of **H. pylori** was not considered before a normal blood sugar curve was achieved.

All patients were middle-eastern citizens, living in a developing country life style and health care standards. Age of patients ranged between 30 and 45 years, they were average to well-built and one of them was overweight. Five patients were having a positive family history of DM; the one with overweight was not having any family history of diabetes. The random blood sugar level upon inclusion of patients in the study ranged between 270 to 330 mg/dl.

Frequency of micturition was a constant feature in all patients and all of them were confirmed positive for **H. pylori** existence by reliable sensitive laboratory tests (**H. pylori** fecal antigen and urea breath tests). None of the patients was undergoing any recent reason of physical or emotional stress, and they were not suffering from any other grave or debilitating illness.

Traditional measures, colon care and colon clear using natural measures were employed for all patients for the relief of dyspeptic symptoms and eradication of **H. pylori** namely vinegar therapy and the potent senna purge leaves extract.[5,6]

A diabetic diet was strictly followed, and extreme carefulness towards re-infection with **H. pylori** via oral intake during the eradication therapy by avoiding outside home meals was seriously needed. The potent senna purge was employed for colon clear while vinegar-mixed yoghurt taken as a salad twice during meals for one week after colon clear was used to behave or get rid of the abnormal behavior gastric **H. pylori** strains. The senna purge and the vinegar therapy were essentially an outpatient treatment. The initial vinegar therapy consisted of one-two table spoonfuls of 5% white vinegar mixed with a small cup of plain yoghurt and taken twice daily during meals for one week.

Successful eradication of **H. pylori** was assessed by the **H. pylori** fecal antigen and urea breath tests. Colon clear, repeated every month with gradual reduction of the dose, was followed during the period of study; while colon care with vinegar-mixed food taken once or twice daily, three to five days a week was considered as a life style during the follow up of patients.

A similar group of patients nearly of similar size (17 patients) who decided to follow oral medical treatment from the start was considered as a control group. They were also of an onset of newly discovered DM with age range of 33-41 years, average built and a random blood sugar of 250-290 mg/dl. They were having no other chronic illness or a family history of diabetes.

Results: All patients became free of any dyspeptic or micturition symptoms, 12 patients (66.7%) resumed a normal blood sugar curve in less than one week. The one with overweight and the five patients with family history of DM were among them. The diabetic condition did not recover except after 10-13 days in 4 patients (22.2%). The glycated hemoglobin (HbA1c) for the above patients ranged between 4.8-5.9% without having any anti-diabetic medical treatment. Failure of follow-up of the case occurred in two patients (11.1%); their diabetic condition did not improve until 2 weeks of therapy, they decided to follow oral medications.

The patients who recovered the diabetic condition were followed up for 18 months; they did not show any recurrence of diabetes. The records of the control group patients were followed for three months. They remained inadequately controlled in spite of medications; the HbA1c was always above 7.0%.

Discussion: DM in developing countries has been lately described as the fire when spreads in hay; giving the title "diabetic epidemic" an actual credibility.[5] Traditional risk factors do not appear fully sufficient to explain this dramatic spread of diabetes in these countries; in a way that further indicates that the traditional measures employed to control the spread of the disease would never be adequate or decisive.

The current study has developed a general impression that the ill-decisiveness and the obvious length of the current ***H. pylori*** eradication treatment courses allowed the chance to the stomach bug to mutate and develop drastic or resistant strains. In addition, the aggression made by antibiotics could have forced this bacterium to hide or migrate where it could influence or compromise the immune system. This impression is being supported by the fact that tonsils and adenoids have been recently discovered as secondary reservoirs for ***H. pylori***.[2,6]

DM which was once considered a disease of the developed world has become a worldwide pandemic, resembling an ocean wave flooding the whole world with two thirds of the diabetic population living in the developing side of the globe.[7,8] As much as the precise statistical revision strongly correlates between the prevalence of ***H. pylori*** and the flare up of DM in developing countries, it also reveals that the diabetic challenge was not as such in these countries before attacking the bug with antibiotics.[7-12]

A lot of controversy has been encountered as concerns the current strategies for ***H. pylori*** eradication. The efficacy of ***H. pylori*** eradication strategies, the appropriate length of treatment and the cost effectiveness; all appear controversial.[13-16] Further reports in literature have devaluated the triple therapy and suggested a quadruple one.[17]

H. pylori recurrence whether it is gastric recurrence from dental plaques, fecal-oral recurrence or recurrence via oral intake is hardly avoidable.[18] The current antibiotic therapies appear to be successful only in forcing ***H. pylori*** outside the stomach to recur later or migrate and hide elsewhere mostly in the colon. The migrated ***H. pylori*** strains in the colon would continue producing ammonia for a reason or no reason leading to accumulation of profuse toxic amounts of ammonia, un-opposed or buffered by any acidity; this constitutes a biological toxic stress to the body that could lead to stress diabetes. Administration of traditional oral hypoglycemic pills to a stressed pancreas means an insistence to flog a tired horse leading to turn a potential condition into an established chronic illness with consequent dramatic flare up of the diabetic phenomena.

Dietary vinegar (acetic acid 5%) has been recently shown to be an effective and decisive measure for the clinical eradication of ***H. pylori*** infection with an immediate dramatic relief of patient's symptoms.[4,19-21] The complex nutritional requirements of ***H. pylori*** are achieved mainly via utilization of pyruvate. As acetate is demonstrated as an end product among the metabolic pathway of ***H. pylori*** and the activity of the pyruvate dehydrogenase complex is controlled by the rules of product inhibition and feedback regulation; this means that addition of acetic acid to the medium could compromise the energy metabolism of ***H. pylori*** or interfere with the organism's respiratory chain metabolism.[22-26]

As long the matter includes interference with the energy metabolism and the respiratory chain metabolism of ***H. pylori***; an immediate paralysis of the organism could be considered, which explains the dramatic immediate symptomatic relief expressed by patients included in this study upon having a vinegar-mixed food. This decisive influence of acetic acid on the activity of ***H. pylori*** allows no chance for the organism to resist the treatment, mutate and develop resistant strains or even get the opportunity to migrate.

Clearing of the colon was considered the integral element of this natural therapy for elimination of all the migrated colonic ***H. pylori*** strains in order to help recovery of a potential diabetic condition that developed consequent to a stressful toxic colonic error.

Follow up of patients of the study was extended to 18 months as those patients are susceptible disadvantaged population and they are liable for recurrence of the diabetic condition in consequence to colonic troubles. They have to keep watching their outside home meals and their colonic condition; they should return to colon clear and regular vinegar therapy whenever they develop any dyspeptic troubles associated with micturition symptoms. They are expected to tolerate and overcome their susceptibility to this toxic biological stress with repeated colon care/colon clear and maintaining carefulness about their colonic condition.

The records of the control group of patients were followed for three months only because they were considered as being candidates of already established diabetes. This could refer to the concept that administration of oral hypoglycemic pills in newly discovered diabetes without ruling out an underlying stress element might constitute a therapeutic malpractice.

Conclusion: In the light of the accurate determination of recent findings and statistics, a revision of the current guidelines for the management of ***H. pylori*** and newly discovered DM may be needed. It may be incorrect that the current world's burden of DM is on the account of type II diabetes. It seems that the antibiotic violence has obliged a domestic bug to become wild in attitude and sequels instead of getting rid of it. The stress element considered in this study in leading to an onset of diabetes is not just hypothetical as upon the basis of this concept the diabetic condition has been successfully and permanently corrected in most patients of the study by mere eradication of the abnormal colonic ***H. pylori*** strains. The patients included in this study should be considered susceptible predisposed individuals and they are liable for recurrence; they should keep watching their meals, their colonic condition and they should return to colon care and colon clear whenever they develop any frank dyspeptic symptoms.

REFERENCES:

1. **Volk WA, Gebhardt BM, Hammarskjold M-L, et al.** Essential of Medical Microbiology. Lippincott-Raven. 1996; 5th Ed: 377.

2. **Farinha P, Gascoyne RD. Helicobacter pylori and MALT Lymphoma.** Gastroenterology 2005 May; 128 (6): 1579-605.

3. **Garcia-Altes a, Jovell AJ, Serra-Part M, et al. Management of Helicobacter pylori in duodenal ulcer: a cost-effectiveness analysis.** Aliment Pharmacol Ther 2000 Dec; 14 (12): 1631-8.

4. **Nasrat AM. The world misconception and misbehavior towards Helicobacter pylori is leading to major spread of illness.** The 7th Anti-Aging Medicine World Congress, Monte-Carlo, Monaco, 2009 Mar. **Available from URL,** www.euromedicom.com

5. **Al-Nozha MM, Al-Maatouq MA, Al-Mazrou YY, et al. Diabetes mellitus in Saudi Arabia.** Saudi Med J 2004 Nov; 25 (11): 1603-10.

6. **Cirak MY, Ozdek A, Yilmaz D, et al. Detection of Helicobacter pylori and its CagA gene in tonsil and adenoid tissues by PCR.** Arch Otolaryngol Head Neck Surg. 2003 Nov; 129 (11): 1225-9.

7. **Katulanda P, Sheriff MH, Matthews DR. The diabetes epidemic in Sri Lanka-a growing problem.** Ceylon Med J 2006 Mar; 51 (1): 26-8.

8. **Wissow LS. Diabetes, poverty and Latin America.** Patient Educ Couns 2006 May; 61 (2): 169-70. Epub 2006 Apr 18.

9. **Hossain P, Kawar B, El Nahas M. Obesity and diabetes in developing world-a growing challenge.** *N Engl J Med 2007 Jan 18; 356 (3): 213-5.*

10. **Einecke D. Like a tsunami: diabetes wave floods the whole world.** *MMC 2006 Apr 6; 148 (14): 4-6.*

11. **Yach D, Stuckler D, Brownell KD. Epidemiologic and economic consequences of the global epidemics of obesity and diabetes.** *N Med 2006 Jan; 12 (1): 62-6.*

12. **Narayan K, Zhang P, Williams D, et al. How should developing countries manage diabetes?** *CMAJ 2006 Sep 26; 175 (7): 733.*

13. **McColl K, Murray L, el-Omar E, et al. Symptomatic benefit from eradicating Helicobacter pylori infection in patients with nonulcer dyspepsia.** *N Eng J Med 1998; 339: 1869-74.*

14. **Laheij RJ, Van Rossum LG, Verbeek AL, et al. Helicobacter pylori infection treatment for nonulcer dyspepsia: An analysis of meta-analysis** *. J Clin Gastroenterol 2003 Apr; 36 (4): 315-20.*

15. **Ikeda S, Tamamuro T, Hamashima C, et al. Evaluation of the cost-effectiveness of Helicobacter pylori eradication triple therapy vs. conventional therapy for ulcers in Japan.** *Aliment Pharmacol Ther 2001 Nov: 15 (11): 1777-85***.**

16. **Mason J, Axon AT, Forman D, et al. The cost-effectiveness of population Helicobacter pylori screening and treatment: a Markov model using economic data from a randomized controlled trial.** *Aliment Pharmacol Ther 2002 Mar; 16 (3): 559-68.*

17. **Songür Y, Senol A, Balkarl A, et al. Triple or quadruple tetracycline-based therapies versus standard triple treatment for Helicobacter pylori treatment.** *Am J Med Sci 2009 May 26.* **[Epub ahead of print]**

18. **McPhee SJ, Lingappa VR, Ganong WF. Pathophysiology of Disease, An introduction to Clinical Medicine.** *Lange Medical Books/McGraw-Hill. 1996; 4*[th] *Ed: 361.***.**

19. **Nasrat AM. The dramatic spread of diabetes mellitus and influence of Helicobacter pylori.** *J Clinic and Appl Res and Educ 2012; 9 (4): 53.*

20. **Nasrat AM. An answer for the controversy of insulin cardioprotection in dysglycemia.** *The 1st American Diabetes Association Congress in the Middle East, Dubai, 2012 Dec.* **Available from URL,** *www.ADA-me.org*

21. **Nasrat AM. Atopic skin pathology; influence of Helicobacter pylori and effect combined colon clear with seroclearance therapy.** *The Aesthetic Dermatology& Anti-Aging Medicine World Congress, Bangkok, Thailand, 2013 Jan.* **Available from URL,** *www.euromedicom.com*

22. **Nasrat AM. An alternative approach for the rising challenge of hypertensive illness via Helicobacter pylori eradication.** *The International Cardiology Symposium, Dubai, 2013 May.* **Available from URL,** *www.ics2013.com*

23. **Mendz GL, Hazell SL, Burns BP. Glucose utilization and lactate production by Helicobacter pylori.** *J Gen Microbiol 1993 Dec; 139 (Pt 12): 3023-8.*

24. **Mendz GL, Hazell SL, van Gorkom L. Pyruvate metabolism in Helicobacter pylori.** *Arch Microbiol. 1994; 162 (3):187-92.*

25. **Berg JM, Tymoczko JL, Stryer L. Biochemistry.** *WH Freeman and Company. 2002; 5th Ed: 480.*

26. **Ge Z. Potential of fumarate reductase as a novel therapeutic target in Helicobacter pylori infection.** *Expert Opin Ther Targets 2002 Apr; 6 (2): 135-46.*

THE CHALLENGE OF CHILDHOOD DIABETES DURING LATE DECADES

The Truth in the Challenge of Childhood Diabetes during Late Decades

Introduction: The frequency of ketoacidosis at onset of childhood in the world particularly in developing countries is significant. Prevention of diabetic ketoacidosis and control of its rising frequency should be a healthcare target.[1] The epidemic of childhood diabetes is a worldwide challenge that could be directly related to the whole world challenging epidemic of childhood obesity or it is simply part of the dramatic spread of adulthood diabetes Mellitus (DM) worldwide.[2-4] _

Similar to the adult DM, *Helicobacter pylori* could represent a major environmental reason that could be directly related to the medical challenge of childhood diabetes. It has been referred to a possible relation between *H. pylori* and DM in children in some studies, while this relation has been denied by other reports.[5,6] *H. pylori* has got an extreme widespread world prevalence; if the organism does not exist in the stomach of all the population in developing countries, the latest knowledge is that 80-90% of adults are estimated to be affected with *H. pylori* in these countries.[7] The flare up of a lot of worldwide medical problems related to *H. pylori* should attract the attention towards the possibility that the stomach bacterium could be lying there behind the problem of DM in children. This possibility deserves to be seriously considered, particularly if autoimmune pancreatitis comes among the medical dilemmas related to *H. pylori*. Moreover, this suggestion is further supported by the fact that tonsils and adenoids have been recently discovered as secondary reservoirs for *H. pylori* in children.[8,9] In addition, the diabetic condition was successfully corrected in adults by mere eradication of colonic *H. pylori* strains. Different reports in literature have confirmed the association of adenotonsillar hypertrophy in children with cytotoxin-associated gene A (cagA) positive *H. pylori* strains, and emphasized that cagA of *H. pylori* encodes a highly immunogenic and virulence-associated protein; the presence of this virulent gene in the body could affect the clinical outcome in many children.[10,11]

The clinical presentation of type 1 childhood DM was studied by some researchers in developing countries, it was emphasized that the clinical picture of type 1 childhood diabetes in developing countries seems to differ from that in developed countries;[12] the difference in *H. pylori* prevalence might be a reason. The world literature does not have sufficient explanation for the rising burden of diabetes among children,[2,3] in the same way, pediatricians do not possess good reasons for this matter in developing countries.[13] The world literature refers with concern to the association and role of *H. pylori* in the adult metabolic syndrome. It was also shown that prevention of the metabolic syndrome was achieved by *H. pylori* eradication in adults.[14,15] In spite of that, the world literature lacks information as concerns the role of *H. pylori* in childhood metabolic syndrome (childhood obesity and childhood diabetes).

H. pylori colonized the stomach since an immemorial time; existence of ***H. pylori*** in children starts trans-familial during early childhood, and the ***H. pylori*** strain is often identical with that of parents. Interestingly, children maintain the same strain genotype even after moving to a different enviroment.[9,10] The challenge lies in the emergence of antibiotic-resistant ***H. pylori*** strains, which is most probably due to inefficiency of the current eradication strategies.[16,17] It would not be scientifically sound to cost the child's delicate physical or immune structure the drastic side-effects of repeated antibiotic eradication therapies upon every detection of ***H. pylori***; revision of the current guidelines for the management of ***H. pylori*** might be urgently required.

H. pylori could migrate or get forced to migrate to the colon; it will continue producing ammonia unopposed or buffered by any acidity, leading to accumulation of profuse toxic amounts of ammonia that could lead to toxic pancreatitis causing an onset of diabetes.[9,10]

REFERENCES:

1. **Habib HS.** Frequency and clinical presentation of ketoacidosis at onset of childhood type 1 diabetes mellitus in Northwest Saudi Arabia. *Saudi Med J 2005 Dec; 26 (12): 1936-9.*

2. **Sabin MA, Shield JP. Childhood obesity.** *Front Home Res 2008; 36: 85-96.*

3. **De Ferranti SD, Osganian SK. Epidemiology of pediatric metabolic syndrome and type 2 diabetes mellitus.** *Diab Vasc Dis Res 2007 Dec; 4 (4): 285-96.*

4. **Al-Nozha MM, Al-Maatouq MA, Al-Mazrou YY, et al. Diabetes mellitus in Saudi Arabia.** *Saudi Med J 2004 Nov; 25 (11): 1603-10.*

5. **Salardi S, Cacciari E, Menegatti M, et al. Helicobacter pylori and type 1 diabetes mellitus in children.** *J Pediatr Gastroenterol Nutr 1999 Mar; 28 (3): 307-9.*

6. **Dore MP, Bilotta M, Malatty HM, et al. Diabetes mellitus and Helicobacter pylori infection.** *Nutrition 2000 Jun; 16 (6): 407-10.*

7. **Baron S. Baron's medical microbiology.** *Churchill Livingstone. 2000; 4ᵗʰ Ed: 346.*

8. **Kountouras J, Zavos C, Chatzopoulos D. A concept on the role of Helicobacter pylori infection in autoimmune pancreatitis.** *J Cell Mol Med 2005 Jan-Mar; 9 (1):196-207.*

9. **Farinha P, Gascoyne RD. Helicobacter pylori and MALT Lymphoma.** *Gastroenterology 2005 May; 128 (6): 1579-605.*

10. **Nasrat SAM, Nasrat RM, Nasrat MN, et al. The dramatic spread of diabetes mellitus worldwide and influence of Helicobacter pylori.** *General Med. 2015; 3 (1): 159-62.*

11. **Bulut Y, Agacayak A, Karlidag D, et al. Association of CagA+ Helicobacter pylori with adenotonsillar hypertrophy.** *Tohoku J Exp Med. 2006 Jul; 209 (3): 229-33.*

12. **12. Kulaylat NA, Narchi H. Clinical picture of childhood type 1 diabetes mellitus in the Eastern Province of Saudi Arabia.** *Pediatr Diabetes 2001 Mar; 2 (1): 43-7.*

13. **Salman H, Abanamy A, Ghassan B, et al. Childhood diabetes in Saudi Arabia.** *Diabet Med 1991 Feb-Mar; 8 (2): 176-8.*

14. **Nabipour I, Vahdat K, Jafari SM, et al. The association of metabolic syndrome and Chlamydia pneumoniae, Helicobacter pylori, cytomegalovirus, and herpes simplex type 1: the Persian Gulf Healthy Heart Study.** *Cardiovasc Diabetol 2006 Dec1; 5: 25.*

15. **Longo-Mbenza B, Nkondi Nsenga J, Vangu Ngoma D. Prevention of metabolic syndrome insulin resistance and the atherosclerotic diseases in Africans infected by Helicobacter pylori infection and treated by antibiotics.** *Int J Cardiol 2007 Oct 18; 121 (3): 229-38. Epub 2007 Mar 26.*

16. **Ge Z. Potential of fumarate reductase as a novel therapeutic target in Helicobacter pylori infection.** *Expert Opin Ther Targets 2002 Apr; 6 (2): 135-46.*

17. **Gasbarrini A, Franceschi F. Does Helicobacter pylori play a role in idiopathic thrombocytopenic purpura and in other autoimmune diseases?** *Am J Gastroenterol 2005 Jun; 100 (6):1265-70.*

SCIENTIFIC EVIDENCES ON THE CHALLENGE OF CHILDHOOD DIABETES DURING LATE DECADES

Scientific Evidences on the Truth of Childhood Diabetes during Late Decades

The *Challenge of Childhood Diabetes:* Published in Journal of General Medicine 2015; 3 (4): 193. (Open Access): Nasrat et al. The challenge of childhood diabetes. *General Med 2015; 3 (4): 193.* [doi: 10.4172/2327-5146.1000193]

Background: The rising frequency of childhood diabetes mellitus (DM) in the world should not be taken in separate consideration from the true scientific facts concerning the worldwide epidemic of adult DM.[1] The correlation between diabetes and the increased incidence of obesity in children should be also considered.[2-4]

Helicobacter pylori was suggested as one of the environmental reasons that could be directly related to the problem of childhood DM. The challenge lies mainly in the emergence of drastic resistant *H. pylori* strains due to the antibiotic violence against the stomach bacterium; these strains can travel from parents during early childhood to kids leading to a state of biological stress that could lead to stress diabetes; interestingly, children maintain the same strain genotype of *H. pylori* lifelong even they move to a different environment unless it is eradicated.[1,2,5-7]

The current eradication treatments of *H. pylori* have shown a lot of controversy;[3,4,8] it would be a plea to cost the child's delicate structure the drastic side effects of repeated antibiotic eradication therapies upon every detection of *H. pylori*.

Objective: Demonstration of a possible correlation between the worldwide challenge of *H. pylori* prevalence and the challenging spread of childhood diabetes in the world._

Design& Setting: A multiple-case clinical study done in Balghsoon Clinics in Jeddah/Saudi Arabia during the period May 2012-October 2013. The protocol of the study was approved and the study followed the research committee ethics of Balghsoon Clinics.

Patients& Methods: The study included 10 children with average body built and an average age range of 6-9 years old, they were discovered with an early onset of hyperglycemia (wasting of weight and diuresis); a blood sugar level above 270 mg/dl confirmed the onset of diabetes. Appearance and spontaneous disappearance of the diabetic condition in 6 children among them was the motive to attract the attention towards the possibility of a potential condition causing temporary insult to the pancreas that recovers spontaneously. An influence of *H. pylori* was suggested; accordingly existence of *H. pylori* was tested in children and their parents using specific tests (urea breath test and *H. pylori* fecal antigen).[9]

Immediate natural therapy for *H. pylori* eradication that consisted of colon clear employing the natural senna leaves purge together with colon care using bio-organic acids; lactic and acetic, were done for children and their parents.[10,11]

Results: All children and their parents were found positive for ***H. pylori*** existence; they became free of ***H. pylori*** strains in the stomach and the colon after the natural therapy as confirmed by specific sensitive tests; urea breath and ***H. pylori*** fecal antigen tests, except parents of three families who needed revision of colon clear for complete eradication of ***H. pylori***. The diabetic condition has been successfully corrected in 9 children (90%) without any insulin therapy while one diabetic child failed to respond to the natural therapy. The diet of children and their bowel motion habits were carefully watched, meanwhile their medical condition was followed up for 18 months. Recurrence of the diabetic condition within 3-5 months occurred in 3 children (30%) which was corrected in 2 of them.

The results of this study was compared with that of other 7 children of rather similar body built and rather similar age range (6-10 years) who newly developed DM and their parents preferred to put them on insulin medication. Their diabetic condition remained inadequately controlled in spite of regular assessment of therapy and carefulness about their diet.

Ethical Considerations: An informed signed consent was taken from all parents; children were allowed to lead their routine style of life except strict follow up of diabetic diet and extreme carefulness about outside-home food intake. Parents were free to make their children quit the study at any time or whenever they feel negative towards the natural therapy.

Discussion: The clinical presentation of type 1 childhood DM was studied by some researchers in developing countries, it was emphasized that the clinical picture of type 1 childhood diabetes in developing countries seems to differ from that in developed countries;[12,13] the difference in ***H. pylori*** prevalence might be a reason. The world literature does not have sufficient explanation for the rising burden of diabetes in children.[2,3] In the same way, pediatricians do not possess good reasons for that matter in developing countries.[14] The world literature refers with concern for the association and role of ***H. pylori*** in the adult metabolic syndrome. It was also shown that prevention of the metabolic syndrome was achieved by ***H. pylori*** eradication in adults.[15,16] In spite of that, the world literature lacks any information as concerns the role of ***H. pylori*** in childhood metabolic syndrome (childhood obesity and childhood diabetes).

H. pylori colonized the stomach since an immemorial time; existence of ***H. pylori*** in children starts trans-familial during early childhood, and the ***H. pylori*** strain is often identical with that of parents. Interestingly, children maintain the same strain genotype even after moving to a different enviroment.[9,10] The challenge lies in the emergence of antibiotic-resistant drastic or abnormal behavior ***H. pylori*** strains, which is most probably due to the abuse of antibiotics or inefficiency of the current eradication strategies.[17] It would not be scientifically sound to cost the child's delicate physical structure or his immune system the drastic side-effects of repeated ***H. pylori*** antibiotic eradication therapies upon detection of ***H. pylori*** each time; revision of the current guidelines for the management of ***H. pylori*** may be needed.[18]

H. pylori could migrate or get forced to migrate to the colon; it will continue producing ammonia for a reason or no reason, unopposed or buffered by any acidity, leading to accumulation of profuse toxic amounts of ammonia that could lead to toxic biological stress or toxic pancreatitis causing an onset of diabetes.[9,10]

Dietary vinegar (acetic acid 5%) has been recently demonstrated as dramatic, effective and decisive solution for all the challenges and medical problems related to ***H. pylori*** infection including eradication and re-infection. The cure rate of vinegar therapy reaches above 97% with negligible incidence of failure of treatment or recurrence of infection. The vinegar therapy is simply based on a definite pathophysiologic principle that can open the gate for wonderful solutions for many patients rendering this dietary stuff worthy to change the whole world attitude in dealing with the challenge known as ***H. pylori*** infection.[19] The complex nutritional requirements of ***H. pylori*** are achieved through its unique energy metabolism, which exhibits characteristic sites. These sites can be considered as targets that should attract any attempts to fight the organism.[12] As acetate is demonstrated as an end product among the metabolic pathway of ***H. pylori***; this means that acetic acid could compromise the energy metabolism of ***H. pylori***, or interfere with the organism's respiratory chain. This suggestion is supported by the fact that the major routes of generation of energy for *H. pylori* are via pyruvate and the activity of the pyruvate dehydrogenase complex is controlled by product inhibition and feedback regulation. It is further supported by the observation that addition of pyruvate to different solid culture media was found to inhibit bacterial growth, and this inhibition was attributed to accumulation of acetate and formate.[12,19,20] As the matter includes interference with the energy metabolism and the respiratory chain of *H. pylori*; an immediate paralysis of the organism could be considered with dramatic relief of patient's symptoms. The fast immediate influence of acetic acid on *H. pylori* gives no chance for the organism to resist the treatment with vinegar or to mutate and develop resistant strains.

In *Conclusion:* The challenge of childhood diabetes could be simply part of the *H. pylori*-related worldwide dramatic spread of DM. Natural colon clear should be regarded as safe and effective measure for eradication of the abnormal-habitat colonic *H. pylori* strains. Revision of the guide lines of the newly discovered childhood diabetes should be considered.

Conflict of Interest: There is no conflict of interest existing.

REFERENCES:

1. **Habib HS.** Frequency and clinical presentation of ketoacidosisat onset of childhood type 1 diabetes mellitus in Northwest Saudi Arabia. *Saudi Med J 2005 Dec; 26 (12): 1936-9.*

2. **Sabin MA, Shield JP. Childhood obesity.** *Front Home Res 2008; 36: 85-96.*

3. **De Ferranti SD, Osganian SK. Epidemiology of pediatric metabolic syndrome and type 2 diabetes mellitus.** *Diab Vasc Dis Res 2007 Dec; 4 (4): 285-96.*

4. **Al-Nozha MM, Al-Maatouq MA, Al-Mazrou YY, etal. Diabetes mellitus in Saudi Arabia.** *Saudi Med J 2004 Nov; 25 (11): 1603-10.*

5. **Salardi S, Cacciari E, Menegatti M, et al. Helicobacter pylori and type 1 diabetes mellitus in children.** *J Pediatr Gastroenterol Nutr 1999 Mar; 28 (3): 307-9.*

6. **Dore MP, Bilotta M, Malatty HM, et al. Diabetes mellitus and Helicobacter pylori infection.** *Nutrition 2000 Jun; 16 (6): 407-10.*

7. **Kountouras J, Zavos C, Chatzopoulos D. A concept on the role of Helicobacter pylori infection in autoimmune pancreatitis.** *J Cell Mol Med 2005 Jan-Mar; 9 (1): 196-207.*

8. **Ge Z. Potential of fumarate reductase as a novel therapeutic target in Helicobacter pylori infection.** *Expert Opin Ther Targets 2002 Apr; 6 (2): 135-46*

9. **Farinha P, Gascoyne RD. Helicobacter pylori and MALT Lymphoma.** *Gastroenterology 2005 May; 128 (6): 1579-605.*

10. **Nasrat SAM, Nasrat RM, Nasrat MN, et al. The dramatic spread of diabetes mellitus worldwide and influence of Helicobacter pylori.** *General Med. 2015; 3 (1): 159-62.*

11. **Nasrat AM. The world misconception and misbehavior towards Helicobacter pylori is leading to major spread of illness.** *The 7th Anti-Aging Medicine World Congress, Monte-Carlo, Monaco, 2009 Mar.* **Available from URL,** *www.euromedicom.com*

12. **Bulut Y, Agacayak A, Karlidag D, et al. Association of CagA+ Helicobacter pylori with adenotonsillar hypertrophy.** *Tohoku J Exp Med. 2006 Jul; 209 (3): 229-33.*

13. **Kulaylat NA, Narchi H. Clinical picture of childhood type 1 diabetes mellitus in the Eastern Province of Saudi Arabia.** *Pediatr Diabetes 2001 Mar; 2(1): 43-7.*

14. **Salman H, Abanamy A, Ghassan B, et al. Childhood diabetes in Saudi Arabia.** *Diabet Med 1991 Feb-Mar; 8 (2): 176-8.*

15. **Nabipour I, Vahdat K, Jafari SM, et al. The association of metabolic syndrome and Chlamydia pneumoniae, Helicobacter pylori, cytomegalovirus, and herpes simplex type 1: the Persian Gulf Healthy Heart Study.** *Cardiovasc Diabetol 2006 Dec1; 5: 25.*

16. **Longo-Mbenza B, Nkondi Nsenga J, Vangu Ngoma D. Prevention of metabolic syndrome insulin resistance and the atherosclerotic diseases in Africans infected by Helicobacter pylori infection and treated by antibiotics.** *Int J Cardiol 2007 Oct 18; 121 (3): 229-38. Epub 2007 Mar 26.*

17. **Ge Z. Potential of fumarate reductase as a novel therapeutic target in Helicobacter pylori infection.** *Expert Opin Ther Targets 2002 Apr; 6 (2): 135-46.*

18. **Gasbarrini A, Franceschi F. Does Helicobacter pylori play a role in idiopathic thrombocytopenic purpura and in other autoimmune diseases?** *AM J Gastroenterol 2005 Jun; 100 (6):1265-70.*

19. **Nasrat AM. A new approach for the hematologic challenges of Helicobacter pylori infection in children. The** *International Symposium of the Egyptian Society of Pediatric Hematology/Oncology, 2006 Mar. Available from URL,* *www. espho.org*

20. **Cirak MY, Ozdek A, Yilmaz d, et al. Detection of Helicobacter pylori and its CagA gene in tonsil and adenoid tissues by PCR.** *Arch Otolaryngol Head Neck Surg 2003 Nov; 129 (11): 1225-9.*

HOW SHOULD THE WORLD MANAGE THE CHALLENGE OF DIABETES!!

ow Should the World Manage the Challenge of Diabetes Mellitus!! Published in Journal of General Medicine 2016; 4 (1): 223. (Open Access). Nasrat AM. How should the world manage the challenge of diabetes mellitus!! *Gen Med 2016; 4 (1): 223. [doi: 10.4172/2327-5146.1000223]*

The last three decades have shown prevalence of abnormal-behavior ***Helicobacter pylori*** strains and rising figures of many medical challenges related to these strains of the bacterium. It means that the last three decades demonstrated rediscovery of ***H. pylori***, the antibiotic aggression towards it, the prevalence of its abnormal-behavior strains instead of getting rid of them, and the flare up of a lot of medical challenges related to these ***H. pylori*** strains.[1,2] A medical study which does not correlate between these obvious findings is definitely not employing a clinical sense.

H. pylori colonized the stomach since an immemorial time;[1] as if both the stomach wall and the bacterium used to live together in peace harmless to each other. ***H. pylori*** in the stomach leads a physiological behavior identical with that of natural bacteria; namely its existence since an immemorial time, having mostly-harmless long history inside the stomach before being attacked by antibiotics, its huge biological talents of survival inside the stomach and its gastric recurrence is being unavoidable. In addition to that, ***H. pylori*** is protective against reflux disease and the development of low acidity-related carcinoma of the cardia of stomach.[1,2]

Although eradications regimens seem to efficiently eradicate ***H. pylori*** from the stomach; the emergence of antibiotic-resistant ***H. pylori*** strains and the severe side effects are major drawbacks of these treatments.[1] Apparently ***H. pylori*** is not eradicated from the stomach but forced to migrate elsewhere as evidenced by its re-appearance in unusual existence exceeding limits of the stomach together with the development of new unusual symptoms.[1,2] More efficient, economic and friendly drugs should be developed.

H. pylori could migrate or get forced to migrate to the colon under the influence of antibiotics where it will continue to produce ammonia for a reason or no reason leading to accumulation of profuse amounts of ammonia un-opposed or buffered by any acidity. Accumulation of profuse amounts of ammonia is toxic and constitutes a biological stress to the body that could lead to stress diabetes in predisposed individuals. Administration of oral hypoglycemic pills to a stressed pancreas means an insistence to flog a tired horse turning a potential condition into an established chronic illness with consequent flare up of the diabetic phenomena all over the world.[1-3]

Colon clear with the senna leaves extract purge and vinegar-mixed food therapy have been recently demonstrated to effectively deal with the challenge of ***H. pylori*** including eradication of colonic and abnormal-behavior gastric ***H. pylori*** strains in addition to prevention of recurrence via interference with re-setting up of further abnormal-behavior colonization via oral intake.[2,3]

H. pylori, being a natural bacterium,[1,2] travels from stomach to stomach via meals. As rich people tour in poor countries and poor people travel to work in rich countries; therefore, bad ***H. pylori*** strains can travel from stomach to stomach and navigate from country to country.

Accumulation of acidic metabolites and inflammatory mediators in the tissues and circulation is a fact that has been documented and reported. Glucose/insulin disproportion is a major reason for accumulation of these toxic elements in the body. These substances can induce vascular spasm and other effects on vascular endothelium.[4,5] Therefore; a dysglycemic patient might no way face a cardiac event, leg ischemia or diabetic foot complication in his life. Elimination of these toxic elements is a challenge that would definitely help to correct an underlying micro-circulatory error.

Therefore; countries should follow a strategy towards ***H. pylori*** dyspepsia and ***H. pylori***-related dysglycemia or diabetes:

Newly discovered diabetes should be first considered a potential condition not an established illness and should be treated as stress diabetes until proved otherwise. Patients should be immediately investigated for existence of colonic ***H. pylori*** strains with immediate employment of colon clear for positive cases using the senna leaves purge once, then followed by vinegar therapy mixed with food once or twice daily for one week. The senna purge could be employed empirically for patients who were found negative for colonic ***H. pylori*** strains. Patients with inadequate improvement of blood sugar level after colon care and colon clear by the vinegar and senna could repeat the senna purge monthly for further two times. Patients who remain hyperglycemic in spite of these measures should be given one week physical rest together with physiological rest of the pancreas by administration of fractionated regular insulin doses for one week; they must not receive oral pills for hyperglycemia. Patients who do not recover after these measures can be considered established diabetic patients (type II diabetes) and can receive the anti-diabetic medication as appropriate to their condition.

Patients who recover a potential diabetic condition should practice extreme carefulness towards outside-home meals and should return to colon care and colon clear whenever they develop frank colonic troubles. They should guard against gastric recurrence by regular dental hygiene and dental plaques cleaning or mouth wash with diluted dietary white vinegar twice weekly; it was observed that cleaning of dental plaques was associated with improvement of dyspeptic symptoms. Washing hands with vinegar and water after washing with soap is necessary when visiting the toilet in order to avoid fecal-oral recurrence as soap alone does kill ***H. pylori***.

The antibiotic aggression against ***H. pylori*** should be stopped and gastric sedatives including anti-urease activity should be subjected to severe revision and accurate re-determination.

Stop searching/researching after ***H. pylori***; save these funds and direct them towards raising the life standards and water supply quality in poor and developing countries.

Patients and family education as concerns misbehavior in food habits and antibiotic use.

Orientation in health care units as concerns natural manures towards ***H. pylori*** dyspepsia.

Food handlers should strictly and frequently disinfect hands with vinegar and travelers should make vinegar a friend with their meals while touring.

Development of the awareness about the need of a diabetic patient to undergo blood-let out cupping therapy once a year or once during the course of his diabetes in order to guard against coronary and peripheral ischemic issues as withdrawal of the ischemic mediators from the body and circulation is not feasible through the available clinical measures but only via cupping therapy.[6-8]

REFERENCES:

1. **Farinha P, Gascoyne RD.** Helicobacter pylori and MALT Lymphoma. *Gastroenterology 2005 May; 128 (6): 1579-605.*

2. **Nasrat AM. The world misconception and misbehavior towards Helicobacter pylori is leading to major spread of illness.** *The 7th Anti-Aging Medicine World Congress, Monte-Carlo, Monaco, 2009 Mar.* **Available from URL,** *www.euromedicom.com*

3. **Nasrat SAM, Nasrat RM, Nasrat MM, et al. The dramatic spread of diabetes mellitus worldwide and influence of Helicobacter pylori.** *General Med 2015; 3 (1): 159-62*

4. **Yu Q, Gao F, Ma XL. Insulin says NO to cardiovascular disease.** *Cardiovasc Res 2011 Feb 15; 89 (3): 516-24.Epub 2010 Nov 4. Review*

5. **Ozben B, Erdogan O. The role of inflammation in acute coronary syndromes.** *Inflamm Allergy Drug Targets 2008 Sep; 7 (3):136-44.*

6. **Nasrat AM, Nasrat SAM, Nasrat RM, et al. Role of blood-let out cupping therapy in taming the wild hepatitis B virus.** *Int J Recent Sci Res 2015 Jul; 6 (7): 5049-5051.*

7. **Nasrat AM, Nasrat RM, Nasrat MM, et al. A therapeutic answer for the controversy of insulin cardio-protection among dysglycemic patients.** *General Med 2015; 3 (6): 1000216.*

8. **Nasrat AM, Nasrat SAM, Nasrat RM, et al. Diabetic leg critical ischemia; early clinical detection and therapeutic cupping prophylaxis.** *General Med 2015; 3 (4): 1000201.*

ILLNESS VIA HELICOBACTER PYLORI ERADICATION
Most Patients Could Quit Medications and Maintain Normal BP Values after Colon Clear

Introduction: The prevalence of hypertension continues to rise across the world, and most patients who receive medical treatment are inadequately controlled. It has been reported that tackling the global challenge of hypertension will require partnerships among multiple centers and constituencies.[1] Hypertension, a disease of rich, is now flaring up as a challenge among poor population. Some reports consider hypertension in developing countries a consequence of progress and life style changes.[2] In spite of that, traditional risk factors do not appear fully sufficient to explain the rising figures of hypertensive illness which further indicates that attempts to control the problem depending upon traditional measures alone can never be adequate, decisive or successful. *Helicobacter pylori* remains a challenging worldwide medical problem due to its extreme widespread prevalence, the lost quality of life of patients, the economic burden associated with its upper gastrointestinal symptoms and its close relation to acid peptic disease, gastric carcinoma and lymphoma.[3-6] About 50% of adults in the developed and 80-90% in the developing countries are estimated to be affected by *H. pylori*.[7,8] Affection with *H. pylori* is typically life-long unless treated. It has got a clear age-related prevalence, increasing from 10% in those younger than 30 until it reaches a plateau of about 60% in those older than age of 60 or even to about 70% at 50 years of age in higher risk areas.[3,9] Although the eradication regimens do eradicate *H. pylori* from the stomach, the emergence of antibiotic-resistant *H. pylori* strains, the severe side effects and high costs are major drawbacks of these treatments.[10] More efficient, economic and friendly drugs need to be developed. Moreover, the flare up of a lot of challenges related to *H. pylori* through immune or different unknown reasons indicates that the current combined antibiotic therapy is not an effective measure to control all the problems caused by the stomach bug. Idiopathic hypertension and atherosclerotic stroke lie among these challenges.[11-13] Arterial hypertension is a risk factor for atherosclerosis which itself is of obscure pathogenesis; growing evidences demonstrate the causative role of endothelial dysfunction. A possible association between *H. pylori* and cardiovascular disorders has been found. The release of cytotoxic substances either of a bacterial origin or produced by the host may represent mediators of these systemic sequelae.[11] Different reports have confirmed the development and association of cytotoxin-associated gene A (cagA) positive *H. pylori* strains with many clinical problems. These reports emphasized that cagA of *H. pylori* encodes a highly immunogenic and virulence-associated protein; the presence of this virulent gene in the body could affect the clinical outcome in many patients.[14] Concerning the pathologic behavior of *H. pylori*, the organism resides and colonizes under the mucus layer overlying gastric mucosa. Although gastric acid plays an important bactericidal role, survival of *H. pylori* inside the stomach is achieved through various defense mechanisms, mainly the profuse buffering capacity of ammonia produced by the organism and the high motility of *H. pylori* even in the extremely viscid gastric mucus that also offers the organism wide range of pH gradients.[6,15-18] In vitro inhibition of *H. pylori* growth was demonstrated due to the effect of some organic acids, lactic, formic and acetic with the lactic acid demonstrating the greatest inhibition due to the effect of feedback regulation and product inhibition as the main product of glucose utilization by *H. pylori* is recognized as lactate.[19]

REFERENCES:

1. **Bakris G, Hill M, Mancia G, et al.** Achieving blood pressures goals globally: five core actions for health-care professionals. A worldwide call to action. *J Hum Hypertens 2008 Jan; 22 (1): 63-70.*

2. **Reddy KS, Naik N, Prabhakaran D. Hypertension in developing world: a consequence of progress.** *Curr Cardiol Rep 2006 Nov; 8 (6); 399-404.*

3. **Andreoli TE. Cecil Essentials of Medicine.** *WB Saunders Company. 2001; 5th Ed: 334.*

4. **Fendrick AM. The role of economic evaluation in the diagnosis and treatment of Helicobacter pylori infection**. *Gastroenterol Clin North Am 2000 Dec; 29 (4): 837-51.*

5. **Groeneveld PW, Lieu TA, Fendrick AM, et al. Quality of life measurement clarifies the cost-effectiveness of Helicobacter pylori eradication in peptic ulcer disease and uninvestigated dyspepsia**. *Am J Gastroenterol 2001 Feb; 96 (2): 338-47.*

6. **Baron S. Baron's medical microbiology.** *Churchill Livingstone. 2000; 4th Ed: 346.*

7. **Versalovic J. Helicobacter pylori. Pathology and diagnostic strategies**. *Am J Clin Pathol 2003 Mar; 119 (3); 403-12.*

8. **Strand M, Presecki V, Babus V, et al. Epidemiology of Helicobacter pylori infection.** *Lijec Vjesn 2002 Sep; 124 Suppl 1: 5-9.*

9. **Asaka M. Epidemiology of Helicobacter pylori infection in Japan.** *Nippon Rinsho 2003 Jan; 61 (1): 19-24.*

10. **Ge Z. Potential of fumarate reductase as a novel therapeutic target in Helicobacter pylori infection.** *Expert Opin Ther Targets 2002 Apr; 6 (2): 135-46.*

11. **Migneco A, Ojetti V, Specchia L, et al. Eradication of Helicobacter pylori infection improves blood pressure values in patients affected by hypertension.** *Helicobacter 2003 Dec; 8 (6): 585-9.*

12. **Diomedi M, Pietroiusti A, Silvestrini M, et al. CagA-positive Helicobacter pylori strains may influence the natural history of atherosclerotic stroke.** *Neurology 2004 Sep; 63 (5):800-4.*

13. **Pietroiusti A, Diomedi M, Silvestrini M, et al. Cytotoxin-associated gene-A-positive Helicobacter pylori strains are associated with atherosclerotic stroke.** *Circulationy 2002 Jul 30; 106 (5):580-4.*

14. **Bulut Y, Agacayak A, Karlidag D, et al. Association of CagA+ Helicobacter pylori with adenotonsillar hypertrophy.** *Tohoku J Exp Med. 2006 Jul; 209 (3): 229-33.*

15. **Zentilin P, Iiritano E, Vingale C, et al. Helicobacter pylori infection is not involved in the Pathogenesis of either erosive or non-erosive gastro-oesophageal reflux disease.** *Aliment Pharmacol Ther 2003 Apr; 17 (8): 1057-64.*

16. **Volk WA, Gebhardt BM, Hammarskjold M-L, et al. Essential of Medical Microbiology. Lippincott–Raven. 1996; 5th Ed: 377.**

17. **Cotran RS, Kumar V, Collins T. Robins Pathologic Basis of Disease.** *WB Saunders Company. 1999; 6th Ed: 790.*

18. **Sleigh JD, Timbury MC. Notes on Medical Microbiology**. *Churchill Livingstone. 1998; 5th Ed: 232.*

19. **Midolo PD, Lambert JR, Hull R, Luo F, et al. In vitro inhibition of Helicobacter pylori NCTC 11637 by organic acids and lactic acid bacteria.** *J Appl Bacteriol. 1995 Oct; 79 (4); 475-9.*

CIENTIFIC EVIDENCES ON THE ROLE OF HELICOBACTER PYLORI IN FLARE UP OF HYPERTENSIVE ILLNESS

A*n Alternative Approach for the Rising Challenge of Hypertensive Illness via Helicobacter pylori Eradication:* Published in Journal of Cardiology Research; 2015; 6 (1): 221-225. (Open Access). Nasrat et al. An alternative approach for the rising challenge of hypertensive illness via Helicobacter pylori eradication. *J Cardiol Res 2015; 6 (1): 221-225. [doi: 10.14740/cr382e]*

Background: The prevalence of hypertension in developing countries has been considered by some reports a consequence of progress and life style changes. In spite of that, traditional risk factors do not appear fully sufficient to explain the rising figures of hypertensive illness which further indicates that attempts to control the problem depending upon traditional measures can never be adequate or decisive.[1,2] ***Helicobacter pylori*** could migrate or get forced to migrate to the colon; it will continue producing ammonia for a reason or no reason leading to accumulation of profuse toxic amounts of ammonia, unopposed or buffered by any acidity, which could lead to multiple colonic and a high rectal spasm. A colonic re-absorptive error is established with excessive fluid and salt retention in the body that would definitely lead to hypertension which is supposed to remain inadequately controlled without correction of the underlying pathological error.[3-9] the flare up of a lot of challenges related to ***H. pylori*** through immune or different unknown reasons indicates that the current combined antibiotic therapy is not an effective measure to control all the problems caused by the stomach bug. Idiopathic hypertension and atherosclerotic stroke lie among these challenges.[10-13] Arterial hypertension is a risk factor for atherosclerosis which itself is of obscure pathogenesis; growing evidences demonstrate the causative role of endothelial dysfunction. A possible association between ***H. pylori*** and cardiovascular disorders has been found.[11,13-18] In vitro inhibition of ***H. pylori*** growth was demonstrated due to the effect of some bio-organic acids, lactic, formic and acetic.[19]

Objective: Demonstration of the effect of natural ***H. pylori*** eradication from the colon on blood pressure (BP) values in patients with hypertension under medication associated with ***H. pylori*** dyspepsia.

Design & Setting: Prospective study was held in Balghsoon Polyclinic, Saudi Arabia during the period from May 2011 to October 2013.

Patients and Methods: Hypertensive patients under medication with frank history of ***H. pylori*** dyspepsia were randomly included in this study without any selection except smokers and those with an associated chronic illness like diabetes who were excluded. The study included 99 different nationality male patients living in Saudi Arabia. The age of patients ranged between 25 and 55 years and they were receiving different groups of antihypertensive medications. Their body weight ranged between average to well-built; seven patients (7.07%) were slim and three patients (3.03%) were overweight. The range of their systolic BP under medication was 140 - 155 mm Hg, and the diastolic range was 90 - 105 mm Hg. The following ***H. pylori***-related dyspeptic symptoms were considered, hyperacidity, stomach upsets, acid reflux, indigestion, abdominal distension after meals and constipation. The lipid profile for all patients had been within normal range without any medical treatment. Their hypertensive illness was essential and was not secondary to any organic disorder. ***H. pylori*** serum antibody test, though non-specific, was used for screening of all patients as being cost effective. ***H. pylori***

existence was confirmed in all patients by reliable specific tests, urea breath test and *H. pylori* fecal antigen.[20] Routine colonoscopy was done for all patients in order to exclude colonic pathology. Patients demonstrating significant colonic pathology such as diffuse ulcerations or multiple polyposis were preferably excluded as they would not tolerate or feel easy with the natural remedies used in the study. The *H. pylori* serum antibodies test was available from Semen Co., USA with Batch No. 104132 while the urea breath test was available from Helicap Co., Sweden with Batch No. HCO1150108-E10. The *H. pylori* fecal antigen test was obtained from Acon Laboratory, USA, Batch No. HP8040008. A colon clear by the natural senna leaves purge was employed for all patients as a primary step in order to eradicate the migrated colonic *H. pylori* strains.[21-22] All patients followed a natural remedy for gastric and colon care to complete eradication of the abnormal-behavior *H. pylori* strains; 20 cc of dietary white vinegar 5-6% mixed with a food staff (white cheese, mashed potato or yoghurt which is the best preferred food stuff for the vinegar to be mixed with), two times daily during meals for 7 - 10 days.[21] Confirmation of *H. pylori* eradication by urea breath test and *H. pylori* fecal antigen was done at end of natural therapy [20]. All individuals included in the study were treated as outpatients.

Ethical considerations: An informed signed consent was taken from all patients, and they were free to quit the study whenever they like. All patients were allowed to follow their usual diet, medications and to lead their routine life style. The research proposal was approved and the study followed the rules of the Research Ethics Committee of King Abdul-Aziz University (KAAU) in Jeddah, Saudi Arabia.

Results: Dyspepsia constituted a major disturbance to the quality of life for all patients. Severe constipation manifested by passage of small pieces of dried stool together with pitting edema opposite the shaft of the leg were constant features in all patients. All patients were positive for *H. pylori* serum antibodies, while urea breath test and *H. pylori* fecal antigen confirmed this diagnosis. A high rectal spasm was demonstrated by proctoscopy or sigmoidoscopy in all patients while colonoscopy showed multiple colonic spasms in most patients. None of them demonstrated any further significant colonic pathology. Data from pre-treatment observational findings showed that patients were having better BP readings whenever they had regular comfortable bowel motions, while their BP was badly controlled when they suffer from indigestive troubles or abdominal distension. All patients expressed dramatic relief concerning their dyspeptic symptoms and constipation was relieved in all patients after 3 - 5 days of treatment. All patients were confirmed negative for *H. pylori* after the natural therapy. Fifty-seven patients (57.6%) were able to quit their medications and maintain normal BP values after the vinegar therapy. Thirty-three patients (33.3%) needed an additional 1 week of therapy with vinegar in order to resume a normal BP and quit medication. Six patients (6.06%) failed to get their BP lowered after therapy with both the vinegar and the purge; the three with overweight were not among them. Their failure to respond to therapy was attributed possibly to gaining new H. pylori strains due to misbehavior in food habits via outside-home meals. Three patients (3.03%) did not complete the study. Patients who responded to the natural therapy were followed up after 1 month, 3 months, 6 months, 1 year and 18 months. Their BP remained controlled within normal levels without any medications. They had been made aware that they should watch their outside-home meals and their condition of the colon as they might need to return to the natural purge and vinegar in their food whenever they develop any dyspeptic symptoms or whenever they feel upset after any query meal. An equal group of patients of an equal size, similar age range, body built, range of BP, associated *H. pylori* dyspepsia and nearly most of other circumstances as not having nor receiving any medication for any other chronic illness was considered as control and was followed up for the same duration. They were not interested in the natural therapy with senna purge and vinegar and they decided to follow medical treatment with antihypertensive pills. They mostly remained inadequately controlled in spite of regular follow-up of medications and carefulness about their life style.

Discussion: Hypertension is considered a major health problem worldwide; it is one of the leading causes of death and disability in many countries. The public health response towards this ongoing pandemic challenge must be promoted and the policies of health organizations need to be re-oriented to include this chronic disease within their prior attention.[1,2] Functional dyspepsia is a clinical syndrome defined by chronic or recurrent pain or discomfort in the upper abdomen of a variable origin. A general agreement exists on the irrelevant role played by *H. pylori* in the pathophysiology of functional dyspepsia. *H. pylori* represents one of the most common and prominent topics worldwide; it is becoming exceedingly a challenging medical problem.[3] A remarkable association between *H. pylori* and cardiovascular disease was documented in literature and it was suggested to be due to a higher prevalence of more virulent *H. pylori* strains. It has been reported that *H. pylori* eradication improves BP values in patients affected by hypertension. The link between hypertensive disease and *H. pylori* was related to a possible activation of the cytokine cascade with the release of vasoactive substances from the primary site of H. pylori colonization.[11-13] Concerning the clinical picture of *H. pylori*, acute conditions include upper gastrointestinal pain, burping, gastric distension, halitosis, hyperacidity and later hypochlohydria, while chronic cases could be asymptomatic. Gastric acid secretion is stimulated during early stages by the inflammatory process and by the juxtamucosal ammonia produced by the organism, while hypochlorhydria develops later due to mucosal atrophy.[6,16] It seems that the medical problems related to *H. pylori* creep up under the silence of chronic existence of the bacterium. The controversy about the efficacy of *H. pylori*-antibiotic eradication strategies and the emergence of antibiotic-resistant *H. pylori* strains have been illustrated in literature;[10,20] the apparent length of antibiotic therapy per se could be the reason to allow the chance for the stomach bug to develop resistance or to escape from the stomach. Antibiotics are seldom effective in patients harboring extra-gastric *H. pylori* strains.[22] *H. pylori* could migrate to the colon,[20] or the antibiotic violence itself does force it to migrate where antibiotics will become ineffective against it. Migration of *H. pylori* to the colon is a fact that has been documented in literature and colonic colonization with these abnormal-behavior *H. pylori* strains would be life-long unless eradicated.[9,10,20] The organism will continue producing ammonia for a reason or no reason with consequent accumulation of profuse toxic amounts of ammonia in the colon, unopposed or buffered by any acidity. As ammonia in residual amounts is smooth muscle tonic and smooth muscle spastic in profuse amounts, its accumulation in the colon would lead to development of multiple colonic and a high rectal spasm. A colonic re-absorptive error could be established with excessive fluid and salt retention in the body that would definitely lead to hypertension which is supposed to remain inadequately controlled without correction of the underlying etiologic pathological error.[21] The passage of small pieces of dry stool as expressed by the patients and the pitting edema demonstrated over their legs were explained by the development of colonic spasms and the colonic re-absorptive error with fluid and salt retention in the body. In this study, high rectal spasms were demonstrated by proctoscopy or sigmoidoscopy while the colonic spasms were confirmed by colonoscopy. It has been demonstrated in literature findings that the incidence of *H. pylori*-associated medical problems is higher in developing countries than in developed ones due to the higher prevalence of *H. pylori* in developing communities,[20] possibly because of the hygienic and life standards and/or the abuse of antibiotics. The matter that *H. pylori* is a sanitary conflict before it is a medical challenge has been confirmed in literature.[8,23-25] The patients included in this study were from different countries; there was no exclusion of patients because of nationality so long they were living sufficient years in the same community, as the matter of the sanitary conflict is food habits and community-related rather than racial or nationality-related. Observational findings in this study have shown that the body weight of patients has got insignificant influence on the degree of their *H. pylori*-associated hypertension; therefore, the body mass indices of patients were not taken into detailed consideration or discussion in the study. The matter is apparently dependent mainly upon the degree of fluid and salt retention in the body which should be related to the rate of colonization of abnormal behavior *H. pylori* strains in the colon rather than the body weight of the patient.

The follow-up of patients was rather long as those patients are susceptible disadvantaged population liable for recurrence whenever they develop colonic troubles; therefore, they were instructed to care for their colon and watch their meals from outside home. Dietary vinegar has been recently demonstrated as an effective natural remedy against *H. pylori* including symptomatic relief and eradication.[19,21] The complex nutritional requirements of *H. pylori* are achieved through its unique energy metabolism, which exhibits characteristic dislocation sites. These sites can be considered as targets that should attract any attempts to fight the organism.[10,26] The major routes of generation of energy of **H. pylori** are via pyruvate and the activity of the pyruvate dehydrogenase complex is controlled by the rules of product inhibition and feedback regulation. As acetate is demonstrated as an end product among the metabolic pathway of **H. pylori**, this means that addition of acetic acid to the atmosphere around the organism could compromise the energy metabolism of **H. pylori** or interfere with the organism's respiratory chain metabolism.[27-30] This fact is further supported by the observation that addition of pyruvate to different solid culture media was found to inhibit bacterial growth, and this inhibition was attributed to accumulation of acetate and formate.[19,27] As the matter includes interference with the energy metabolism and the respiratory chain of **H. pylori**, an immediate paralysis of the organism can be considered which further explains the dramatic symptomatic relief that has been mostly expressed by all patients taking a vinegar-mixed food. The fast immediate influence of acetic acid on **H. pylori** gives no chance for the organism to resist the treatment with vinegar and migrate or develop resistant strains. In vitro inhibition of **H. pylori** growth was demonstrated due to the effect of some bio-organic acids such as lactic, formic and acetic with the lactic acid demonstrating the greatest inhibition as the main product of glucose utilization by **H. pylori** is recognized as lactate.[19] Therefore, yoghurt was chosen in this study as the best food stuff for the vinegar to be mixed with, as it will assist the inhibitory effect of vinegar on **H. pylori** according to the rules of feedback regulation and product inhibition. In this study, the effect of pyruvate, 20 times dilutions of dietary vinegar (acetic acid 6%) and three times dilution of the senna purge preparation added to **H. pylori** solid culture media was studied. Addition of pyruvate demonstrated a delayed inhibitory effect on the motility of **H. pylori**, while addition of the diluted vinegar and the diluted senna leaves extract showed an immediate lethal influence on **H. pylori**.

Conclusion: The concept of the colonic re-absorptive error considered in this study is not just hypothetical as upon the basis of this concept; most of the patients of the study (90.9%) were able to quit their medications and maintain normal BP values by mere natural eradication of **H. pylori**, colon care and colon clear, although they were inadequately controlled in spite of regular follow-up of medications and extreme carefulness about their style of life.

Revision of the current guidelines of **H. pylori** eradication and management of hypertension may be needed. Therapy with dietary vinegar and natural senna purge is a promising remedy and is worthy of further accurate determination and wider practical applications.

Acknowledgement: The study appreciates the facilities offered by the laboratory departments of KAAU and Al-Borg laboratories in Jeddah, Saudi Arabia. The continuous support offered by Abdul-Aziz Al-Sorayai Investment Company (ASIC) in Jeddah, Saudi Arabia is extremely appreciated.

Conflict of Interest: There is no conflict of interest existing.

REFERENCES:

1. **Bakris G, Hill M, Mancia G, et al.** Achieving blood pressures goals globally: five core actions for health-care professionals. A worldwide call to action. *J Hum Hypertens 2008 Jan; 22 (1): 63-70.*

2. **Reddy KS, Naik N, Prabhakaran D. Hypertension in developing world: a consequence of progress.** *Curr Cardiol Rep 2006 Nov; 8 (6); 399-404.*

3. **Andreoli TE. Cecil Essentials of Medicine.** *WB Saunders Company. 2001; 5th Ed: 334.*

4. **Fendrick AM. The role of economic evaluation in the diagnosis and treatment of Helicobacter pylori infection**. *Gastroenterol Clin North Am 2000 Dec; 29 (4) : 837-51.*

5. **Groeneveld PW, Lieu TA, Fendrick AM, et al. Quality of life measurement clarifies the cost-effectiveness of Helicobacter pylori eradication in peptic ulcer disease and uninvestigated dyspepsia**. *Am J Gastroenterol 2001 Feb; 96 (2): 338-47.*

6. Baron S. Baron's medical microbiology. *Churchill Livingstone. 2000; 4th Ed: 346.*

7. Versalovic J. Helicobacter pylori. Pathology and diagnostic strategies. *Am J Clin Pathol 2003 Mar; 119 (3); 403-12.*

8. Strand M, Presecki V, Babus V, et al. Epidemiology of Helicobacter pylori infection. *Lijec Vjesn 2002 Sep; 124 Suppl 1: 5-9.*

9. Asaka M. Epidemiology of Helicobacter pylori infection in Japan. *Nippon Rinsho 2003 Jan; 61 (1): 19-24.*

10. Ge Z. Potential of fumarate reductase as a novel therapeutic target in Helicobacter pylori infection. *Expert Opin Ther Targets 2002 Apr; 6 (2): 135-46.*

11. Migneco A, Ojetti V, Specchia L, et al. Eradication of Helicobacter pylori infection improves blood pressure values in patients affected by hypertension. *Helicobacter 2003 Dec; 8 (6):585-9.*

12. Diomedi M, Pietroiusti A, Silvestrini M, et al. CagA-positive Helicobacter pylori strains may influence the natural history of atherosclerotic stroke. *Neurology 2004 Sep; 63 (5):800-4.*

13. Pietroiusti A, Diomedi M, Silvestrini M, et al. Cytotoxin-associated gene-A-positive Helicobacter pylori strains are associated with atherosclerotic stroke. *Circulationy 2002 Jul 30; 106 (5):580-4.*

14. Bulut Y, Agacayak A, Karlidag D, et al. Association of CagA+ Helicobacter pylori with adenotonsillar hypertrophy. *Tohoku J Exp Med. 2006 Jul; 209 (3): 229-33.*

15. Zentilin P, Iiritano E, Vingale C, et al. Helicobacter pylori infection is not involved in the Pathogenesis of either erosive or non-erosive gastro-oesophageal reflux disease. *Aliment Pharmacol Ther 2003 Apr; 17 (8): 1057-64.*

16. Volk WA, Gebhardt BM, Hammarskjold M-L, et al. Essential of Medical Microbiology. Lippincott–Raven. 1996; 5th Ed: 377.

17. Cotran RS, Kumar V, Collins T. Robins Pathologic Basis of Disease. *WB Saunders Company. 1999; 6th Ed: 790.*

18. Sleigh JD, Timbury MC. Notes on Medical Microbiology. *Churchill Livingstone. 1998; 5th Ed: 232.*

19. Midolo PD, Lambert JR, Hull R, et al. In vitro inhibition of Helicobacter pylori NCTC 11637 by organic acids and lactic acid bacteria. *J Appl Bacteriol. 1995 Oct; 79 (4); 475-9.*

20. Farinha P, Gascoyne RD. Helicobacter pylori and MALT Lymphoma. *Gastroenterology 2005 May; 128 (6): 1579-605.*

21. Nasrat AM. The world misconception and misbehavior towards Helicobacter pylori is leading to major spread of illness. *The 7th Anti-Aging Medicine World Congress, Monte-Carlo, Monaco, 2009 Mar.* Available from URL, *www.euromedicom.com*

22. Grünberger B, Wöhrer S, Streubel B, et al. Antibiotic treatment is not effective in patients infected with Helicobacter pylori suffering from extragastric MALT lymphoma. *J Clin Oncol 2006 Mar 20; 24 (9):1370-5.*

23. **Valenzuela J. Helicobacter pylori: two decades later.** *Rev Med Chil 2004 Nov; 132 (11): 1339-44.*

24. **Zaterka S, Eisig JN, Chinzon D, et al. Factors related to Helicobacter pylori prevalence in an adult population in Brazil.** *Helicobacter 2007 Feb; 12 (1):82-8.*

25. **Cataldo F, Simpore J, Greco P, et al. Helicobacter pylori infection in Burkina Faso: an enigma within an enigma.** *Dig Liver Dis 2004 Sep; 36 (9): 589-93.*

26. **Mendz GL, Hazell SL, Burns BP. Glucose utilization and lactate production by Helicobacter pylori.** *J Gen Microbiol 1993 Dec; 139 (Pt 12): 3023-8.*

27. **Mendz GL, Hazell SL. Fumarate catabolism in Helicobacter pylori.** *Biochem Mol Biol Int. 1993 Oct; 31 (2): 325-32.*

28. **Mendz GL, Hazell SL, van Gorkom L. Pyruvate metabolism in Helicobacter pylori.** *Arch Microbiol. 1994; 162 (3):187-92.*

29. **Hughes NJ, Clayton CL, Chalk PA, et al. Helicobacter pylori porCDAB oorDABC genes encode distinctpyruvate: flavodoxin and 2-oxoglutarate: acceptor oxidoreductases which mediate electron transport to NADP.** *J Bacteriol 1998 Mar; 180 (5): 1119-28.*

30. **Mendz GL, Ball GE, Meek DJ, Pyruvate metabolism in Campylobacter spp.** *Biochim Biophys Acta 1997 Mar 15; 1334 (2-3): 291-302.*

IMPROVEMENT OF IDIOPATHIC CARDIOMYOPATHY AFTER COLON CLEAR

Not All Cardiomyopathy in Late Decades is related to Viral Myocarditis but Mostly Toxic Myocarditis which is Curable

Introduction: The widespread prevalence and the medical challenges constituted by ***Helicobacter pylori***, namely its close relation to acid peptic disease, gastric carcinoma and lymphoma have led to the widely established medical concept that ***H. pylori*** eradication should be a necessary attempt.[1,2] ***H. pylori*** colonized the stomach since an immemorial time,[2] as if both the stomach and the bacterium used to live together in peace harmless to each other. ***H. pylori*** could migrate or get forced to migrate to the colon due to the influence of antibiotic violence;[2-4] antibiotics are seldom effective against extra-gastric ***H. pylori*** strains.[5] The latest reports in literature demonstrate a definite flare up of many medical challenges related to ***H. pylori*** through immune or different unknown reasons.[6-9] The association of ***H. pylori*** and some cardiovascular diseases like myocarditis and cardiomyopaty has been sufficiently mentioned in literature. The role played by the increased mucosal production of inflammatory mediators (cytokines) induced by ***H. pylori*** among patients with ischemic heart diseases has been also clearly illustrated.[10-12] The clinical association of gastritis and carditis is controversial; opinions are currently divided as whether it is the result of gastro-esophageal reflux or a proximal extension of ***H. pylori*** infection from the stomach.[10] Active lymphocytic myocarditis manifested by intractable ventricular tachycardia, non-specific intra-ventricular block, and myocardial dysfunction has been described in a young woman infected with ***H. pylori***; an immune influence has been emphasized in that patient as a possible etiology behind the development of autoimmune myocarditis.[11] It has been also reported in literature that a possible role of autoimmunity induced by ***H. pylori*** in cardiomyopathy cannot be excluded.[12] Different reports in literature have confirmed the association of cytotoxin-associated gene A (cagA) positive ***H. pylori*** strains with many medical problems, and emphasized that cagA of ***H. pylori*** encodes a highly immunogenic and virulence-associated protein; the presence of this virulent gene in the body could affect the clinical outcome in many patients.[2,13]

REFERENCES:

1. **Ge Z.** Potential of fumarate reductase as a novel therapeutic target in Helicobacter pylori infection. *Expert Opin Ther Targets 2002 Apr; 6 (2): 135-46.*

2. **Farinha P, Gascoyne RD. Helicobacter pylori and MALT Lymphoma.** *Gastroenterology 2005 May; 128 (6): 1579-605.*

3. **Matsuo S, Mizuta Y, Hayashi T, et al. Mucosa-associated lymphoid tissue lymphomaof the transverse colon: a case report. World** *J Gastroenterol 2006 Sep 14; 12 (34): 5573-6.*

4. **Nasrat AM. The world misconception and misbehavior towards Helicobacter pylori is leading to major spread of illness.** *The 7th Anti-Aging Medicine World Congress, Monte-Carlo, Monaco, 2009 Mar.* **Available from URL,** *www.euromedicom.com*

5. **Grünberger B, Wöhrer S, Streubel B, et al. Antibiotic treatment is not effective in patients infected with Helicobacter pylori suffering from extragastric MALT lymphoma.** *J Clin Oncol 2006 Mar 20; 24 (9):1370-5.*

6. **Segni M, Borrelli O, Pucarelli I, et al. Early manifestations of gastric autoimmunity in patients with juvenile autoimmune thyroid disease.** *J Clin Endocrinol Metab 2004 Oct; 89 (10): 4944-8.*

7. **Kountouras J, Zavos C, Chatzopoulos D. A concept on the role of Helicobacter pylori infection in autoimmune pancreatitis.** *J Cell Mol Med 2005Jan-Mar; 9 (1):196-207.*

8. **Kountouras J, Deretzi G, Zavos C, et al. Association between Helicobacter pylori infection and acute inflammatory demyelinating polyradiculoneuropathy.** *Eur J Neurol 2005 Feb; 12 (2):139-43.*

9. **Veneri D, Krampera M, Franchini M. High prevalence of sustained remission of idiopathic thrombocytopenic purpura after   Helicobacter pylori eradication: a long-term follow-up study.** *Platelets 2005 Mar; 16 (2):117-9.*

10. **Owen DA. Gastritis and casrditis.** *Mod Pathol 2003 Apr; 16 (4):325-41. Review.*

11. **Bilinska ZT, Grzybowski J, Szajewski T, et al. Active lymphocytic myocarditis treated with murine OKT3 monoclonal antibody in a patient presenting with intractable ventricular tachycardia.** *Tex Heart Inst J 2002; 29 (2): 113-7.*

12. **Klausz G, Tiszai A, Lénárt Z, et al. Helicobacter pylori-induced immunological responses in patients with duodenal ulcer and in patients with cardiomyopathies.** *Acta Microbiol Immunol Hung. 2004; 51 (3): 311-20.*

13. **Pietroiusti A, Diomedi M, Silvestrini M, et al. Cytotoxin-associated gene-A-positive Helicobacter pylori strains are associated with atherosclerotic stroke.** *Circulationy 2002 Jul 30; 106 (5):580-4.*

SCIENTIFIC EVIDENCES ON THE IMPROVEMENT OF IDIOPATHIC CARDIOMYOPATHY AFTER COLON CLEAR

Improvement of Idiopathic Cardiomyopathy after Colon Clear: Published in Journal of Cardiology Research 2015 Apr; 6 (2): 249-254. Nasrat et al. Improvement of idiopathic cardiomyopathy after colon clear. *J Cardiol Res 2015 Apr; 6 (2): 249-254.* [doi: 10.14740/cr398e]

Background: Helicobacter pylori colonized the stomach since an immemorial time, as if both the stomach and the bacterium used to live together in peace harmless to each other. ***H. pylori*** could migrate or get forced to migrate to the colon; antibiotics are seldom effective against extra-gastric ***H. pylori*** strains.[1-5] The association of ***H. pylori*** and some cardiovascular diseases like myocarditis and cardiomyopaty has been sufficiently mentioned in literature. The role played by the increased mucosal production of inflammatory mediators (cytokines) induced by ***H. pylori*** among patients with ischemic heart diseases has been also clearly illustrated. The clinical association of gastritis and carditis is controversial.[6-10] Active lymphocytic myocarditis manifested by intractable ventricular tachycardia, non-specific intra-ventricular block, and myocardial dysfunction has been described in a young woman infected with ***H. pylori***; an immune influence has been emphasized in that patient as a possible etiology behind the development of autoimmune myocarditis. It has been reported also in literature that a possible role of autoimmunity induced by ***H. pylori*** in cardiomyopathy cannot be excluded.[2,11-13]

Objective: Illustration of the effect of colon clear on idiopathic myocardial dysfunction.

Design and setting: Multiple-case clinical study was done in Balghsoon Outpatient Clinics in Jeddah/ Saudi Arabia during October 2012 – May 2013.

Patients and Methods: Three female patients with frank long history of ***H. pylori*** dyspepsia and an age range of 41 -47 years have developed palpitation, chest tightness and breathing discomfort with frequent extra-systoles in the echocardiography (ECG). Shortly, two of them developed ventricular extra-systoles; an initial diagnosis of viral myocaditis complicated with idiopathic cardiomyopathy was made based upon ECG and magnetic resonance imaging (MRI). Their left ventricular ejedtion fraction was ranging between 29% and 30%. They were advised for insertion of an automated implantable cardioverter defibrillator (AICD) but they hesitated towards this procedure; therefore, they were put on medical treatment. Ventricular extra-systoles disappeared on medications but their distressing symptoms showed no improvement. ***H. pylori*** existence in the colon was confirmed by a reliable specific test, ***H. pylori*** fecal antigen.[2] Colon clear with the potent natural senna leaves purge was employed for them. Successful ***H. pylori*** eradication was confirmed by ***H. pylori*** fecal antigen test.[2-4] ***H. pylori*** fecal antigen test was available from Acon Laboratory, USA, Batch No. HP8040008.

Ethical considerations: An informed signed consent was taken from all patients, and they were free to quit the study whenever they like. All patients were allowed to follow their usual diet, medications and to lead their routine style of life. They were not requested to stop their medications but they did that gradually by their own because of physical uneasiness upon intake of pills. One of them stopped her medications all of a sudden

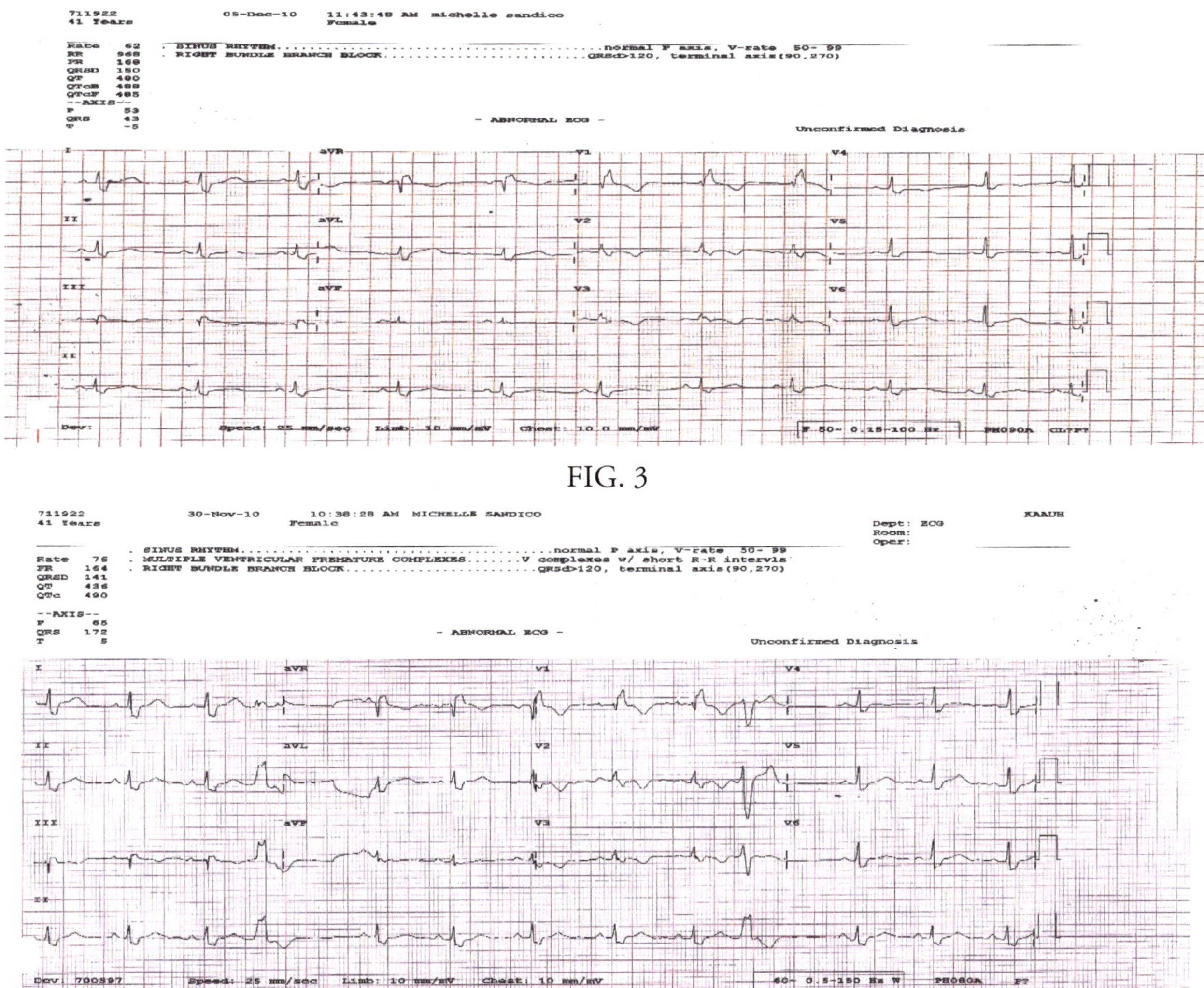

FIG. 3

FIG. 4

as she missed them while traveling by road; she gave the expression of suddenly feeling health and freedom. The research proposal was approved and the study followed the rules of the Research Ethics Committee of King Faisal Specialized Hospital and Research Center in Jeddah, Saudi Arabia.

Results: The three patients expressed immediate dramatic improvement after colon clear; they became free of any symptoms instantly after diarrhea was complete and they were able to exercise walking for continuous 1 h without fatigue or doing more than 400 m walk exercise in less than 6 min. One patient expressed "I am back myself again" while another patient said "now I can count my pulse". Their ECG resumed a sinus rhythm with few supra-ventricular extra-systoles, around 7 - 9/min. The left ventricular ejection fraction became 47-49%. The three patients achieved complete recovery within 3 - 4 weeks; their left ventricular function improved to 53-55% and the ECG tracing became straight forward normal.

Patients were not obliged to stop medications but later they did that by their own because of feeling uneasy with medications and they kept maintaining their condition stable even they were feeling better expressing further physical relief upon quit of medications. Patients were followed up for 12 months showing no recurrence as they were watching carefully their colonic condition.

The results of this study were compared with the records of seven female patients of rather similar age range (40 - 49 years) and rather similar physical and clinical parameters who have developed myocarditis and cardiomypathy confirmed by ECG and MRI, they were put on the following several medications: amiodarone hydrochloride 200 mg once daily, carvedilol 6.25 mg once daily and candesartan cilexetil 8 mg once daily together with two diuretic drugs (furosemide and spironolactone), a gstric sedative and aspirin in order to reduce symptoms and burden on the heart, while one patient was obliged to undergo AICD insertion because of risk on life. In spite of these measures, those patients were not getting much better as concerns palpitation, easy fatigability and chest discomfort.

The results of this study were further compared and confirmed also by the clinical study of one female patient aged 49.5 years who developed myocarditis and cardiomyopathy manifested with ventricular extra-systoles following a long history of **H. pylori** dyspepsia. She was advised for AICD insertion because of risk on her life but she was not able to afford the cost of this procedure, and she disappeared to reappear after 1 month symptom-less; she mentioned that she just followed camel milk intake with honey for 1 month. Her ECG was restored normal and her left ventricular ejection fraction improved from 31% to 49%.

Figures 1 and 2 show parts of the Holter monitor tracing of one of the patients of the study before undergoing colon clear.

Figure 3 shows the ECG tracing of the same patient before colon clear, while Figure 4 shows her ECG tracing after colon clear.

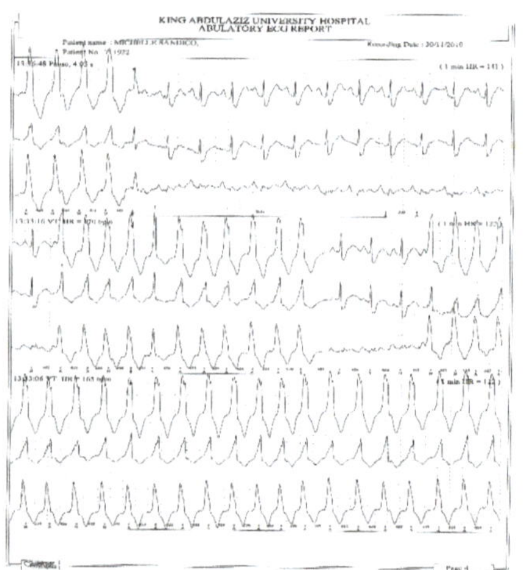
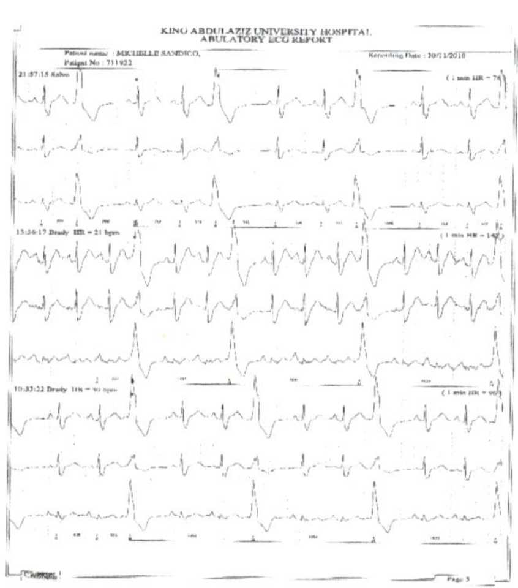

Discussion: Migration of **H. pylori** to the colon is a fact that has been reported in literature.[2-4] It was suggested that the antibiotic violence could have forced the stomach bacterium to migrate to the colon rather than eradicating it from the stomach.[2,4] This suggestion is supported by the finding that pseudomembranous toxic colitis and toxic megacolon have developed after eradication of **H. pylori** from the stomach by antibiotic therapy.[14,15] **H. pylori** in the colon will continue producing ammonia for a reason or no reason leading to accumulation of profuse toxic amounts of ammonia, unopposed or buffered by any acidity. Ammonia is known to be toxic and colon spastic;[16] a colonic re-absorptive error could establish leading to excessive fluid and salt retention in the body with subsequent burden on blood pressure and heart rate. Accumulation of ammonia in the colon could lead to adverse toxic effects on the myocardium in susceptible people; toxic myocarditis and cardiomyopathy could be integral sequences of these toxic effects.[11,12] The results of this study confirm the concept of improvement of cardiomyopathy after colon clear due to elimination of a potential source of toxins from the colon as the wonderful senna purge is potent and is known to effectively kill and/or expel the migrated colonic **H. pylori** strains.[4,17] This concept is further supported by the results achieved by the patient who followed the camel milk/honey therapeutic remedy; camel milk is a known potent colon clear measure while acetate which is directly lethal to **H. pylori** is existing among the end products of glucose utilization by the body.[17-19] In this study, the effect of the senna leaves extract on the growth of **H. pylori** was studied; addition of three times dilution of the senna leaves purge preparation to solid culture of **H. pylori** was found directly lethal to it. The records of the seven female patients who followed medical treatment and AICD insertion in one of them failed to provide information about any history of **H. pylori** for those patients although it was expected as existence of abnormal *H. pylori* strains is common particularly in developing countries,[2,4,17] and because of their failure to respond to adequate medications, most probably due to persistence of an underlying etiologic pathology. Toxic myocarditis rather than viral myocarditis could have been the pathological etiology behind many cases diagnosed as idiopathic cardiomyopathy during the last three decades. The value of this study is gained from the true promising opportunity that many cases of cardiomyopathy could be avoided and that many cases of the newly discovered condition could be cured or at least progress of the disease could be stopped. A general impression has been developed that those patients developing cardiomyopathy due to the influence of colonic *H. pylori* strains are disadvantaged susceptible individuals; they should watch their colonic condition and employ colon care and colon clear whenever they develop frank dyspeptic symptoms. It was also observed that females are more predisposed than males to these adverse toxic effects produced by the abnormal-behavior colonic *H. pylori* strains; therefore, further comparative studies concerning this regard including both male and female patients are recommended.

Conclusion: The senna leaves purge should be considered as a recognized potent colon clear measure. Toxic myocarditis rather than viral could be the pathologic etiology behind many cases of idiopathic cardiomyopathy; hence it could be prevented, the newly discovered conditions could be cured or at least progress of the disease could be stopped. Eradication of *H. pylori* from the colon via colon clear could lead to improvement of cardiomyopathy due to elimination of colonic *H. pylori* strains below its pathologic level. Colon clear could be a simple and safe measure to improve changes in cardiac rhythm, heart rate and myocardial function developing in association with *H. pylori* due to inflammatory, toxic or immune reasons.

Acknowledgement: The study appreciates the facilities and time allowed by Balghsoon Clinics in Jeddah, Saudi Arabia. The continuous encouragement of Abdul-Aziz Al-Sorayai Investment Company (ASIC) in Jeddah, Saudi Arabia and the scientific emotional support of Dr Ahmed S. Balghsoon are extremely valued and appreciated.

Conflict of Interest: There is no conflict of interest existing.

REFERENCES:

1. **Ge Z.** Potential of fumarate reductase as a novel therapeutic target in Helicobacter pylori infection. *Expert Opin Ther Targets 2002 Apr; 6 (2): 135-46.*

2. **Farinha P, Gascoyne RD. Helicobacter pylori and MALT Lymphoma.** *Gastroenterology 2005 May; 128 (6): 1579-605.*

3. **Matsuo S, Mizuta Y, Hayashi T, et al. Mucosa-associated lymphoid tissue lymphomaof the transverse colon: a case report. World** *J Gastroenterol 2006 Sep 14; 12 (34): 5573-6.*

4. **Nasrat AM. The world misconception and misbehavior towards Helicobacter pylori is leading to major spread of illness.** *The 7th Anti-Aging Medicine World Congress, Monte-Carlo, Monaco, 2009 Mar.* **Available from URL,** *www.euromedicom.com*

5. **Grünberger B, Wöhrer S, Streubel B, et al. Antibiotic treatment is not effective in patients infected with Helicobacter pylori suffering from extragastric MALT lymphoma.** *J Clin Oncol 2006 Mar 20; 24 (9):1370-5.*

6. **Segni M, Borrelli O, Pucarelli I, et al. Early manifestations of gastric autoimmunity in patients with juvenile autoimmune thyroid disease.** *J Clin Endocrinol Metab 2004 Oct; 89 (10): 4944-8.*

7. **Kountouras J, Zavos C, Chatzopoulos D. A concept on the role of Helicobacter pylori infection in autoimmune pancreatitis.** *J Cell Mol Med 2005Jan-Mar; 9 (1): 196-207.*

8. Kountouras J, Deretzi G, Zavos C, et al. Association between Helicobacter pylori infection and acute inflammatory demyelinating polyradiculoneuropathy. *Eur J Neurol 2005 Feb; 12 (2):139-43.*

9. Veneri D, Krampera M, Franchini M. High prevalence of sustained remission of idiopathic thrombocytopenic purpura after Helicobacter pylori eradication: a long-term follow-up study. *Platelets 2005 Mar; 16 (2): 117-9.*

10. Owen DA. Gastritis and casrditis. *Mod Pathol 2003 Apr; 16 (4): 325-41. Review.*

11. Bilinska ZT, Grzybowski J, Szajewski T, et al. Active lymphocytic myocarditis treated with murine OKT3 monoclonal antibody in a patient presenting with intractable ventricular tachycardia. *Tex Heart Inst J 2002; 29 (2): 113-7.*

12. Klausz G, Tiszai A, Lénárt Z, et al. Helicobacter pylori-induced immunological responses in patients with duodenal ulcer and in patients with cardiomyopathies. *Acta Microbiol Immunol Hung. 2004; 51 (3):311-20.*

13. Pietroiusti A, Diomedi M, Silvestrini M, et al. Cytotoxin-associated gene-A-positive Helicobacter pylori strains are associated with atherosclerotic stroke. *Circulationy 2002 Jul 30; 106 (5):580-4.*

14. Kubo N, Kochi S, Ariyama I, et al. Pseudomembranous colitis after Helicobacter pylori eradication therapy. *Kansenshogaku Zasshi 2006 Jan; 80 (1): 51-5.*

15. Schweigart U, Franck H, Schepp W, et al. Toxic megacolon after Helicobacter pylori eradication therapy. *Internist (Berl) 1997 Apr; 38 (4): 352-4.*

16. Andreoli TE. Cecil Essentials of Medicine. *WB Saunders Company. 2001; 5th Ed: 334.*

17. Nasrat SAM, Nasrat RM, Nasrat MM, et al. The dramatic spread of diabetes mellitus worldwide and influence of Helicobacter pylori. *General Med 2015; 3 (1): 159-62.*

18. Mendz GL, Hazell SL, Burns BP. Glucose utilization and lactate production by Helicobacter pylori. *J Gen Microbiol 1993 Dec; 139 (Pt 12): 3023-8.*

19. Habib HM, Ibrahim WH, Schneider-Stock R, et al. Camel milk lactoferrin reduces the proliferation of colorectal cancer cells and exerts antioxidant and DNA damage inhibitory activities. *Food Chemistry 2013 Nov 1; 141 (1): 148-162.*

AN INFLUENCE OF HELICOBACTER PYLORI ON THROMBOCYTOPENIA IN CHILDREN

This Article does not have a digital object identification (DOI) but it is available on Google as an Open Access; it has been included due to the importance of its results for patients, families and practitioners.

This article was already published in the International Journal of Recent Scientific Research and was available on line but lately it is not available in the journal site search records probably because of some technical reasons of the journal, revision with the journal board did not help. It was decided to remove this article and its related criteria for sake of credibility of the book, however it was finally decided to keep it as such as it is a real original work of the research team and the knowledge included within it could be of useful value for patients, families and practitioners. Therefore; the downloaded PDF is posted on the BlogSpot site of the New Concepts in Medicine via the following link https://newmedicineconcepts.blogspot.com/ and the article is still available on Google search via the following link:

http://www.recentscientific.com/sites/default/files/2853_0.pdf

Introduction: Immune or idiopathic thrombocytopenic purpura (ITP) can be simply classified into primary or secondary to an underlying condition.[1] It is characterized by a reduced platelet count due to impaired both platelet survival and production representing a frequent cause of improper cellular haemostasis in clinical practice. Information about the incidence and prevalence of ITP is limited. Recent reports have confirmed earlier studies suggesting that the disease occurs in 5.8-6.6 per 100,000 children per year, and that spontaneous recovery is typical. The incidence in adults is roughly two in 100,000 per year and may be more common in older adults than previously recognized. A female predominance occurs only among middle-aged patients, and there is no racial variation in incidence. Spontaneous remission rate varies and ranges from 5 to 11%.[2-4] Splenectomy remains the best curative treatment for adults with chronic disease, while steroids and other treatments might allow the decision of splenectomy to be postponed, possibly indefinitely, if haemostatic platelet count is attained.[5]

Childhood ITP in the western world is essentially an acute self-limited disorder. In contrast, the clinical expression of the disease in developing countries is heterogeneous including the acute self-limited, the intermediate, and the chronic adulthood-like form. Some Arab areas are famous of various forms of hemoglobinopathies where splenectomy is performed rather frequently, ITP is being represented among these disorders.[6,7]

Several recent reports have suggested that a strong association exists between ***Helicobacter pylori*** and ITP and successful eradication is followed with improvement in platelet count. Further recent reports have revealed common limitations of some studies that underestimated the link between ITP and ***H. pylori***; these reports has described ITP as the disease for which the strongest association with ***H. pylori*** has been shown.[8,9] The high prevalence of ***H. pylori*** in patients with ITP and the marked sustained platelet recovery after mere eradication therapy rendered some investigators to emphasize that the management of ITP, especially with a recent onset of the disease, should include an investigation and eradication of *H. pylori*.[8]

Existence of *H. pylori* starts in children trans-familial during early childhood, and the *H. pylori* strain is often identical with that of parents. Interestingly, children maintain the same strain genotype even after moving to a different enviroment.[10] The challenge lies in the emergence of antibiotic-resistant *H. pylori* strains, which is probably due to the frequent abuse of antibiotics or inefficiency of the current eradication strategies.[11] These facts put a great responsibility upon the parent's misbehavior in their food habits or antibiotic abuse.

The overrepresentation of specific *H. pylori* genotypes with ITP has led to the development of a concept that strain genotyping may be a good predictor of platelet recovery in ITP patients after eradication of *H. pylori*.[12] Different reports have confirmed the association of cytotoxin-associated gene A (cagA) positive *H. pylori* strains with many clinical problems, and emphasized that cagA of *H. pylori* encodes a highly immunogenic and virulence-associated protein; the presence of this virulent gene in the body could affect the clinical outcome in many children.[13]

Bio-organic acids (lactic, formic and acetic) and the senna leaves extract purge have been recently demonstrated as effective measures for symptomatic relief *H. pylori* dyspepsia and natural eradication of *H. pylori*.[14-16]

REFERENCES:

1. **Liebman H.** Other immune thrombocytopenias. *Semin Hematol 2007 Oct; 44 (4 Suppl 5): S24-34.*

2. **Gernsheimer T. Epidemiology and pathophysiology of immune thrombocytopenic purpura.** *Eur J Hematol Suppl 2008 Feb; (69): 3-8.*

3. **Fogarty PF, Segal JB. The epidemiology of immune thrombocytopenic purpura.** *Curr Opin Hematol 2007 Sep; 14 (5): 515-9.*

4. **Sachs UJ. Diagnosis of idiopathic thrombocytopenic purpura.** *Hamostaseologie 2008; 28 (1): 72-76.*

5. **Godeau B, Provan D, Bussel J. Immune thrombocytopenic purpura in adults.** *Curr Opin Hematol 2007 Sep; 14 (5): 535-56.*

6. **Afifi AM, Adnan M, Guindi MM. Childhood idiopathic thrombocytopenic purpura in Egypt and the neighboring Arab countries: a regional form with three different patterns of clinical expression.** *Acta Hematol 1981; 65 (3): 211-6.*

7. **Al-Salem AH, Naserullah Z, Qaisaruddin S, et al. Splenectomy for hematological diseases: The Qatif Central Hospital experience.** *Ann Saudi Med 1999 Jul-Aug; 19 (4): 325-30.*

8. **Rostami N, Keshtkar-Jahromi M, Rahnavardi M, etal. Effect of eradication of Helicobacter pylori on platelet recovery in patients with chronic idiopathic thrombocytopenic purpura: A controlled trial.** *Am J Hematol 2008 May; 83 (5): 376-81.*

9. **de Korwin JD. Does Helicobacter pylori play a role in extragastric diseases?** *Presse Med 2008 Mar; 37 (3 Pt 2): 525-34. Epub 2008 Feb 4.*

10. **Farinha P, Gascoyne RD. Helicobacter pylori and MALT Lymphoma.** *Gastroenterology 2005 May; 128 (6): 1579-605.*

11. 11. Ge Z. Potential of fumarate reductase as a novel therapeutic target in Helicobacter pylori infection. *Expert Opin Ther Targets 2002 Apr; 6 (2): 135-46.*

12. Suzuki T, Matsushima M, Shirakura K, et al. Association of inflammatory cytokine gene polymorphisms with platelet recovery in idiopathic thrombocytopenic purpura patients after the eradication of Helicobacter pylori. *Digestion. 2008; 77 (2): 73-8. Epub 2008 Mar 20.*

13. Bulut Y, Agacayak A, Karlidag D, et al. Association of CagA+ Helicobacter pylori with adenotonsillar hypertrophy. *Tohoku J Exp Med. 2006 Jul; 209 (3): 229-33.*

14. Nasrat SAM, Nasrat RM, Nasrat MM, et al. The dramatic spread of diabetes mellitus worldwide and influence of Helicobacter pylori. *General Med 2015; 3 (1): 159-62.*

15. Nasrat SAM, Nasrat AM. An alternative approach for the rising challenge of hypertensive illness via Helicobacter pylori eradication. *J Cardiol Res 2015; 6 (1): 221-225.*

16. Nsarat RM, Nasrat MM, Nasrat AM, et al. Improvement of idiopatic cardiomyopathy after colon clear. *J Cardiol Res 2015 Apr; 6 (2): 249-254.*

SCIENTIFIC EVIDENCES ON THE INFLUENCE OF HELICOBACTER PYLORI ON THROMBOCYTOPENIA IN CHILDREN

An Influence of Helicobacter pylori in Thrombocytopenia in Children, this article has been published in an Indian Medical Journal without DOI but it is available on Google as an Open Access (Available Online at *http://www.recentscientific.com*): Published in the International Journal of Recent Scientific Research 2015 Jul; 6 (7): 5052-5054. Nasrat et al. An influence of Helicobacter pylori in thrombocytopenia in children. *Int J Recent Sci Res 2015 Jul; 6 (7): 5052-5054. [http://www.recentscientific.com/sites/default/files/2853_0.pdf]*

This article was already published in the International Journal of Recent Scientific Research and was available on line but lately it is not available in the journal site search records probably because of some technical reasons of the journal, revision with the journal board did not help. It was decided to remove this article and its related criteria for sake of credibility of the book, however it was finally decided to keep it as such as it is a real original work of the research team and the knowledge included within it could be of useful value for patients, families and practitioners. Therefore; the downloaded PDF is posted on the BlogSpot site of the New Concepts in Medicine via the following link https://newmedicineconcepts.blogspot.com/ and the article is still available on Google search via the following link:

http://www.recentscientific.com/sites/default/files/2853_0.pdf

Background: Information about the incidence and prevalence of idiopathic thrombocytopenic purpura (ITP) is rather limited.[1] The recent knowledge signifies a rising incidence of ITP in developing countries where splenectomy is performed rather frequently for various forms of hemoglobinopathies; ITP is being represented among these disorders.[2-7]

Several recent reports have suggested that a strong association exists between *Helicobacter pylori* and ITP and that successful eradication of *H. pylori* is accompanied with marked and sustained platelet recovery. The overrepresentation of specific *H. pylori* genotypes with ITP could indicate that strain genotyping may be a good predictor of platelet recovery in ITP patients after eradication.[8-12] Different reports have confirmed the association of cytotoxin-associated gene A (cagA) positive *H. pylori* strains with many clinical problems, and emphasized that cagA of *H. pylori* encodes a highly immunogenic and virulence-associated protein; the presence of this virulent gene in the body could affect the clinical outcome in many children.[13] Bio-organic acids (lactic, formic and acetic) and the senna leaves extract purge have been recently demonstrated as effective measures for symptomatic relief *H. pylori* dyspepsia and natural eradication of *H. pylori*.[14-16]

Objective: demonstration of a link between ITP in children and *H. pylori*.

Design& Setting: Single-case clinical study (October 2012), Balghsoon Clinics, Jeddah, Saudi Arabia

Patients& Methods: A boy aged 6 years old was on symptomatic and therapeutic medications for six months because of bleeding tendency events and a platelet level of 6000/Cmm. His platelet count never improved above 9000/Cmm in spite of adequate medications. Parents did not seek for an alternative therapy until splenectomy appeared among treatment suggestions. Both parents and the child were tested for *H. pylori* fecal antigen and DNA extraction was done for *H. pylori* strain genotyping. Colon clear with the senna leaves extract purge was employed for both parents for eradication of colonic *H. pylori* strains; a calculated dose of the senna purge was given also to the child. Colon care was maintained by intake of vinegar-mixed food or salad, once or twice daily during meals for 5 days every week. Confirmation of *H. pylori* eradication from the colon was done using *H. pylori* fecal antigen test.[10]

Results: Both parents and their child were found positive for *H. pylori* fecal antigen; the child has got the same *H. pylori* strain genotype as his parents. They became negative for colonic *H. pylori* strains after colon clear. The platelet count of the child jumped to 19000/Cmm few days after his colon is cleared, it became 96000/Cmm one week later and it became 169000/Cmm after further one week.

Ethical Considerations: An informed signed consent was taken from the parets, they were made aware about safety of the natural remedies employed for them and they were free to make their kid quit the natural therapy whenever they like. Their child was allowed to continue his conventional medications and to lead his routine style of life except restriction of outside-home meals.

Discussion: *H. pylori* could migrate or get forced to migrate to the colon; *H. pylori* in the colon will continue producing ammonia for a reason or no reason leading to accumulation of profuse toxic amounts of ammonia, unopposed or buffered by any acidity. Accumulation of profuse amounts of ammonia in the colon is toxic to the body and could lead to adverse toxic effects in disadvantaged susceptible individuals; ITP is one of these adverse sequels in children.[10,17,18]

The association of cytotoxin-associated gene A (cagA) positive *H. pylori* strains with many clinical problems could encode high immunogenicity and virulence; which could in turn affect the clinical outcome in many children.[13] In the light of these recent findings, a revision of the current guidelines for the management of *H. pylori* may be needed; as it would be a plea to cost the child's fragile construction a repeated drastic antibiotic eradication therapy upon every detection of *H. pylori*.

It has been demonstrated that addition of three times dilutions of the senna leaves extract or 20 times dilutions of the dietary white vinegar (acetic acid 6%) to *H. pylori* culture media was directly lethal to the bacterium.[15,16]

Dietary vinegar (acetic acid 5%) has been recently demonstrated as dramatic, effective and decisive solution for all the challenges and medical problems related to *H. pylori* infection including eradication and re-infection. The cure rate of vinegar therapy reaches around 90.1% with negligible incidence of failure of treatment or recurrence. The vinegar therapy is simply based on a definite pathophysiologic principle offering in this way wonderful promises for many patients.[17] The complex nutritional requirements of *H. pylori* are achieved through its unique energy metabolism, which exhibits characteristic dislocation sites. These sites can be considered as targets that should attract any attempts to fight the organism.[11] As acetate is demonstrated as an end product among the metabolic pathway of *H. pylori*; this means that addition of acetic acid in the atmosphere around *H. pylori,* it could compromise the energy metabolism of *H. pylori*, or interfere with the organism's respiratory chain metabolism. This suggestion is supported by the fact that the major routes of generation of energy for *H. pylori* are via pyruvate and the activity of the pyruvate dehydrogenase complex is controlled by the rules of product inhibition and feedback regulation. It is further supported by the observation that addition of pyruvate to different solid culture media was found to inhibit bacterial growth, and this inhibition was attributed to accumulation of acetate and formate.[11,17] As the matter includes interference with the energy metabolism and the respiratory chain of *H. pylori*; an immediate paralysis of the organism can be considered with dramatic relief of patient's symptoms. The fast immediate influence of acetic acid on *H. pylori* gives no chance for the bacterium to resist the treatment with vinegar or to mutate and develop resistant strains.

Although the role of auto-immunity in *H. pylori*-associated ITP has been widely emphasized in literature,[17] the rapid dramatic response to *H. pylori* eradication from the colon in this case study should attract the attention towards a toxic effect played by the ammonia produced by colonic *H. pylori* strains. It was surprising to discover during the observation of the diet habits of this child that he was, like his parents, fond of eating chilly green pepper which could have been an additional factor that forced *H. pylori* to escape to the colon.

Conclusion: A toxic element rather than an auto-immune alone should not be overlooked in cases of ITP in children associated with *H. pylori*. Children may pay an expensive bill due to their parent's misbehavior in food habits and antibiotic abuse.

Acknowledgement: The study appreciates the facilities and time allowed by Balghsoon Clinics in Jeddah/Saudi Arabia. The continuous support offered by Abdul-Aziz Al-Sorayai Investment Company (ASIC) in Jeddah/Saudi Arabia, the scientific and emotional support of Dr Ahmed S. Balghsoon are extremely valued and appreciated.

Conflict of Interest: No conflict of interest is existing.

REFERENCES:

1. **Liebman H.** Other immune thrombocytopenias. *Semin Hematol 2007 Oct; 44 (4 Suppl 5): S24-34.*

2. **Gernsheimer T. Epidemiology and pathophysiology of immune thrombocytopenic purpura.** *Eur J Hematol Suppl 2008 Feb; (69): 3-8.*

3. **Fogarty PF, Segal JB. The epidemiology of immune thrombocytopenic purpura.** *Curr Opin Hematol 2007 Sep; 14 (5): 515-9.*

4. **Sachs UJ. Diagnosis of idiopathic thrombocytopenic purpura.** *Hamostaseologie 2008; 28 (1): 72-76.*

5. **Godeau B, Provan D, Bussel J. Immune thrombocytopenic purpura in adults.** *Curr Opin Hematol 2007 Sep; 14 (5): 535-56.*

6. **Afifi AM, Adnan M, Guindi MM. Childhood idiopathic thrombocytopenic purpura in Egypt and the neighboring Arab countries: a regional form with three different patterns of clinical expression.** *Acta Hematol 1981; 65 (3): 211-6.*

7. **Al-Salem AH, Naserullah Z, Qaisaruddin S, et al. Splenectomy for hematological diseases: The Qatif Central Hospital experience.** *Ann Saudi Med 1999 Jul-Aug; 19 (4): 325-30.*

8. **Rostami N, Keshtkar-Jahromi M, Rahnavardi M, etal. Effect of eradication of Helicobacter pylori on platelet recovery in patients with chronic idiopathic thrombocytopenic purpura: A controlled trial.** *Am J Hematol 2008 May; 83 (5): 376-81.*

9. **de Korwin JD. Does Helicobacter pylori play a role in extragastric diseases?** *Presse Med 2008 Mar; 37 (3 Pt 2): 525-34. Epub 2008 Feb 4.*

10. **Farinha P, Gascoyne RD. Helicobacter pylori and MALT Lymphoma.** *Gastroenterology 2005 May; 128 (6): 1579-605.*

11. Ge Z. **Potential of fumarate reductase as a novel therapeutic target in Helicobacter pylori infection.** *Expert Opin Ther Targets 2002 Apr; 6 (2): 135-46.*

12. Suzuki T, Matsushima M, Shirakura K, et al. **Association of inflammatory cytokine gene polymorphisms with platelet recovery in idiopathic thrombocytopenic purpura patients after the eradication of Helicobacter pylori.** *Digestion. 2008; 77 (2): 73-8. Epub 2008 Mar 20.*

13. Bulut Y, Agacayak A, Karlidag D, et al. **Association of CagA+ Helicobacter pylori with adenotonsillar hypertrophy.** *Tohoku J Exp Med. 2006 Jul; 209 (3): 229-33.*

14. Nasrat SAM, Nasrat RM, Nasrat MM, et al. **The dramatic spread of diabetes mellitus worldwide and influence of Helicobacter pylori.** *General Med J 2015; 3 (1): 159-62.*

15. Nasrat SAM, Nasrat AM. **An alternative approach for the rising challenge of hypertensive illness via Helicobacter pylori eradication.** *J Cardiol Res 2015; 6 (1): 221-225.*

16. Nsarat RM, Nasrat MM, Nasrat AM, et al. **Improvement of idiopatic cardiomyopathy after colon clear.** *J Cardiol Res 2015 Apr; 6 (2): 249-254.*

17. Nasrat AM. **A new approach for the hematologic challenges of Helicobacter pylori infection in children. The** *International Symposium of the Egyptian Society of Pediatric Hematology/Oncology, 2006 Mar. Available from URL, www. espho.org*

18. Nasrat AM. **The world misconception and misbehavior towards Helicobacter pylori is leading to major spread of illness.** *The 7th Anti-Aging Medicine World Congress, Monte-Carlo, Monaco, 2009 Mar.* **Available from URL,** *www.euromedicom.com*

MALE PELVIC CONGESTION AND ERECTILE DYSFUNCTION; OBSCURE REASONS FOR AN OBVIOUS PHENOMENON AMONG THE YOUNG

Introduction: Erectile dysfunction (ED) has got its impact on the quality of life of both partners. Erectile function (EF), as a neurovascular phenomenon, is characterized by penile engorgement that results from local arousal induced-release of neuronal and endothelial-derived nitric oxide (NO). ED can arise from arterial etiology, venous leakage or psychogenic reasons.[1,2]

Consistent with the fact that the cavernous tissue is a complex extension of the vasculature; risk factors that affect the vasculature have been shown to affect cavernous function as well.[3] Therefore; ED can be adequately prevented and improved by reduction of cardiovascular disease (CVD) risk factors, regular exercise, weight loss and abstinence from smoking.[2]

An apparent role of the cytokines in the pathophysiology of ED has been emerging; these substances can induce vascular spasm and affect vascular endothelial function including endothelial-derived NO production. Demonstration of high levels of tumor necrosis factor-alpha, which is a member of the cytokine family, in patients with ED supports the suggestion of a potential influence of cytokines in the pathogenesis of this sexual conflict.[3,4] The association of male pelvic congestion and prostatitis or prostatism with the frequency of male sexual dysfunction has been documented also in literature.[5-7]

Cyclic guanosine monophosphate (cGMP), by inducing activation of protein kinase G, mediates the effects of NO by enhancing calcium sequestration and activating large-conductance calcium-sensitive potassium channels. Phosphodiesterase-5 (PDE5) inhibitors (sildenafil, tadalafil and vardenafil) were found to increase cGMP levels in erectile tissue. These agents are effective in 80% of arterial ED, even with CVD and can be used safely.[2] Penile prosthesis implantation is a safe and effective measure for management of ED due to venous leak.[7]

 Pelvic congestion syndrome has been widely studied in the female sex, while there are not many publications on the male equivalent. Prostatitis represents the most frequent affections of the genito-urinary male tract but in the majority of cases, the etiology of such affections remains unknown.[8] The pathophysiology of prostatodynia (chronic prostatitis-like syndrome) is still remaining unknown. Recently, it was reported that intra-pelvic venous congestion especially around the prostate was found predominantly in patients with prostatodynia.[9] The insufficient circulation of the internal pudendal vessels is a characteristic sign observed in patients with intra-pelvic venous congestion syndrome.[10]

Helicobacter pylori has been found associated with many medical challenges and having different influence in these conditions. Colonic ***H. pylori*** strains were found frequently associated with pelvic congestion due to accumulation of profuse toxic amounts of ammonia in the colon; **_H. pylori_** was considered as a possible underlying etiologic pathology in cases of pelvic pathology in general.[11-13]

REFERENCES:

1. **Zhu YC, Zhao JL, Wu YG, et al.** Clinical features and treatment options for Chinese patients with severe primary erectile dysfunction. _Urology 2010 Mar 16._ [Epub ahead of print]

2. **Archer SL, Gragasin FS, Webster L, et al. Aetiology and management of male erectile dysfunction and female sexual dysfunction in patients with cardiovascular disease.** _Drugs Aging 2005; 22 (10): 823-44._

3. **Carneiro FS, Webb RC, Tostes RC. Emerging Role for TNF-alpha in Erectile Dysfunction.** _J Sex Med 2010 Mar 15._ **[Epub ahead of print]**

4. **Ozben B, Erdogan O. The role of inflammation in acute coronary syndromes.** _Inflamm Allergy Drug Targets 2008 Sep; 7 (3): 136-44._

5. **Davis SN, Binik YM, Carrier S. Sexual dysfunction and pelvic pain in men: a male sexual pain disorder?** _J Sex Marital Ther. 2009; 35 (3):182-205. Review._

6. **Rosen RC, Link CL, O'Leary MP, et al. Lower urinary tract symptoms and sexual health: the role of gender, lifestyle and medical comorbidities.** _BJU Int. 2009 Apr; 103 Suppl 3:42-7._

7. **Permpongkosol S, Kongkakand A, Ratana-Olarn K, et al. Increased prevalence of erectile dysfunction (ED): results of the second epidemiological study on sexual activity and prevalence of ED in Thai males.** _Aging Male. 2008 Sep; 11 (3):128-33._

8. **Sarteschi LM, Simi S, Turchi P, et al. Echo-color Doppler in male pelvic congestion syndrome.** _Arch Ital Urol Androl 2002 Dec; 74 (4): 166-70._

9. **Minamiguchi N. Epidemiological study of intrapelvic venous congestion syndrome (IVCS) using new IVCS symptom score.** _Nippon Hinyokika Gakkai Zasshi 1998 Nov; 89 (11): 863-70._

10. **Kamoi K. Pathologic significance of the internal pudendal vein in the development of intrapelvic venous congestion syndrome.** _Nippon Hinyokika Gakkai Zasshi 1996 Nov; 87 (11): 1214-20._

11. **Farinha P, Gascoyne RD. Helicobacter pylori and MALT Lymphoma.** _Gastroenterology 2005 May ; 128 (6) : 1579-605._

12. **Nasrat AM. The world misconception and misbehavior towards Helicobacter pylori is leading to major spread of illness.** _The 7th Anti-Aging Medicine World Congress, Monte-Carlo, Monaco, 2009 Mar._ **Available from URL,** _www.euromedicom.com_

13. **Nasrat AM, Nasrat SAM, Nasrat RM, et al. Misconception and misbehavior towards Helicobacter pylori is leading to major spread of illness.** _GM 2015; S1: 002._ **[Open Access]**

SCIENTIFIC EVIDENCES ON THE INFLUENCE OF HELICOBACTER PYLORI ON MALE PELVIC CONGESTION AND ERECTILE DYSFUNCTION

M*ale Pelvic Congestion and Erectile Dysfunction; Obscure Reasons for an Obvious Phenomenon Among the young:* Published in Journal of General Medicine 2016; 4 (2): 1000236. (Open Access). Nasrat et al. Male Pelvic Congestion and Erectile Dysfunction; Obscure Reasons for an Obvious Phenomenon Among the young. *Gen Med 2016; 4 (2): 1000236. [doi: 10.4172/2327-5146.1000236]*

Background: Erectile dysfunction (ED) has got its impact on the quality of life of both partners. Erectile function (EF) is due to local arousal induced by release of nitric oxide (NO). ED can be adequately prevented and improved by reduction of cardiovascular disease risk factors, regular exercise, weight loss and abstinence from smoking. An apparent role for cytokines in the pathophysiology of ED has been emerging; this substance can induce vascular spasm and affect vascular endothelial function including endothelial-derived NO production. The association of male pelvic congestion with the frequency of male sexual dysfunction has been documented in literature. As concerns therapeutic modalities, medicines work essentially by mediating or enhancing the effect of NO.[1-7]

Colonic ***Helicobacter pylori*** strains were found frequently associated with pelvic congestion; ***H. pylori*** was considered as a possible underlying etiologic pathology in cases of pelvic pathology in general. The increased mucosal production of inflammatory cytokines of ***H. pylori*** could play an integral role in the pathogenesis of ED.[8-10]

The association of the colonic ***H. pylori*** strains with pelvic pathology, the role played by the inflammatory cytokines and the therapeutic effect of NO in ED were the scientific reasons to employ colon clear and blood-let out (BLO) cupping therapy in cases of ED.[11-13]

Objective: Demonstration of recent environmental reasons behind the rising phenomena of erectile dysfunction among young ages during late decades.

Design & Setting: A multiple clinical-case prospective study done in Balghsoon Clinics in Jeddah/Saudi Arabia between May 2012 and October 2014.

Patients& Methods: Forty patients scheduled in two equal different age groups with an onset of different grades of ED. The age of patients of the first group ranged between 50 and 55 years while age of patients of the second group ranged between 30 and 35 years. Patients were selected so as to have sufficient recent duration of erectile un-satisfaction (6-8 months) that did not improve in spite of seeking adequate medical advice. The purpose of the young age group was to illustrate an enviromental reason that may affect EF in those who should not generally suffer such problem, while the purpose of the older age group was demonstration of the efficacy of the natural methods employed in this study on ED in an age group that may normally start to feel uneasy about this matter. The patient's complaint was mostly incomplete or soft erection which does not last enough making penetration of the vagina uneasy; attempts to restore or improve erection ends ultimately by premature ejaculation. Validated self-report measures, (the International Prostate Symptom Score and International Index of Erectile Function), have been considered.[6] Existence of colonic *H. pylori* strains was confirmed by the specific test, *H. pylori* fecal antigen.[11] The potent natural senna leaves extract purge was employed for all patients monthly for three months in order to achieve adequate eradication of colonic *H. pylori* strains. One week after the last purge, all patients had undergone a traditional therapeutic procedure of suction blood-let out cupping therapy with skin scratching and suction of blood on the upper back for the purpose of sero-clearance followed by a further cupping session few time later on the lower back for the purpose of pelvic decongestion. This traditional therapy can be described as *"functional modified multiple mini fasciotomy"*.[14-16]

Results: 90% of patients were found positive for colonic *H. pylori* strains; eradication of *H. pylori* from the colon was confirmed by the same specific test (*H. pylori* fecal antigen test). 17 patients of the first older group with ED restored 75% at least of their usual erectile satisfaction after completing colon clear and 85% of EF few days after cupping therapy. 19 patients of the second younger group restored 80% of EF after colon clear and 90% of EF after cupping therapy. All patients of both groups who responded to therapy expressed their satisfaction of restoring nearly their usual sexual health and having no problem with intercourse. They were followed up for few months and then left to lead their normal life without interference; they were instructed to care for their colon and food habits in order to avoid recurrence of colonic *H. pylori* strains.

The three patients from first group and two patient from second group who did not respond to therapy were not happy because of inability to achieve or maintain an erection adequate for sexual intercourse; they were referred to psychiatric andrologists to exclude psychogenic reasons before revision of natural therapy.

Ethical Considerations: An informed signed consent was taken from all patients, they were made aware about safety of the natural colon clear remedy and the procedure of cupping therapy employed for them; they were free to quit the study whenever they like. The research proposal was approved and the study followed the rules of the Research Ethics Committee of Balghsoon Clinics in Jeddah, Saudi Arabia.

Discussion: ED is lately a common occurrence and its incidence is expected to increase significantly along with the increase in various lifestyle diseases. It constitutes an increasing obvious phenomenon during latest decades; the reasons of spreading of this phenomena lately even among younger men are obscure to explain.[17] As man grows older, sexual and non-sexual symptoms of testosterone deficiency can negatively affect the quality of life and cause considerable general health concerns but not in young age generations and not in such fast scenario.[18]

Concerning pathogenesis of ED, inflammatory cytokines has been frankly and majorly considered in this topic.[3,4] As regards risk factors in ED, cardiovascular risk factors may constitute the same risk in ED also.[2,3] As concerns therapeutic modalities, the immediate objective of PDE5 inhibitor treatments is to restore the ability of man to achieve a maintained erection adequate for sexual satisfaction.[2] Penile prosthesis implantation has been employed as well in ED caused by venous leak.[7]

H. pylori could migrate or get forced to migrate to the colon under the influence of antibiotic violence leading to accumulation of profuse amounts of ammonia unopposed or buffered by any acidity.[11,12] Accumulation of profuse amounts of ammonia in the colon is toxic and could lead to pelvic congestion. In addition, the increased mucosal production of inflammatory cytokines of colonic *H. pylori* strains could play also an integral role in the pathogenesis of ED.[19,20]

Depending upon these facts, and upon the fact that cytokines accumulate in the body with or without apparent vascular insufficiency,[21] together with the findings that male pelvic congestion is associated with male sexual dysfunction;[22,23] colon clear and cupping therapy have been employed in cases of male ED for eradication of colonic *H. pylori* strains, decongestion of the pelvis and elimination of the undesired elements from the pelvis such as trapped blood and inflammatory cytokines which are functionally obliged to this blood.[12,15]

The expected role of colon clear in ED for eradication of colonic *H. pylori* strains is getting rid of the reasons of pelvic congestion due to accumulation of profuse ammonia in the area of the pelvis and withdrawal of the inflammatory cytokines produced due to existence of *H. pylori* in the colon.[11,12,19,20] The expected role of cupping blood-letting out therapy in cases of ED is withdrawal of the congested blood in the pelvis, elimination of the interstitial cytokines trapped with this blood in the pelvis and encouragement of pelvic circulation due histamine release at the scratch sites and liberation of endothelial-derived NO owing to the act of repeated suction.[15,23,24]

Antibiotics are seldom effective against extra-gastric *H. pylori* strains,[25] therefore; the senna leaves extract purge was used for colon clear. In addition to the adequate clearance of the colonic contents, the senna extract is the only available traditional measure that can kill and expel all bacteria in the colon including colonic *H. pylori* strains as documented by *H. pylori* fecal antigen testing. It was found that addition of three times dilution of the senna purge extract has got a direct lethal effect on *H. pylori* culture media.[26-29]

The traditional blood-letting out cupping therapy can be described as a sort of *"functional modified multiple mini fasciotomy"*. It is functional modified as it does not include actual anatomical fasciotomy, but elimination of the trapped subfascial and subcutaneous interstitial elements is achieved under the effect of skin scratching and suction.[14,30]

Figure 1 shows a deep thigh hematoma visualized by MRI (1.1), its response towards the skin suction (1.2), and its disappearance after skin scratching and repeat suction (1.3).

Conclusion: Employment of combined colon clear and cupping therapy in cases of ED is promising and is not just hypothetical as upon the basis of this combined traditional natural cure most of the patients of the study have achieved satisfactory improvement. Hence, it is safely logic to correlate the un-explained prevalence of ED among young age groups during late decades to the prevalence of colonic *H. pylori* strains during the same periods.

Conflict of Interest: There is no conflict of interest existing.

REFERENCES:

1. **Zhu YC, Zhao JL, Wu YG, et al.** Clinical features and treatment options for Chinese patients with severe primary erectile dysfunction. *Urology 2010 Mar 16.* [Epub ahead of print]

2. **Archer SL, Gragasin FS, Webster L, et al. Aetiology and management of male erectile dysfunction and female sexual dysfunction in patients with cardiovascular disease.** *Drugs Aging 2005; 22 (10): 823-44.*

3. **Carneiro FS, Webb RC, Tostes RC. Emerging Role for TNF-alpha in Erectile Dysfunction.** *J Sex Med 2010 Mar 15.* **[Epub ahead of print]**

4. **Ozben B, Erdogan O. The role of inflammation in acute coronary syndromes.** *Inflamm Allergy Drug Targets 2008 Sep; 7 (3): 136-44.*

5. **Davis SN, Binik YM, Carrier S. Sexual dysfunction and pelvic pain in men: a male sexual pain disorder?** *J Sex Marital Ther. 2009; 35 (3):182-205. Review.*

6. **Rosen RC, Link CL, O'Leary MP, et al. Lower urinary tract symptoms and sexual health: the role of gender, lifestyle and medical comorbidities.** *BJU Int. 2009 Apr; 103*

Suppl 3:42-7.

7. **Permpongkosol S, Kongkakand A, Ratana-Olarn K, et al. Increased prevalence of erectile dysfunction (ED): results of the second epidemiological study on sexual activity and prevalence of ED in Thai males.** *Aging Male. 2008 Sep; 11 (3): 128-33.*

8. **Sarteschi LM, Simi S, Turchi P, et al. Echo-color Doppler in male pelvic congestion syndrome.** *Arch Ital Urol Androl 2002 Dec; 74 (4): 166-70.*

9. **Minamiguchi N. Epidemiological study of intrapelvic venous congestion syndrome (IVCS) using new IVCS symptom score.** *Nippon Hinyokika Gakkai Zasshi 1998 Nov; 89 (11): 863-70.*

10. **Kamoi K. Pathologic significance of the internal pudendal vein in the development of intrapelvic venous congestion syndrome.** *Nippon Hinyokika Gakkai Zasshi 1996 Nov; 87 (11): 1214-20.*

11. **Farinha P, Gascoyne RD. Helicobacter pylori and MALT Lymphoma.** *Gastroenterology 2005 May ; 128 (6) : 1579-605.*

12. **Nasrat AM. The world misconception and misbehavior towards Helicobacter pylori is leading to major spread of illness.** *The 7th Anti-Aging Medicine World Congress, Monte-Carlo, Monaco, 2009 Mar.* **Available from URL,** *www.euromedicom.com*

13. **Nasrat AM, Nasrat SAM, Nasrat RM, et al. Misconception and misbehavior towards Helicobacter pylori is leading to major spread of illness.** *GM 2015; S1 (002).* **[Open Access]**

14. **Nasrat AM. It is neither re-implantation nor implantation, it is hair plantation.** *The International Congress of Aesthetic Dermatology, Bangkok, Thailand, 2010 Jan.* **Available from URL,** *www.euromedicom.com*

15. **Nasrat AM. Role of blood-let out cupping therapy in angina and angina risk management, emergency Vs elective.** *The 22nd International scientific session of Saudi Heart Association, Riyadh, 2011 Jan.* **Available from URL,** *www.sha.org.sa*

16. **Nasrat AM, El-Sayed SM, Nasrat SAM. Role of blood-let out cupping therapy in angina and angina risk management.** *GM 2015; 3 (3).* **[Open Access]**

17. **Mutha AS, KulKarni VR, Bhagat SB, et al. An observational study to evaluate the prevalence of erectile dysfunction (ED) and prescribing pattern of drugs n patients with ED visiting an Andrology Specialty Clinic, Mumbai: 2012-2014.** *J Clin Diagn Res.* **[Epub 2015 Jul 1]**

18. **Aversa A, Morgentater A. The practical management of testosterone deficiency in men.** *Nat Rev Urol 2015 Oct 13.* **[Epub ahead of print] Revew.**

19. **Owen DA. Gastritis and casrditis.** *Mod Pathol 2003 Apr; 16 (4):325-41. Review.*

20. **Klausz G, Tiszai A, Lénárt Z, et al. Helicobacter pylori-induced immunological responses in patients with duodenal ulcer and in patients with cardiomyopathies.** *Acta Microbiol Immunol Hung. 2004; 51 (3):311-20.*

21. **Ganeshan A, Upponi S, Hon LQ, et al. Chronic pelvic pain due to pelvic congestion syndrome: the role of diagnostic and interventional radiology.** *Cardiovasc Intervent Radiol. 2007 Nov-Dec; 30 (6):1105-11.* **Epub 2007 Sep 6. Review.**

22. **Loffredo V. Clinical aspects and complementary tests in pelvic congestive states.** *Rev Fr Gynecol Obstet. 1991 Feb 25; 86 (2 Pt 2):191-4.* **Review.**

23. **Charles G. Congestive pelvic syndromes.** *Rev Fr Gynecol Obstet. 1995 Feb; 90 (2):84-90.* **Review.**

24. **Nasrat AM, Nasrat SAM, Nasrat RM, et al. Role of blood-let out cupping therapy in female pelvic congestion syndrome.** *GM 2015;* **S1: 3.**

25. **Grünberger B, Wöhrer S, Streubel B, et al. Antibiotic treatment is not effective in patients infected with Helicobacter pylori suffering from extragastric MALT lymphoma.** *J Clin Oncol 2006 Mar 20; 24 (9):1370-5.*

26. **Nasrat AM, Nasrat SAM, Nasrat RM, et al. The definitive eradication of Helicobacter pylori from the colon.** *GM 2015; S1 (1).* **[Open Access]**

27. **Nasrat AM, Nasrat SAM, Nasrat RM, et al. A comparative study of natural eradication of Helicobacter pylori Vs antibotics.** *GM 2015; S1 (1).* **[Open Access]**

28. **Nasrat SAM, Nasrat AM. An alternative approach for the rising challenge of hypertensive illness via Helicobacter pylori eradication.** *J Cardiol Res 2015; 6 (1): 221-225.*

29. **Nsarat RM, Nasrat MM, Nasrat AM, et al. Improvement of idiopatic cardiomyopathy after colon clear.** *J Cardiol Res 2015 Apr; 6 (2): 249-254.*

30. **Nasrat AM, Nasrat SAM, Nasrat RM, et al. Therapeutic effect of combined colon clear and cupping therapy on idiopathic skin pathology.** *GMJ 2015; 3 (5).* **[Open Access]**

WHY DO PHYSICIANS DIAGNOSE GOUT IN YOUNG ADULTS WITH PERFECT KIDNEY FUNCTION!!

Introduction: Gout is a very old disease which exists for thousands of years with joint swelling, pain or tenderness; the first description of symptoms of gout was found in the Egyptian medical papyri dating to 3000 years BC.[1] Hyperuricema has long been established as the major etiologic factor in gout.[2] Gout has recently become the most common presentation of arthritis in developed countries; however, studies indicate that treatment of gout is still unsatisfactory.[3]

As much as hyperuricemia increases the risk of gout, it is also a risk factor of cardiovascular diseases. The relationship between hyperuricemia and cardiovascular disease risk has been also clearly emphasized in literature; elevated serum uric acid was found strongly associated with obesity and hyperlipidemia in both men and women. These findings indicate that attention towards cardiovascular complications should be paid among hyperuricemic patients to the extent that lowering the level of serum uric acid might provide a novel target for cardiovascular protection.[4,5]

In addition to the inflammatory state triggered by urate crystal deposition in the joints, hyperuricemia constitutes additional pathophysiologic sequences due to tissue inflammation mainly in the vascular wall leading to endothelial dysfunction contributing in turn in the pathogenesis of diabetes, hypertension, arteriosclerosis and chronic heart failure.[2] These reasons made physicians anxious to rush in the immediate assessment and treatment of gout once elevated levels of uric acid were detected.

On the contrary, patients try to hesitate accepting that they are becoming candidates of gouty illness particularly if they are young and their renal function is normal. Severe joint pain combined with no obvious signs of physical trauma or injury caused confusion to patients who try to interpret their symptoms. Self-diagnosis or self-medication, financial and work pressure constitute the main reasons for delayed consultation or reluctance to seek medical attention. Delayed diagnosis after consultation was due to misdiagnosis as per confusion towards attacks in joints other than the first metatarso-phalangeal joint. Resistance to the diagnosis was related to the response of patient's belief about the causes of gout and characteristics of individuals likely to be affected.[6]

Although gout is potentially curable with long-term urate lowering therapy; confusion about the details of urate measurement has contributed to suboptimal care of patients.[7] As cytokines are the most important soluble mediators of inflammation; new discoveries has considered gout as an auto-inflammatory disease and included a role of inflammatory cytokines in the pathogenesis of gout allowing further understanding and enabling the use of new therapies for the disease that could reduce patient's resistance to existing procedures.[3,8-10] The association of *Helicobacter pylori* with disease spread during late decades through immune, inflammatory, toxic or different unknown reasons has been sufficiently reported in literature.[11]

REFERENCES:

1. **Alusik T, Alusik S.** Gout and its manifestations, description and treatment in ancient times. *Cas Lek Cesk 2015; 154 (4): 194-5.*

2. **Gliozzi M, Malara N, Muscoli S, et al. The treatment of hyperuricemia.** *Int J Cardiol 2015 Aug 8.* **[Epub ahead of print]**.

3. **Cal-Kocikowska J, Nawrocka M, Bogdanski P. Gout – from pathogenesis to treatment – progress in the XXI century.** *Pol Merkur Lekarski 2015 Jun; 38 (228): 354-9.* **Review.**

4. **Derosa G, Maffioli P, Sahebkar A. Plasma uric acid concentrations are reduced by fenofibrate: a systematic review and meta-analysis of randomized placebo-controlled trials.** *Pharmacol Res 2015 Sep 15. 31 (1): 36-42.* **[Epub ahead of print] Review.**

5. **Su P, Hong L, Zhao Y, et al. Relationship between hyperuricemia and cardiovascular disease risk factors in a Chinese population: a cross-sectional study.** *Med Sci Monit 2015 Sep 12; 21: 2707-17.*

6. **Liddle J, Roddy E, Mallen CD, et al. Mapping patients' experiences from initial symptoms to gout diagnosis.** *BMJ Open 2015 Sep 14; 5 (9): e008323.*

7. **Dalbeth N, Winnard D, Gow PJ, et al. Urate testing in gout: why, when and how.** *NZMed J 2015 Aug 21; 128 (1420): 65-8.*

8. **Marcuzzi A, Piscianz E, Valencic E, et al. To extinguish the fire from outside the cell or to shutdown the gas valve insde? Novel trend in anti-inflammatory therapies. Int** *J Mol Sci 2015 Sep 7; 16 (9): 21277-93.*

9. **Owen DA. Gastritis and carditis.** *Mod Pathol 2003 Apr; 16 (4):325-41. Review.*

10. **Klausz G, Tiszai A, Lénárt Z, et al. Helicobacter pylori-induced immunological responses in patients with duodenal ulcer and in patients with cardiomyopathies.** *Acta Microbiol Immunol Hung. 2004; 51 (3):311-20.*

11. **Farinha P, Gascoyne RD. Helicobacter pylori and MALT Lymphoma.** *Gastroenterology 2005 May; 128 (6): 1579-605.*

SCIENTIC EVIDENCES ON THE ROLE OF HELICOBACTER PYLORI IN THE INCREASED INCIDENCE OF GOUT

Why Do Physicians Diagnose Gout in Young Adults with Perfect Kidney Function!! Published in the Journal of General Medicine 2015; 3 (5): 208. (Open Accesss) Nasrat et al. Why do physicians diagnose gout in young adults with perfect kidney function!!. *General Med 2015; 3 (5): 208. [doi: 10.4172/2327-5146.1000208]*

Background: Gout is a very old disease which exists for thousands of years with joint swelling, pain or tenderness. Hyperuricema has long been established as the major etiologic factor in gout. Gout has recently become the most common presentation of arthritis in developed countries. Hyperuricemia increases the risk of gout and is also a risk factor of cardiovascular diseases. Hyperuricemia could contribute to diabetes, hypertension and arteriosclerosis due to endothelial dysfunction triggered by vascular wall tissue inflammation because of urate crystals deposition. These reasons are sufficient to render physicians anxious in immediate assessment and treatment of elevated serum uric acid levels. On the contrary, patients hesitate to accept the decision of their pre-gouty illness due to elevation of serum urate particularly if they are young and having perfect renal function.[1-7]

Helicobacter pylori could migrate or get forced to migrate to the colon leading to colonic re-absorptive error with excess accumulation of fluids and salts in the body; uric acid could be among these reabsorbed elements giving a picture of elevated serum uric acid level that would have no relation to age of the individual or the integrity of his renal function. Furthermore, gout has been recently considered as one of the auto-inflammatory diseases, hence cytokines are the most common mediators of inflammation; therefore, the role played by the increased mucosal production of inflammatory mediators (cytokines) induced by ***H. pylori*** is supposed to contribute in the pathogenesis of gout. In this situation, hyperuricemia is not expected to be adequately or successfully improved by traditional urate lowering measures regardless of the age of patient or the state of his kidney function.[3,8-11]

Objective: Demonstration that detection of high levels of serum uric acid in young adults should not be considered final diagnosis of hyperuricemia pre-gouty illness so long kidney function is normal.

Design& Setting: Prospective study done in Balghsoon Clinics in Jeddah, Saudi Arabia between May 2011 and October 2013.

Patients& Methods: Thirty three patients aged between 31-40 years, having normal kidney function and frank history of ***H. pylori*** dyspepsia were included in the study due to newly discovered elevated levels of serum uric acid regardless of their body built or any associated chronic illness.

5 patients were overweight, 3 patients were obese but none of them were having any other illness than hyperuricemia while the remaining patients were average built. Among those patients with average built, 5 patients were diabetic, 7 patients were hypertensive and all of them were inadequately controlled on oral anti-

diabetic and anti-hypertensive medications. Serum uric acid level ranged between 6.5-7.3 mg/dl while existence of colonic *H. pylori* strains was proved by sensitive specific tests (*H. pylori* fecal antigen test).[11]

All patients underwent colon clear employing the potent natural senna purge once and colon care was maintained by vinegar-mixed food therapy for one week.[12]

Patients were free to lead their regular life style except restriction of out-side home meals in order to avoid recurrence of abnormal-behavior *H. pylori* strains. Eradication of *H. pylori* from the colon was confirmed by the same specific test.

Results: All patients were found positive for existence of colonic *H. pylori* strains and its eradication from the colon after the natural therapy was confirmed by using *H. pylori* fecal antigen test.

The serum uric acid levels dropped below 4 mg/dl within 3 days after colon clear in 30 patients while the remaining 3 patients showed the same drop at end of the first week of natural therapy.

Interestingly, all diabetic and hypertensive patients became adequately controlled on their own medications while 6 hypertensive patients were able to quit their medications and maintain normal blood pressure values although they were inadequately controlled in spite of regular follow up of medications and carefulness about their style of life.

Patients were followed up for 12 months and they maintained normal uric acid levels as long as they maintained carefulness about their colonic condition.

Ethical Considerations: An informed signed consent was taken from all patients; they were made aware about safety of the natural remedies employed for them. They were free to quit the study whenever they like.

Discussion: Traditional risk factors do not appear fully sufficient to explain the rising figures of chronic disease spread all over the world; in a way that further indicates that traditional measures employed to control disease spread can never be adequate or decisive. The spreading incidence of gout in young adults around 30 years of age or even below 40 years particularly if they are having a normal kidney function is one of these medical conditions which can not be explained by traditional risk rules. The latest decades demonstrated flare up of a lot of medical challenges associated or directly related to *H. pylori* existence. [11,12] Different reports in literature have confirmed the association of cytotoxin-associated gene A (cagA) positive *H. pylori* strains, and emphasized that cagA of *H. pylori* encodes a highly immunogenic and virulence-associated protein; the presence of this virulent gene in the body could affect the clinical outcome in many patients.[13] In addition, gout has been recently considered as one of the auto-inflammatory diseases; and hence cytokines are the most common mediators of inflammation,[3,8] therefore; the increased mucosal production of inflammatory cytokines of *H. pylori* could play an integral role in the pathogenesis of gout regardless of the age of patient or the state of his kidney function.[9,10]

H. pylori could migrate or get forced to migrate to the colon under the influence of antibiotic violence leading to accumulation of profuse toxic amounts of ammonia unopposed or buffered by any acidity. Ammonia is smooth muscle tonic and in profuse amounts can cause multiple colonic spasms leading to colonic re-absorptive error with excess accumulation of fluids and salts in the body;[11,12] uric acid could be among theses reabsorbed elements giving a picture of elevated serum uric acid level that would have no relation to age of the individual or the integrity of his renal function. Therefore; it is vital to emphasize that urate lowering therapies are not definitive treatment in this situation as they do no treat the pathology and hence are not expected to adequately control the resulting hyperuricemia.

It is interesting to notice the obvious improvement on the clinical condition of chronic illness associated with cases of this study after employment of the natural *H. pylori* eradication therapy. A simple conclusion could directly jump up that it is not necessary that gout is always a risk factor for many diseases but *H. pylori* itself could be mostly the main pathogenic risk of many of the diseases spreading during latest decades like diabetes, hypertension, cardiovascular diseases and of course gout amongst them.[11,12,14-16]

It is worthy to mention that antibiotics are seldom effective against extra-gastric *H. pylori* strains.[17] A potent natural purgative is the only measure to eradicate *H. pylori* strains migrated to the colon, otherwise; these *H. pylori* strains would remain in the colon for life.[11,12,16]

Conclusion: Revision of the guidelines of diagnosis and treatment of *H. pylori* and many chronic diseases associated with it may be needed. Detection of high levels of uric acid in young adults should not be considered final diagnosis of pre-gouty illness unless kidney function is assessed and association of *H. pylori* is excluded by specific tests.

Acknowledgement: The study appreciates the facilities and time allowed by Balghsoon Clinics in Jeddah/ Saudi Arabia. The continuous support offered by Abdul-Aziz Al-Sorayai Investment Company (ASIC) in Jeddah/ Saudi Arabia, the scientific and emotional support of Dr Ahmed S. Balghsoon and the true brotherhood friendly encouragement of Mr. Abdul-Aziz Al-Sorayai are extremely valued and appreciated.

Conflict of Interest: No conflict of interest exists.

REFERENCES:

1. **Alusik T, Alusik S.** Gout and its manifestations, description and treatment in ancient times. *Cas Lek Cesk 2015; 154 (4): 194-5.*

2. **Gliozzi M, Malara N, Muscoli S, et al. The treatment of hyperuricemia.** *Int J Cardiol 2015 Aug 8.* **[Epub ahead of print]**

3. **Cal-Kocikowska J, Nawrocka M, Bogdanski P. Gout – from pathogenesis to treatment – progress in the XXI century.** *Pol Merkur Lekarski 2015 Jun; 38 (228): 354-9.* **Review.**

4. **Derosa G, Maffioli P, Sahebkar A. Plasma uric acid concentrations are reduced by fenofibrate: a systematic review and meta-analysis of randomized placebo-controlled trials.** *Pharmacol Res 2015 Sep 15; 31 (1): 36-42.* **[Epub ahead of print] Review**.

5. **Su P, Hong L, Zhao Y, et al. Relationship between hyperuricemia and cardiovascular disease risk factors in a Chinese population: a cross-sectional study.** *Med Sci Monit 2015 Sep 12; 21: 2707-17.*

6. **Liddle J, Roddy E, Mallen CD, et al. Mapping patients' experiences from initial symptoms to gout diagnosis.** *BMJ Open 2015 Sep 14; 5 (9): e008323.*

7. **Dalbeth N, Winnard D, Gow PJ, et al. Urate testing in gout: why, when and how.** *NZMed J 2015 Aug 21; 128 (1420): 65-8.*

8. **Marcuzzi A, Piscianz E, Valencic E, et al. To extinguish the fire from outside the cell or to shutdown the gas valve insde? Novel trend in anti-inflammatory therapies. Int** *J Mol Sci 2015 Sep 7; 16 (9): 21277-93.*

9. **Owen DA. Gastritis and casrditis.** *Mod Pathol 2003 Apr; 16 (4):325-41. Review.*

10. **Klausz G, Tiszai A, Lénárt Z, et al. Helicobacter pylori-induced immunological responses in patients with duodenal ulcer and in patients with cardiomyopathies.** *Acta Microbiol Immunol Hung. 2004; 51 (3):311-20.*

11. **Farinha P, Gascoyne RD. Helicobacter pylori and MALT Lymphoma.** *Gastroenterology 2005 May; 128 (6): 1579-605.*

12. **Nasrat AM. The world misconception and misbehavior towards Helicobacter pylori is leading to major spread of illness.** *The 7th Anti-Aging Medicine World Congress, Monte-Carlo, Monaco, 2009 Mar.* **Available from URL,** *www.euromedicom.com*

13. Bulut Y, Agacayak A, Karlidag D, et al. Association of CagA+ Helicobacter pylori with adenotonsillar hypertrophy. *Tohoku J Exp Med. 2006 Jul; 209 (3): 229-33.*

14. Nasrat SAM, Nasrat RM, Nasrat MM, et al. The dramatic spread of diabetes mellitus worldwide and influence of Helicobacter pylori. *General Med 2015; 3 (1): 159-62.*

15. Nasrat SAM, Nasrat AM. An alternative approach for the rising challenge of hypertensive illness via Helicobacter pylori eradication. *J Cardiol Res 2015; 6 (1): 221-225.*

16. Nsarat RM, Nasrat MM, Nasrat AM, et al. Improvement of idiopatic cardiomyopathy after colon clear. *J Cardiol Res 2015 Apr; 6 (2): 249-254.*

17. Grünberger B, Wöhrer S, Streubel B, et al. Antibiotic treatment is not effective in patients infected with Helicobacter pylori suffering from extragastric MALT lymphoma. *J Clin Oncol 2006 Mar 20; 24 (9):1370-5.*

ENDOMETRIOSIS AND OVARIAN CYSTIC DISEASE; WHY SO LINKED AS IF BORN SIMULTANEOUS!!

SCIENTIFIC EVIDENCES ON THE PATHOGENESIS SIMILARITY OF BOTH ENDOMETRIOSIS AND OVARIAN CYSTIC DISEASE

Endometriosis and Ovarian Cystic Disease; why so Linked as if Born Simultaneous!! *Letter to Editor:* Published in Journal of General Medicine 2016; 4 (1): 1000221. (Open Access). Nasrat AM. Endometriosis and ovarian cystic disease; why so linked as if born simultaneous!! *General Med 2016; 4 (1): 1000221.* *[doi:10.4172/2327-5146.1000221]*

Helicobacter pylori colonized the stomach since an immemorial time. More than 160 years before in 1852, it was reported that there is ammonia in the stomach. In 1930s, it was reported that the ammonia demonstrated in the stomach is due to the effect of a urease enzyme. In 1960s, it was confirmed that urease activity in the stomach is not a property of the stomach but it is due to the activity of a bacterium in the stomach. Early in 1980s, it was clearly emphasized that the ammonia detected in the stomach is not toxic or not in toxic amounts but it is even useful. In 1985, *H. pylorus* was rediscovered or as claimed by two Australian physicians; "I got it, a bacterium surviving in the stomach". They accused it for causing gastric ulcers and cancer; hence, they started the antibiotic violence against this stomach bacterium in 1986.[1] Via personal communications between 2002 and 2003, some scientific research centers in the west and the author expressed to each other their inconvenience about the story claimed by the two Australian doctors; hence, a research investigation team and the author started an extensive work on the confusing subject of *H. pylori*.

The last three decades have shown prevalence of abnormal-behavior *H. pylori* strains and the rising figures of many medical challenges related to it. Therefore; the last three decades demonstrated rediscovery of *H. pylori*, the antibiotic aggression towards it, the prevalence of its abnormal-behavior strains instead of getting rid of it, and the flare up of a lot of medical challenges related to these *H. pylori* strains.[1,2] A medical study which does not correlate between these well-established findings is definitely not employing a clinical sense.

In the same way, the latest decades demonstrate un-explained rising incidence of endometriosis and ovarian cystic disease (OCD) in a pattern that as if they behave like twins; endometriosis is a common condition affecting a significant population of women during their reproductive life. Endometriosis is a modern syndrome with complex pathogenesis and increasing evidences indicating that it is part of a uterine reproductive dysfunction syndrome; while polycystic ovarian syndrome is a common endocrine disorder among women of reproductive age also caused by estrogen and progesterone dysfunction with an often increase in the levels of androgen. Although endometriosis is recognized as benign gynecologic condition, its association with ovarian cancer has been frequently reported. Ovarian endometrioma is the most common form of endometriosis and endometriosis may be a precursor lesion for some epithelial ovarian cancers, while polycystic ovarian disease increases the potential risk of endometrial cancer.[2-8]

The introduction of laparoscopy in early 1960s allowed distinguishing three different clinical presentations of endometriosis: peritoneal, deep adenomyotic and cystic ovarian. The easy access to the pelvis via laparoscopy has led to an appreciable increase in the diagnosis of endometriosis and OCD in women with infertility or chronic pelvic pain.[4-9] In a study of the effect of blood-let out cupping therapy on cases of female pelvic congestion syndrome, it was found that most patients with endometriosis do have ovarian cysts and most patients with OCD have got endometriosis [10]. The current theories of pathogenesis and the current therapeutic strategies of both endometriosis and OCD vary;[5,7,9] hence, why they are so linked as if they were born simultaneous in the same pathogenic atmosphere!!

The association of both endometriosis and OCD with *H. pylori* related dyspeptic sequels and pathologic conditions has been sufficiently reported. It has been emphasized that the majority of endometriosis patients experience severe gastrointestinal symptoms to the extent of indicating an existing co-morbidity between endometriosis and irritable bowel syndrome which is frequently found associated with *H. pylori*. Women with OCD were found to have high risk of hypertension, diabetes, high cholesterol and obesity; most cases of these medical conditions were found during latest decades to be either directly related or associated with *H. pylori* existence.[5,10,11] The cease of the disease progress in endometriosis and OCD associated with cases of pelvic pain and congestion was frankly demonstrated during studying the effect of combined natural eradication of *H. pylori* by colon clear and elimination of *H. pylori* -related pelvic congestion by cupping therapy on pelvic inflammatory congestive syndrome.[12,13] This could refer to the possibility that *H. pylori*-related pelvic congestion due to accumulation of profuse toxic amounts of colonic ammonia produced by the abnormal colonic *H. pylori* strains could be a hidden reason behind the rising figures of endometriosis and OCD during late decades. This could further indicate that regular combined colon clear and cupping therapy could be a good prophylactic measure for endometriosis and OCD in susceptible disadvantaged young females. These suggestions are supported by the fact that *H. pylori* could migrate or get forced to migrate to the colon under the influence of antibiotic violence or misbehavior in food habits; *H. pylori* in the colon will continue producing ammonia for a purpose or no purpose, unopposed or buffered by any acidity leading to accumulation of profuse toxic amounts of ammonia in the colon with consequent rising incidence of pelvic congestion.[1,13]

The aim of this review letter is introducing a novel health care predictor for early screening of young females with pelvic pain/ congestion and dyspeptic symptoms for the existence of colonic *H. pylori* strains and starting its early eradication and early management of pelvic congestion by natural measures for the purpose of early prophylaxis from a potential risk of endometriosis and OCD.

REFERENCES:

1. **Farinha P, Gascoyne RD.** Helicobacter pylori and MALT Lymphoma. *Gastroenterology 2005; 128 (6): 1579-605.*

2. **Nasrat AM. The world misconception and misbehavior towards Helicobacter pylori is leading to major spread of illness.** *The 7th Anti-Aging Medicine World Congress, Monte-Carlo, Monaco, 2009 Mar.* **Available from URL,** *www.euromedicom.com*

3. **Mavrelos D, Saridogan E. Treatment of endometriosis in women desiring fertility.** *J Obstet Gynaecol India 2015; 65: 11-16.*

4. **Brosens I, Benagiano G. Endometriosis, a modern syndrome. Indian J Med Res 2011; 133: 581-593.**

5. **Murta EF, Nomelini RS, Ferreira FA. Ovarian clear cell carcinoma associated with endometriosis: a case report with immunohistochemical study.** *Eur J Gynaecol Oncol 2007; 28: 403-405.*

6. **GUO SW. Endometriosis and ovarian cancer: potential benefits and harms of screening and risk-reducing surgery.** *Fertil Steril 2015; 104: 813-830.*

7. **Kaponis A, Taniguchi F, Azuma Y. Current treatment of endometrioma.** *Obstet Gynecol Surg 2015; 70: 183-195.*

8. **Del Carmen MG. Evidence for relationship between endometriosis and epithelial ovarian cancer.** *Obstet Gynecol Surg 2015; 70: 587-595.*

9. **Vercillini P, Bocciolone L, Crosignani PG.** Is mild endometriosis always a disease? *Hum Reprod 1992; 7: 627-629.*

10. **EK M, Roth B, EKstrom P.** Gastrointestinal symptoms among endometriosis-A case-cohort study. *BMC Women's Health 2015; 15: 59.*

11. **Nasrat AM, Nasrat SAM, Nasrat RM, et al.** Misconception and misbehavior towards Helicobacter pylori is leading to major spread of illness. *GM 2015; S1: 002.* [Open Access]

12. **Nasrat AM, Nasrat SAM, Nasrat RM, et al.** Role of bloodlet out cupping therapy in female pelvic congestion syndrome. *Gen Med 2015;* **S1: 3.**

13. **Nasrat AM, Nasrat SAM, Nasrat RM, et al.** The biology of combined colon clear and blood-let out cupping therapy in female health. *Gen Med 2015; 3 (4): 203.*

THE SECRET OF THE SILENCE OF THE SILENT MAXILLARY SINUS SYNDROME

Introduction: Helicobacter pylori colonized the stomach since and immemorial time as both the stomach wall and the bacterium used to live together in peace harmless to each other.[1,2] As prevalence of the migrating abnormal behavior ***H. pylori*** strains due to the antibiotic violence and their existence in unusual secondary reservoirs other than the common gastric habitat is associated with local tissue pathology and symptomatic disorders; therefore, it should be of vital interest to identify the secondary reservoirs of this bacterium. The maxillary sinus is one of the common and most critical sites among the oro-nasal secondary reservoirs for ***H. pylori***.[1-3]

Maxillary sinusitis is a common finding and an important issue in dentistry and maxillofacial surgery.[4] The silent maxillary sinus syndrome or silent maxillary atelectasis is rare but serious clinical event; it is due to accumulation of profuse amounts of mucus leading to obliteration of the sinus cavity. Chronic maxillary collapse is characterized by progressive enophthalmos secondary to maxillary sinus hypoventilation.[5,6] The silent maxillary sinus syndrome presents with unilateral enophthalmos without any particular evidence of sinus pathology. The reason the sinus component of the disease remains mostly asymptomatic and is discovered only after thorough evaluation of enophthalmos is unclear.[6-8] The most effective treatment of the silent maxillary sinus syndrome is endoscopic maxillary antrostomy and reconstruction of the orbital floor.[5,7]

The chewing stick or the Arak stick (miswak) which is an organic natural green toothbrush that requires no toothpaste is obtained from the Salvadora persica (the Arak) tree. Various studies have demonstrated strong antibacterial activity of the chewing stick with immediate effect against oral and cariogenic bacteria. Further reports have emphasized significant in vitro influence of the crude chewing stick extract on the activity and growth of oral pathogens. The world health organization has suggested and encouraged the use of the chewing stick as an effective remedy for oral hygiene. The traditional reputation wisdom recommends the chewing stick for purification of the mouth.[9-12]

Dietary vinegar (acetic acid 5%) has been recently shown to be an effective and decisive measure for the clinical eradication of ***H. pylori*** with an immediate dramatic relief of patient's symptoms.[2,13-15] The complex nutritional requirements of ***H. pylori*** are achieved mainly via utilization of pyruvate. As acetate is demonstrated as an end product among the metabolic pathway of ***H. pylori*** and the activity of the pyruvate dehydrogenase complex is controlled by the rules of product inhibition and feedback regulation; this means that addition of acetic acid to the medium could compromise the energy metabolism of ***H. pylori***, or interfere with the organism's respiratory chain metabolism.[16-19] As long the matter includes interference with the energy metabolism and the respiratory chain metabolism of ***H. pylori***; an immediate lethal effect on the organism could be considered.

REFERENCES:

1. **Farinha P, Gascoyne RD.** Helicobacter pylori and MALT Lymphoma. *Gastroenterology 2005 May; 128 (6): 1579-605.*

2. **Nasrat AM. The world misconception and misbehavior towards Helicobacter pylori is leading to major spread of illness.** *The 7th Anti-Aging Medicine World Congress, Monte-Carlo, Monaco, 2009 Mar.* **Available from URL,** *www.euromedicom.com*

3. **Schein W, Meryn S. Helicobacter pylori and the mouth cavity--overview and perspectives.** *Wien Klin Wochenschr 1994; 106 (17): 547-9.*

4. **Akhlaghi F, Esmaeelinejad M, Safai P. Etiologies and treatments of odontogenic maxillary sinusitis: A systemic review.** *Iran Red Crescent Med J 2015 Dec 27; 17 (12): e25536.*

5. **Claros P, Ahmed H, Minka Ngom, et al. The silent sinus syndrome: A reconstruction of the orbital floor with Medpor implant.** *Rev Laryngol Otol Rhinol (Bord) 2015; 136 (1): 37-40.*

6. **Vnder Meer JB, Harris G, Toohill RJ, et al. The silent sinus syndrome: a case series and literature review.** *Laryngoscope 2001 Jun; 111 (6): 975-8.*

7. **Babinski D, Skorek A, Stankiewicz C. Chronic maxillary atelectasis (silent sinus syndrome). Otolaryngol Pol** *2006; 60 (6): 929-33.*

8. **Rose GE, Sandy C, Hallberg L, et al. Clinical and radiologic characteristics of the imploding antrum, or "silent sinus," syndrome. Ophthalmology** *2003 Apr; 110 (4): 811-8.*

9. **Sofrata AH, Claesson RL, Lingstrom PK, et al. Strong antibacterial effect of miswak against oral microorganisms associated with periodontitis and caries.** *J Periodontol 2008 Aug; 79 (8):1474-9.*

10. **Almas K, Al-Zed Z. The immediate antimicrobial effect of a toothbrush and miswak on cariogenic bacteria: A clinical study.** *J Complementary Dental Practice 2004 Feb 15; 5 (1).*

11. **Abdel Rahman HF, Skaug N, Francis GW, et al. In vitro antimicrobial effects of crude miswak extracts on oral pathogens.** *Saudi Dental J. 2002 Jan-Apr; 14 (1).*

12. **Dahiya P, Kamal R, Luthra RP, et al. Miswak: A periodontist's perspective.** *J Ayurveda Integr Med 2012 Oct-Dec; 3 (4): 184-87.*

13. **Nasrat AM. An alternative approach for the rising challenge of hypertensive illness via Helicobacter pylori erdication.** *The International Cardiology Symposium, Dubai, 2013 May.* **Available from URL,** *www.ics2013.com*

14. **Nasrat SAM, Nasrat AM. An alternative approach for the rising challenge of hypertensive illness via Helicobacter pylori eradication.** *J Cardiol Res 2015; 6 (1): 221-225.*

15. **Nasrat AM, Nasrat RM, Narat MM. Misconception and misbehavior towards Helicobacter pylori is leading to major spread of illness.** *Gen Med 2016; S1: (002).* **[Open Access]**

16. **Mendz GL, Hazell SL, Burns BP. Glucose utilization and lactate production by Helicobacter pylori.** *J Gen Microbiol 1993 Dec; 139 (Pt 12): 3023-8.*

17. **Mendz GL, Hazell SL, van Gorkom L. Pyruvate metabolism in Helicobacter pylori.** *Arch Microbiol. 1994; 162 (3): 187-92.*

18. **Berg JM, Tymoczko JL, Stryer L. Biochemistry.** *WH Freeman and Company. 2002; 5th Ed: 480.*

19. **Ge Z. Potential of fumarate reductase as a novel therapeutic target in Helicobacter pylori infection.** *Expert Opin Ther Targets 2002 Apr; 6 (2): 135-46.*

SCIENTIFIC EVIDENCES ON THE ETIOLOGY OFTHE SILENT MAXILLARY SINUS SYNDROME

The Secret of the Silence of the Silent Maxillary Sinus Syndrome: Published in the American Journal of Medicine and Medical Sciences 2017; 7 (6): 242-247. Nasrat et al. The secret of the silence of the silent maxillary sinus syndrome. *Am J Med Med Sci 2017; 7 (6): 242-247. [doi: 10.5923/j.ajmms.20170706.03]*

Background: Sinusitis is a disease with significant discomfort affecting health and quality of life of the patient; it is one of the most common chronic diseases involving different age groups. Diagnosis of sinusitis is clinical and the standard of choice for the detection of micro-organisms that cause sinusitis is culture of sinus drainage discharge. The etiology of chronic sinusitis is not completely known and due to the fact that there is no standard treatment for the disease, routine cultures are often made to assist empirical antibiotic prescribing therapy. As the etiology of chronic sinusitis is not clearly understood, the frequency of all causative agents of the disease must be adequately determined.[1-8]

Helicobacter pylori could migrate or get forced to migrate to the maxillary sinus under the influence of antibiotic violence leading to local tissue pathology. ***H. pylori*** was detected in the nasal and maxillary sinus tissue specimens of some patients with chronic sinusitis associated with gastric existence of ***H. pylori***. The study of ***H. pylori*** DNA extracted from patients with gastric reflux disease and chronic rhino-sinusitis emphasized prevalence of ***H. pylori*** in the oral and nasal cavities and prevalence of the same ***H. pylori*** strain genotype among the same family but whether the strain genotype of gastric ***H. pylori*** is mostly identical with that of the oro-nasal strains and whether ***H. pylori*** is leading to chronic rhino-sinusitis or its existence in the maxillary sinus is a result of rino-sinusitis remained rather indefinite for some investigators.[1-3]

Various studies have demonstrated strong antibacterial activity of the chewing stick with immediate effect against oral and cariogenic bacteria. Further reports have emphasized significant in vitro influence of the crude chewing stick extract on the activity and growth of oral pathogens.[9-12] Dietary vinegar (acetic acid 5%) has been recently shown to be an effective and decisive measure for the clinical eradication of ***H. pylori*** with an immediate dramatic relief of patient's symptoms.[2,13-19]

Objective: Demonstration of a hidden influence of the bacterium ***H. pylori*** in the pathogenesis of the silent maxillary sinus syndrome.

Design& Setting: Prospective study done in Jeddah, Saudi Arabia between October 2013 and May 2014.

Patient& Methods: Sixteen middle aged patients with resistant symptoms of recurrent maxillary sinusitis in spite of adequate medications and sinus drainage were included in the study. ***H. pylori*** DNA extraction was done for the drained sinus discharge. Patients who proved positive for existence of ***H. pylori*** in the maxillary sinus discharge were encouraged for following the traditional habit of using the chewing stick even after every small bite of food in order to interfere with the nutrition of **H. pylori** from remnants of food particles in the mouth. Inhalation of the smell of white vinegar once or twice per day and daily mouth wash with diluted white vinegar was requested from them in order to disappoint **H. pylori** from the atmosphere of its new secondary habitat in the oro-nasal cavity.

Figure 1: shows veiling of the maxillary antrum, more on the right side, of one patient before starting therapy.

Figure 2: demonstrates persistence of opacity of the maxillary sinus with faint improvement in spite of two weeks of adequate therapy.

Results: H. pylori was detected in the maxillary sinus drainage in fourteen patients. All patients showed improvement of symptoms within three days while twelve of them demonstrated disappearance of all symptoms in one week with clearance of the maxillary sinus in X-ray. Interestingly, the two patients with negative **H. pylori** detection in the sinus preferred to follow the same traditional therapy and they quit the study after improvement of their symptoms in few days.

Figure 3 shows clearance of the maxillary sinus shadow after completing one week therapy with the natural remedy.

Ethical Considerations: An informed signed consent was taken from all patients; they were made aware about safety of the natural remedies employed for them. They were free to quit the study whenever they like.

Discussion: H. pylori colonized the stomach as its main and commonest habitat since an immemorial time. **H. pylori** could migrate or get forced to migrate to the maxillary sinus under the influence of antibiotic violence.[1,2] **H. pylori** escapes from the antibiotic aggression and hides in the maxillary sinus and other secondary sites in the body as antibiotics are seldom effective against extra-gastric **H. pylori** strains.[20] The reason that the investigators miss to detect **H. pylori** in the sinus discharge in cases of chronic sinusitis should be due to the conventional practice of performing routine bacterial cultures without much attention towards the specific tests for detecting **H. pylori** like urease (CLO) test or DNA extraction.[7,8]

H. pylori survives in the stomach since unrecognized time leading the attitude of natural bacteria as if both the gastric wall and the bacterium used to live together in peace harmless to each other. The attitude of **H. pylori** in the stomach simulates the behavior of natural bacteria as supported by the observational facts of its existence since an immemorial time, having majorly harmless long history inside the stomach before the anti-**H. pylori** antibiotics, its huge biological talents of survival among the hell fire of the gastric acid, its unavoidable gastric recurrence,[1,2,15] its protective influence against low acidity-related carcinoma of the cardia of stomach and the possibility of its defensive effect towards esophageal reflux disease.[2,21-24] As long as **H. pylori** can survive in the colon; therefore, what forces this weak bacterium that can not tolerate brief immersion in a weak acid to select by its own a shelter inside the hell fire of the gastric acid unless it is a natural bacterium and is obliged for a natural biological function in the stomach. So long **H. pylori** can survive in the mouth and a brief immersion in a very weak acid is sufficient to kill it, if the matter is up to its own; why it does not choose the mouth and enjoy fun and company with millions of bacteria there!!

Maxillary sinusitis includes the cardinal signs of pathologic inflammatory sequels of the sinus such as pain, fever and bad fetor of mouth.[4] Silence of the sinus syndrome which is related to H. pylori existence should mean absence of these cardinal signs. Actually, the matter is not totally silent as there should be negligible recurrent unilateral nasal obstruction, nasal discharge and recurrent odorless faintly-brownish post-nasal discharge; it is apparently odorless and even leaves a slightly sweetish sensation in the throat due to non-change of its muco-polysaccharide component by any infective pathology. These negligible manifestations (recurrent nasal obstruction/discharge and recurrent post-nasal secretions) could be easily missed or ignored by the attention of patients, even their physicians could miss that these symptoms could overlie a serious sequel.

The reason that **H. pylori** can reside in the maxillary sinus in silence without causing remarkable pathologic signs is the observational finding that it is not essentially pathologic by its own; a normal-behavior **H. pylori** is only recognized by the gastric wall, it is mostly peaceful and useful to the stomach protecting it via ammonia production from the gastric acid if it goes in excess. Migration of *H. pylori* to extra-gastric sites will render it a foreign structure to the tissues that may lead to local tissue pathology or inflammatory reaction.[1,2,15] *H. pylori* in the sinus would continue to be sheltered with ammonia in its immediate vicinity; this ammonia per se is a stimulus for mucus secretion; therefore, existence of *H. pylori* in the maxillary sinus will cause continued stimulation of mucus production until obliteration and collapse of the sinus cavity happens in silence. For the same reason that *H. pylori* is essentially a natural bacterium and non- pathogenic in nature, the mucus produced in the sinus is not infective, hence; it is odorless and is not associated with fever or other constitutional symptoms of sinusitis such as pain, a matter that explains the silent consequence of the sinus syndrome.

Concerning criteria of inclusion of patients, the patients were selected in this study so that their symptoms were limited to recurrent negligible unilateral nasal obstruction which lasts for short periods or few time of the day and post-nasal discharge which did never smell bad. Patients experienced also un-explained occasional recurrent bronchial irritation with smooth or sticky bronchial secretions and transient chocking sensation which usually lasts for few time. The recurrent sensation of light-headedness or as expressed by some patents 'heaviness of the head' and the increased desire to sleep or desire to go back to sleep after short time from waking up were considered part of the constitutional symptoms of the sinus disease. Accordingly, easy fatigue was found constant in those patients; it was attributed to loss of the physiologic nature and function of the sinus or to the original upsets in the colon. These symptoms were persistent in all patients in spite of adequate or aggressive medications and all of them had got used to their symptoms, even some of their physicians considered these symptoms negligible and re-assured the patients that they can survive with these negligible residual symptoms. Those patients were selected in this study in purpose according to this particular clinical history as those patients are the candidates who are possibly expected to proceed and progress into silent collapse of the maxillary sinus.

A smart questionnaire had been raised by an elegant research study as concerns the undesired sequels of existence of oral *H. pylori* strains, a question that still remained without answer by the researcher; "oral *H. pylori*, is it possible to stomach it again!!"[25] That was exactly the actual purpose of this study; *H. pylori* as all living structures needs nutrition, in the stomach it feeds on remnants of food in gastric lumen, when it resides in the maxillary sinus, it must pick up remnants of food particles from the mouth and it escapes back to the sinus,[1,2] this could account for the recurrent irritant bronchial secretions due to spreading of ammonia related to the immediate vicinity of the bacterium while roaming in the mouth. Therefore, this study intended to interfere with nourishment of maxillary sinus *H. pylori* strains via continuous purification of the mouth by using the strong antiseptic chewing stick after any food. In addition, *H. pylori* was also repeatedly rendered disappointed towards the atmosphere of the mouth by inhaling the smell of vinegar and by the mouth wash with diluted vinegar. The expected outcome is that the maxillary sinus would become no longer a favorite shelter for *H. pylori* anymore; this is consistent with the results of this study.[9-12] Hence; the main purpose of employing the chewing stick (miswak) is to ensure purification of the mouth in order to disappoint the bacterium but not elimination of all remnants of food particles from the mouth. In this regard, cleaning the teeth with the stick before meals is as useful as purification of the mouth with the stick after food-intake in case of severe symptoms. Brushing the teeth with the chewing stick at bed times even the tooth paste and brush are being used should be therefore integral.

The principle of employing vinegar in this study was supported by the results of previous literature which reported that a brief exposure to high dilutions of acetic acid (0.03%) is sufficient to suffocate *H. pylori*. It has been also demonstrated that 20 times dilution of acetic acid 6% has got an immediate lethal influence on *H. pylori* culture media;[14,26-29] an intense fast effect that explains why the mere smell of vinegar could be disappointing and terrifying to *H. pylori*. The smell of vinegar is strong and was found in this study directly related to relief of nasal obstruction; whether the relief of nasal symptoms related to the smell of vinegar is due to local physical effect or metabolic influence on *H. pylori* still needs further assessment.

Those disadvantaged patients who developed ***H. pylori***-related maxillary sinusitis should learn that they are liable for recurrences whenever they neglect their colonic condition or mouth hygiene; that is no big matter, all what they do need is referring to colon care/colon clear and returning strictly to oral hygiene care with the chewing stick and white vinegar.[14,15,30]

Persistent sinusitis with recurrent unilateral nasal obstruction and discharge, morning and wake-up brownish odorless post-nasal discharge, recurrent un-explained irritant cough upon having few bites of food that stops with smelling the vinegar or washing the mouth with diluted white vinegar and the recurrent development of sticky bronchial secretions that turn soft easily- producible in brief time upon using the chewing stick are sufficient symptomatic predictors in a person for the possibility of developing silent collapse of the maxillary sinus. ***H. pylori*** DNA detection in the post-nasal discharge for those patients should be a new health care predictor to break the silence in developing a sinus syndrome.

Conclusion: Migration and escape of ***H. pylori*** inside the maxillary sinus hiding from the antibiotic violence towards it could be a definite reason for maxillary sinusitis to creep in silence into obliteration and collapse of the sinus. The world conceptions, medical attitudes and aggressive antibiotic behaviors towards ***H. pylori*** might be in need of serious revision and accurate re-determination. Regular mouth hygiene should be the integral shield to protect from developing silent collapse of the maxillary sinus in association with existing abnormal-behavior oral ***H. pylori*** strains. Improvement of the symptoms of chronic sinusitis upon inhaling the smell of vinegar could be an indication for a new health care predictor to screen patients with persistent nasal discharge and recurrent bronchial secretions for ***H. pylori*** DNA detection for the purpose of employing natural measures suggested in this study in order to protect from development of maxillary sinusitis syndrome in silence.

Acknowledgement: The study appreciates the facilities and time allowed by Balghsoon Clinics in Jeddah/ Saudi Arabia. The continuous support offered by Abdul-Aziz Al-Sorayai Investment Company (ASIC) in Jeddah/ Saudi Arabia, the scientific and emotional support of Dr Ahmed S. Balghsoon and the true brotherhood friendly encouragement of Mr. Abdul-Aziz Al-Sorayai are extremely valued and appreciated.

Conflict of Interest: No conflict of interest exists.

REFERENCES:

1. **Farinha P, Gascoyne RD.** Helicobacter pylori and MALT Lymphoma. *Gastroenterology 2005 May; 128 (6): 1579-605.*

2. **Nasrat AM. The world misconception and misbehavior towards Helicobacter pylori is leading to major spread of illness.** *The 7th Anti-Aging Medicine World Congress, Monte-Carlo, Monaco, 2009 Mar.* **Available from URL,** *www.euromedicom.com*

3. **Schein W, Meryn S. Helicobacter pylori and the mouth cavity--overview and perspectives.** *Wien Klin Wochenschr 1994; 106 (17): 547-9.*

4. **Akhlaghi F, Esmaeelinejad M, Safai P. Etiologies and treatments of odontogenic maxillary sinusitis: A systemic review.** *Iran Red Crescent Med J 2015 Dec 27; 17 (12): e25536.*

5. **Claros P, Ahmed H, Minka Ngom, et al. The silent sinus syndrome: A reconstruction of the orbital floor with Medpor implant.** *Rev Laryngol Otol Rhinol (Bord) 2015; 136 (1): 37-40.*

6. **Vnder Meer JB, Harris G, Toohill RJ, et al. The silent sinus syndrome: a case series and literature review.** *Laryngoscope 2001 Jun; 111 (6): 975-8.*

7. **Babinski D, Skorek A, Stankiewicz C. Chronic maxillary atelectasis (silent sinus syndrome).** *Otolaryngol Pol 2006; 60 (6): 929-33.*

8. **Rose GE, Sandy C, Hallberg L, et al. Clinical and radiologic characteristics of the imploding antrum, or "silent sinus," syndrome. Ophthalmology** *2003 Apr; 110 (4): 811-8.*

9. **Sofrata AH, Claesson RL, Lingstrom PK, et al. Strong antibacterial effect of miswak against oral microorganisms associated with periodontitis and caries.** *J Periodontol 2008 Aug; 79 (8):1474-9.*

10. **Almas K, Al-Zed Z. The immediate antimicrobial effect of a toothbrush and miswak on cariogenic bacteria: A clinical study.** *J Complementary Dental Practice 2004 Feb 15; 5 (1).*

11. **Abdel Rahman HF, Skaug N, Francis GW, et al. In vitro antimicrobial effects of crude miswak extracts on oral pathogens.** *Saudi Dental J. 2002 Jan-Apr; 14 (1).*

12. **Dahiya P, Kamal R, Luthra RP, et al. Miswak: A periodontist's perspective.** *J Ayurveda Integr Med 2012 Oct-Dec; 3 (4): 184-87.*

13. **Nasrat AM. An alternative approach for the rising challenge of hypertensive illness via Helicobacter pylori erdication.** *The International Cardiology Symposium, Dubai, 2013 May.* **Available from URL,** *www.ics2013.com*

14. **Nasrat SAM, Nasrat AM. An alternative approach for the rising challenge of hypertensive illness via Helicobacter pylori eradication.** *J Cardiol Res 2015; 6 (1): 221-225.*

15. **Nasrat AM, Nasrat RM, Narat MM. Misconception and misbehavior towards Helicobacter pylori is leading to major spread of illness.** *Gen Med 2016; S1: 002.* **[Open Access]**

16. **Mendz GL, Hazell SL, Burns BP. Glucose utilization and lactate production by Helicobacter pylori.** *J Gen Microbiol 1993 Dec; 139 (Pt 12): 3023-8.*

17. **Mendz GL, Hazell SL, van Gorkom L. Pyruvate metabolism in Helicobacter pylori.** *Arch Microbiol. 1994; 162 (3):187-92.*

18. **Berg JM, Tymoczko JL, Stryer L. Biochemistry.** *WH Freeman and Company. 2002; 5th Ed: 480.*

19. **Ge Z. Potential of fumarate reductase as a novel therapeutic target in Helicobacter pylori infection.** *Expert Opin Ther Targets 2002 Apr; 6 (2): 135-46.*

20. **Grünberger B, Wöhrer S, Streubel B, et al. Antibiotic treatment is not effective in patients infected with Helicobacter pylori suffering from extragastric MALT lymphoma.** *J Clin Oncol 2006 Mar 20; 24 (9):1370-5.*

21. **Issing WJ. Gastroesophageal reflux – a common illness.** *Laryngorhinootologie 2003 Feb; 82 (2): 118-22.*

22. **Labenz J, Blum AL, Bayerdorffer E, et al. Curing Helicobacter pylori infection in patients with duodenal ulcer may provoke reflux esophagitis.** *Gastroenterology 1997; 112: 1442: 47.*

23. **Sharma P, Vakil N, Review article: Helicobacter pylori and reflux disease.** *Aliment Pharmacol Ther 2003 Feb; 17 (3): 297-305.*

24. **Vakil N. Gastroesophageal reflux disease and Helicobacter pylori infection.** *Rev Gastroenterol Disord 2003 winter; 3 (1):1-7*

25. **Dowsett SA, Kowolik MJ. Oral Helicobacter pylori: can we stomach it?** *Crit Oral Biol Med 2003; 14 (3): 226-33.*

26. **Midolo PD, Lambert JR, Hull R, et al. In vitro inhibition of Helicobacter pylori NCTC 11637 by organic acids and lactic acid bacteria.** *J Appl Bacteriol. 1995 Oct; 79 (4); 475-9.*

27. **Makino SI, Cheun HI, Tabuchi H, et al. Antibacterial activity of chaff vinegar and its practical application.** *J Vet Med Sci. 2000 Aug; 62 (8):893-5.*

28. **Debevere J, Devlieghere F, van Sprundel P, et al. Influence of acetate and CO2 on the TMAO – reduction reaction by Shewanella baltica.** *Int J Food Microbiol 2001 Aug 15; 68 (1-2):115-23.*

29. **Nsarat RM, Nasrat MM, Nasrat AM, et al. Improvement of idiopatic cardiomyopathy after colon clear.** *J Cardiol Res 2015 Apr; 6 (2): 249-254.*

30. **Nasrat AM, Nasrat SAM, Narat RM, et al. Characteristics of Helicobacter pylori-related dysglycemia.** *Gen Med 2015; S1: 004.* **[Open Access]**

AUTISM; AN APPROACH FOR DEFINITE ETIOLOGY ANDDEFINITIVE ETIOLOGIC MANAGEMENT

Autism Might Not be a Disease of Definitive Cure but it is a Typical Disease of Definite Prevention

Introduction: Autism is a brain disorder that limits a person's ability to communicate, correlate and relate to other people. It is a series of neuro-developmental disorders that are characterized by deficits in both social and cognitive functions.[1] It first appears in young children, who fall along a spectrum from mild to severe presentation. Some people can navigate their life; some have exceptional abilities, while others struggle to speak. Autism spectrum disorders (ASD) affect about one child in 68, striking nearly five times as many boys as girls.[2,3] It was concluded that genetic and environmental factors are both responsible for the etiology of ASD. Although epidemiological studies have been conducted to clarify these factors but this conclusion remains unclear.[4,5]

Before turning three, careful observers can discover development of signs of autism in a child. Some children develop normally until 18-24 months of age and then they stop or loose previously acquired skills. Signs of development of ASD could include repeated motions (rocking or spinning), avoiding eye contact or physical touch, delay in learning to talk, repeating words or phrases and getting upset by minor changes.[5,6] _

Young infants are very social even in the first year of age therefore; it is possible to detect early signs of autism as early as how babies interact with their world. At this age, a child with an ASD may not turn to a mother's voice, respond to his own name, look people in the eye, have no babbling or pointing and no smiling or responding to social cues from others.[7-9] _

The signs of autism are more noticeable in a child's second year., other children are forming their first words and pointing to things they want, a child with autism remains detached showing no single words at age of 16 months, no pretend games at age of 18 months, no two-word phrases at age of 2 years, loss of language skills, no interest when adults point out objects, such as a plane flying overhead.[6,7] _

Children with autism may sometimes have physical symptoms including digestive troubles such as constipation and sleep problems. Children may have poor coordination of the large muscles used for running and climbing or the smaller muscles of the hand. Children with autism could also have seizures.[4,10] _

It was long believed that autism affects only those regions of the brain that control social interaction, communication and reasoning; instead it is suggested that the disorder in autism affects the entire brain. It was found that even highly functioning autistic children are having difficulty when asked to perform a wide range of complex tasks involving other areas of the brain. It was suggested that different parts of the autistic brain have difficulty working together to process complex information; this may be the driving component of autism.[11-17] These findings could indicate that a further understanding of autism will not likely come from the study of factors affecting one brain area or system but from the study of factors affecting many systems of the brain. The earlier diagnostic assessment of autism in children and adults was based on three main behaviors; they typically have problems with social interactions, verbal and nonverbal communications. They tend to exhibit repetitive behaviors or narrow, obsessive interests. It is increasingly clear that other areas of brain function are affected as well, including balance, movement and memory.[18-25]

It was reported that autistic adults are having difficulty performing certain complex tasks that involve different areas of the brain working together; this could offer further evidence to support the whole-brain hypothesis in autism. In an effort to confirm the findings of autism, highly-functioning autistic children were compared to non-autistic children with similar IQ, ages and all could speak, read and write. It was found that autistic children did as well as or even better than non-autistic children when asked to perform basic tasks but they scored much less when asked to perform complex tasks.[16,18,22,25] The better the understanding about autism and the brain, the better effective and efficient therapy could be designed. Accordingly, the whole-brain disorder hypothesis in autism could allow new treatment approach for fundamental cure of autism particularly with sufficient opportunity for cognitive growth and development rehabilitation are allowed.

A permanent pathologic sequels involving different areas of the brain which have possibly influenced brain development early during fetal life have been demonstrated by different reports such as specific alterations in white matter structural property.[26,27] Abnormalities of specific components of grey matter structure in early brain growth patterns of autistic children have been reported by some investigators. Children with more autistic traits showed widespread areas of decreased gyrification.[14,15] White matter impairment, dysplasia with abnormal cortical thinning or decreased cortical thickness have been identified among children with autism.[22-24,26]

Most investigators were successful to come in agreement that various gastro-intestinal (GI) factors may contribute to behavior in children with autism,[1,4] but they mostly missed to successfully achieve the real pathology behind these GI factors in contribution to autistic behavior. The last three decades have demonstrated prevalence of abnormal-behavior ***Helicobacter pylori*** strains and the flare up of a lot of medical challenges related to these ***H. pylori*** strains via inflammatory, toxic, immune or different unknown reasons to the extent that the medical world has believed that ***H. pylori*** eradication should be a necessary attempt.[28,29] Accordingly, a research motive for this study has developed with purpose to investigate for a possible correlation or contribution of ***H. pylori*** dyspepsia in leading to ASD among disadvantaged children.

REFERENCES:

1. **Li Q, Zhou JM.** The microbiota-gut-brain axis and its potential therapeutic role in autism spectrum disorder. *Neuroscience 2016 Jun 2; 324: 131-9.*

2. **Woolfenden S, Eapen V, Jalaludin B, et al. Prevalence and factors associated with parental concerns about development detected by the Parents' Evaluation of Developmental Status (PEDS) at 6-month, 12-month and 18-month well-child checks in a birth cohort.** *BMJ 2016 Sep 8; 6 (9): e012144.*

3. **Baio J. Prevalence of autism spectrum disorders - Autism and Developmental Disabilities Monitoring Network, United States, 2006.** *MMWR Surveill Summ 2009 Dec 18; 58 (10): 1-20.*

4. **Galichi F, Ghaemmaghami J, Malek A, et al. Effect of gluten free diet on gastrointestinal and behavioral indices for children with autism spectrum disorders: a randomized clinical trial.** *World J Pediatr 2016 Jun 10; 26 (12): 1936-9. [Epub ahead of print]*

5. **Kiely B, Vettam S, Adesman A. Utilization of genetic testing among children with developmental disabilities in the United States.** *Appl Clin Genet 2016 Jul 11; 9: 93-100. eCollection 2016.*

6. **Allen DA. Autistic spectrum disorders: clinical presentation in preschool children.** *J Child Neurol 1988; 3 Suppl: S48-56.*

7. **Emberti Gialloreti L, Benvenuto A, Battan B, et al. Can biological components predict short-term evolution in Autism Spectrum Disorders? A proof-of-concept study.** *Ital J Pediatr 2016 Jul 22; 42 (1): 70.*

8. **Spjut Jansson B, Miniscalco C, Westerlund J, et al. Children who screen positive for autism at 2.5 years and receive early intervention: a prospective naturalistic 2-year outcome study.** *Neuropsychiatr Dis Treat 2016 Sep 1; 12: 2255-63. eCollection 2016.*

9. **Locke J, Williams J, Shih W, et al. Characteristics of socially successful elementary school-aged children with autism.** *J Child Psychol Psychiatry 2016 Sep 13. doi: 10.1111/jcpp.12636. [Epub ahead of print]*

10. **Schwichtenberg AJ, Hensle T, Honaker S, et al. Sibling sleep-What can it tell us about parental sleep reports in the context of autism?** *Clin Pract Pediatr Psychol 2016 Jun; 4 (2): 137-152.*

11. **Donovan AP, Basson MA. The neuroanatomy of autism - a developmental perspective.** *J Anat 2016 Sep 12. Doi: 10.1111/joa. 12542. [Epub ahead of print]*

12. **Benitez-Burraco A, Lattanzi W, Murphy E. Language Impairments in ASD Resulting from a Failed Domestication of the Human Brain.** *Front Neurosci 2016 Aug 29; 10: 373. eCollection 2016.*

13. **Grecucci A, Rubicondo D, Siugzdaite R, et al. Uncovering the Social Deficits in the Autistic Brain. A Source-Based Morphometric Study.** *Front Neurosci 2016 Aug 31; 10: 388. eCollection 2016.*

14. **Richter J, Henze R, Vomstein K, et al. Reduced cortical thickness and its association with social reactivity in children with autismspectrum disorder.** *Psychiatry Res 2015 Oct 30; 234 (1): 15-24. Epub 2015 Aug 22.*

15. **Blanken LM, Mous SE, Ghassabian A, et al. Cortical morphology in 6- to 10-year old children with autistic traits: a population-based neuroimaging study.** *Am J Psychiatry 2015 May; 172 (5): 479-86. Epub 2015 Jan 13.*

16. **Blatt GJ, Fatemi SH. Alterations in GABAergic biomarkers in the autism brain: research findings and clinical implications.** *Anat Rec (Hoboken) 2011 Oct; 294 (10): 1646-52. Epub 2011 Sep 8.*

17. **Jou RJ, Mateljevic N, Kaisern MD, et al. Structural neural phenotype of autism: preliminary evidence from a diffusion tensor imaging study using tract-based spatial statistics.** *AJNR Am J Neuroradiol 2011 Oct; 32 (9): 1607-13. Epub 2011 Jul 28.*

18. **Jaber M. The cerebellum as a major player in motor disturbances related to Autistic Syndrome Disorders.** *Encephale 2016 Sep 8. doi: 10.1016/1. encep.2016.03.018. [Epub ahead of print]*

19. **Sperdin HF, Schaer M. Aberrant Development of Speech Processing in Young Children with Autism: New Insights from Neuroimaging Biomarkers.** *Front Neurosci 2016 Aug 25; 10: 393. eCollection 2016.*

20. **Happe F, Conway JR. Recent progress in understanding skills and impairments in social cognition.** *Curr Opin Pediatr 2016 Sep 6. [Epub ahead of print]*

21. **Dinan TG, Cryan JF. Gut Instincts: microbiota as a key regulator of brain development, ageing and neurodegeneration.** *J Physiol 2016 Sep 19. Doi: 10.1113/JP273106. [Epub ahead of print]*

22. **Peeva MG, Tourville JA, Agam Y, et al. White matter impairment in the speech network of individuals with autism spectrum disorder.** *Neuroimage 2013 Aug 28; 3: 234-41. eCollection 2013.*

23. **Casanova MF, El-Baz AS, Kamat SS, et al. Focal cortical dysplasias in autism spectrum disorders.** *Acta Neuropathol Commun 2013 Oct 11; 1: 67. Doi: 10.1186/2051.5960.1.67.*

24. **Misaki M, Wallace GL, Dankner N, et al. Characteristic cortical thickness patterns in adolescents with autism spectrum disorders: interactions with age and intellectual ability revealed by canonical correlation analysis.** *Neuroimage 2012 Apr 15; 60 (3): 1890-901. Epub 2012 Feb 3.*

25. **Randolph-Gips M, Srinivasan P. Modeling autism: a systems biology approach.** *J Clin Bioinforma 2012 Oct 8; 2 (1): 17. Doi: 10.1186/2043.9113.2.17.*

26. **Chiang HL, Chen YJ, Lin HY, et al. Disorder-Specific Alteration in White Matter Structural Property in Adults With Autism Spectrum Disorder Relative to Adults with a DHD and Adult Controls.** *Hum Brain Mapp 2016 Sep 15y. doi: 10.1002/hbm.23367. [Epub ahead of print]*

27. **Chang J, Gilman SR, Chiang AH, et al. Genotype to phenotype relationships in autism spectrum disorders.** *Nat Neurosci 2015 Feb; 18 (2): 191-8. Epub 2014 Dec 22.*

28. **Farinha P, Gascoyne RD. Helicobacter pylori and MALT Lymphoma.** *Gastroenterology 2005 May; 128 (6): 1579-605.*

29. **Nasrat AM, Nasrat SAM, Nasrat RM, et al. Misconception and misbehavior towards Helicobacter pylori is leading to major spread of illness.** *Gen Med 2015; S1: 002.* **[Open Access]**

SCIENTIFIC EVIDENCES ON THE DEFINITE ETIOLOGY AND DEFINITIVE ETIOLOGIC MANAGEMENT OF AUTISM

Autism; An Approach for Definite Etiology and Definitive Etiologic Management: Published in the American Journal of Medicine and Medical Sciences; 2017; 7 (5): 108-118. Nasrat et al. Autism; an approach for definite etiology and definitive etiologic management. Am J Med Med Sci 2017; 7 (5): 108-118. *[doi: 10.5923/j.ajmms.20170703.04]*

Background: Autism constitutes a challenging unsolved puzzle affecting disadvantaged children at early age where they grow normal until age of 18-24 months then they begin failure to develop some skills or loose already developed skills. The exact etiology of the condition remains unclear while all promises of complete cure are unsuccessful.[1-10]

Young infants are very social even in the first year of age therefore; it is possible to detect early signs of autism as early as how babies interact with their world. Children with autism may sometimes have physical symptoms including digestive troubles such as constipation and sleep problems.[4,11-17]

It was long believed that autism affects only those regions of the brain that control social interaction, communication and reasoning; instead it is suggested that the disorder in autism affects the entire brain. It was found that even highly functioning autistic children are having difficulty when asked to perform a wide range of complex tasks involving other areas of the brain.[3,18-25]

The association of gastro-intestinal (GI) troubles with autism is frank and the importance of early life gut microbiota in shaping future health was always considered. Disturbances of the structure of microbiota by chronic antibiotic exposure could affect physiology and behavior; therefore, strategies of probiotic supplements were suggested to improve GI symptoms and brain functions in autism.[7,22-27]

Helicobacter pylori was suggested as one of the environmental reasons that could be directly related to many medical challenges. ***H. pylori*** could get forced to migrate to the colon under the influence of antibiotic violence leading to accumulation of excess amounts of ammonia. The accumulated ***H. pylori***-produced ammonia conforms to the observation of elevated serum ammonia among autistic children and its toxic effect with the hypothesis of the entire brain compromise suggested to explain inability of autistic children to perform complex interactions. Ammonia could trigger its toxic effect early on fetal brain due to elevated serum ammonia of ***H. pylori***-dyspeptic pregnant ladies. Interestingly, kids develop the abnormal colonic ***H. pylori*** strains trans-familial at an early age which is the typical timing where children start to develop autistic features or loose already developed skills.[1,4,28,29]

Objective: Demonstration of a possible relationship between ***H. pylori*** and the GI symptoms associated with autism in leading to an impact on the entire brain with purpose to find out an etiologic pathology and definite cure.

Design& Setting: A multiple-case clinical study which was done in Jeddah/Saudi Arabia during the period May 2014 to October 2015. The protocol of the study was approved and the study followed the research committee ethics.

Patients& Methods: The study started with 25 patients while only 19 continued the follow up as most parents of autistic children had lost confidence in possibility of cure. Autistic patients are not identical in symptomatology as they markedly vary in type, grade of symptoms and susceptibility for developing the disease. Hence; the study included 19 autistic children with variable symptoms and different grades of the disease. They were 16 boys and 3 girls, their age ranged between 11 months and 6 years with an average age of 36 months. The study included one boy 2 years old who was seen at a very early onset of the disease; few days of losing the developed skills and included an 11 months girl with typical autistic features but atypical early age of developing autism.

Existence of ***H. pylori*** in the colon was tested for children and parents by employing specific test (***H. pylori*** fecal antigen test).[28,29] Serum ammonia level was tested for all children. ***H. pylori*** fecal antigen test was obtained from Acon Laboratory, USA.

Natural ***H. pylori*** eradication from the colon was done employing the senna leaves purge and intake of vinegar-mixed salad once or twice daily for children and parents.[29]

Results: All children and parents were found positive for colonic ***H. pylori*** strains; they became free of ***H. pylori*** strains in the colon after the natural therapy as confirmed by ***H. pylori*** fecal antigen test and serum ammonia was found elevated in all children. The level of serum ammonia was found ranging between 99-113 umol/L except the boy with newly-discovered onset of the disease who has got a serum ammonia level of 351 umol/L and the eleven-months girl who has got a serum ammonia level of 279 umol/L. The normal reference of ammonia level of this study was 18-72 umol/L for all ages.

All children showed different grades of improvement but none of them was cured after six month of therapy and further six months of follow up except the child seen at a very early onset of the disease who recovered completely. The eleven-momths girl who developed autistic features at early age (7 months) was suggested to develop drastic ***H. pylori*** strains from her mother; therefore, ***H. pylori*** DNA extraction in the stool was done for the girl and parents. This girl also markedly improved but was not completely cured.

Revision of previous records of serum ammonia done one year earlier to this study for a group of 16 non-autistic children studied for their low IQ scores who were free of abdominal symptoms and colonic ***H. pylori*** strains, serum ammonia level was found ranging between 49-57 umol/L. Further revision of the records of a group of 21 children with 2-5 years autistic history who were positive for colonic ***H. pylori*** strains with an age range of 4-7 years studied during the same period of this study in order to demonstrate the effect of the senna purge in clearance of the elevated serum ammonia. Their serum ammonia level ranged between 90-107 umol/L. Colon clear was done for them and the serum ammonia level dropped on next 2 days to a range of 32-41 umol/L.

Ethical Considerations: An informed signed consent was taken from all parents; children were allowed to lead their routine style of life except strict follow up of dietary instruction of colon care and extreme restriction of outside-home food intake. Parents were free to make their children quit the study at any time whenever they feel inconvenience towards the natural therapy or strategy of the study.

Discussion: Although various reports in literature refer with great concern to the role played by ***H. pylori*** in disease pathology,[28,29] research studies seldom indicated directly to the possibility that ***H. pylori*** could be behind the pathogenesis of Autism. Recent clinical studies have revealed a high prevalence of GI symptoms such as inflammation and dysfunction in children with autism. Mild to moderate degrees of inflammation were found in both the upper and lower intestinal tract and decreased digestive enzyme activities were reported in many autistic children. Treatment of digestive problems appeared to have positive effects on autistic behavior; these new observations represent only a piece of the unsolved puzzle "autism" and should stimulate more researches into the brain-gut connection.[30]

As Autism spectrum disorders (ASD) is often associated with different GI disturbances which may also impact behavior; therefore, alterations in autonomic nervous system functions should be also expected frequently in ASD. The relationship between these findings in autism is not clearly known. It was suggested that autonomic functions and GI problems are intertwined in children with ASD.[31] Although the exact etiology and pathology of ASD remain unclear, a disorder of the microbiota-gut-brain axis is emerging as a prominent factor in the generation of autistic behavioral disorders. Different clinical studies have shown that GI symptoms and compositional changes in gut microbiota frequently accompany cerebral disorders in patients with ASD. A disturbance in the gut microbiota which is usually induced by a bacterial infection or chronic antibiotic exposure has been implicated as a potential contributor to ASD. The bi-directional microbiota-gut-brain axis was suggested to be acting mainly through neuro-endocrine, neuro-immune, and autonomic nervous mechanisms. It was reported that application of modulators of the microbiota-gut-brain axis such as probiotics and certain special diets may be a promising strategy for the treatment of ASD. Different observations of disruption of the microbiota-gut-brain axis as concerns the pathogenesis of ASD has therefore suggested its potential therapeutic role in autistic deficits.[1]

A gut to brain interaction in ASD and the role of probiotics on clinical, biochemical and neuro-physiological parameters in autistic individuals have been emphasized and confirmed in further reports. It was adequately reported that the high prevalence of the frequent GI disturbances in patients with autism might be linked to gut dysbiosis representing a phenotype of a "gut-brain axis" disruption. Employment of strategies that can restore normal gut microbiota and reduce the gut production and absorption of toxins such as probiotic supplements in diet may represent a non-pharmacological option in the treatment of GI disturbances in ASD. The effect of probiotic supplements in autistic children is not only specific on GI symptoms but also to improve the core deficits of the brain disorder, cognitive and language development, brain function and connectivity.[32] It was further reported that specific assessment of gut functions including the microbiome would be necessary to evaluate the contribution of gut physiology to functional constipation observed in autistic children.[33] As much as GI symptoms were frequently reported among autistic children; an impact of GI co-morbidity on ASD behavioral problems has been hypothesized. 'Constipated' and 'Not-Eat' were described as the most frequent GI symptoms in autistic individuals.[34] Alteration in intestinal function which was often referred to as a "leaky gut" due to mucosal inflammation has been attributed to children who are on the autism spectrum; this particular symptom was even put into consideration to identify children with autism who have atypical symptoms.[35]

The concept of gut-brain axis, its regulation by the microbiota and its role in the biological and physiological basis of neuro-developmental and neuro-degenerative disorders could constitute a considerable role in the pathogenesis of autism. The importance of early life gut microbiota in shaping future health outcomes should be also considered. Disturbances of this composition by way of antibiotic exposure can result in long-term effects on physiology and behavior.[21,36] *H. pylori* in the stomach is leading the behavior of natural bacteria as it does not exist in the gastric lumen during presence of food and it remains settling juxta-mucosal under the mucus layer of gastric mucosa with the ammonia at its immediate vicinity functioning to protect the gastric wall from its acid if it goes in excess.[28,29] Therefore; the antibiotic violence towards *H. pylori* forcing it to migrate to the colon could definitely disturb its natural microbiotic function with its sequels on human body physiology.

The routes of communication between the microbiota and brain are being unraveled and could include the microbial metabolites such as ammonia.[21,28] As *H. pylori* could migrate or get forced to migrate to the colon under the influence of antibiotics, it will continue producing ammonia for a reason or no reason, unopposed or buffered by any acidity, leading to accumulation of profuse toxic amounts of ammonia. Colonic *H. pylori* strains in their abnormal colonic habitat could lead to adverse toxic effects in the body; certainly the delicate physical structure of a child during early growth could be also severely affected by these aggressive drastic strains and the delicate integrity of the child's growing brain could be further in susceptible children a fragile target to the toxic influence of colonic ammonia.[28,29,37,38]

The hypothesis of the entire brain involvement in autism was designed on the basis of impairment of the histology of whole areas of the brain in order to explain inability of autistic children to perform complex tasks.[11,13-17,21-23] In spite of the finding that many investigators have demonstrated rise of serum ammonia level among autistic children, they missed to indicate the possibility that elevated levels of serum ammonia could influence the entire functions of the whole brain.[39-49] Serum level of ammonia was also found elevated among all children in this study.

H. pylori colonized the stomach since an immemorial time as if both the stomach and the bacterium used to live together in peace harmless to each other and hence *H. pylori* has been considered by some investigators a natural bacterium.[28,29] *H. pylori* when forced to migrate to the colon, mainly under the influence of antibiotic violence, will lead to different dyspeptic symptoms and accumulation of profuse amounts of ammonia in the colon with consequent elevated levels of serum ammonia.[28,29,50,51] It is common that ladies develop dyspepsia during pregnancy; abnormal *H. pylori* strains are responsible for most cases of functional dyspepsia, but it is rarely recognized that this dyspepsia is *H. pylori*-related.[52] Accordingly; serum ammonia would be elevated in both maternal blood of those dyspeptic pregnant ladies and in the fetal blood in turn with the possibility of a toxic influence of ammonia on the delicate structure of the developing fetal brain leading also to sensitization of the fetal brain during early embryonic life to the adverse effect of ammonia. It has been reported that the neuropathology of autism starts early during embryonic life due to heterogeneity.[11,27,53] The sustained elevated ammonia level in fetal blood caused by the colonic *H. pylori* strains of dyspeptic pregnant mothers could constitute a trigger of a causative pathology for neuro-development of autistic disorders confirming accordingly with the suggestion that both environmental and genetic factors are responsible for the etiology of autism.[4,5]

The suggestion that the elevated residual ammonia serum level in fetal blood plays an early causative pathogenic factor in leading to the autistic neuro-developmental disorders since embryonic life is supported by an observational finding in this study expressed by mothers of 7 autistic children during their delivery. The mothers confirmed a frank history of *H. pylori*-related dyspepsia during their pregnancy which had been confirmed by specific laboratory tests, they were just able to follow gastric sedatives. They were astonished that their babies did not cry immediately after delivery and suction of their secretions in spite of their good general condition. Those mothers continued to have *H. pylori* dyspepsia after delivery because of a contraindication for eradication therapy or failure of therapies as antibiotics are seldom effective against extra-gastric *H. pylori* strains.[28,29,54] Later, their kids developed autism between the age of 2-3 years.

Existence of *H. pylori* in children occurs trans-familial via food at an early age; this matter is confirmed by the fact that *H. pylori* strain of children is often identical with that of their parents. Interestingly, children maintain the same strain genotype life-long even after moving to a different environment unless eradicated. *H. pylori* travels between parents via oral to oral route while transmission to kids occurs via meals.[37,38] The kids develop the abnormal-behavior colonic *H. pylori* strains at the time of their weaning when they start to share the dining table with their parents; that is typically the critical timing where children begin to develop autistic features or loose already developed skills.[5,6,28,29]

Migration of *H. pylori* to the colon occurs mainly under the influence of antibiotic exposure. Existence of *H. pylori* in the colon is typically life-long unless eradicated as antibiotics are seldom effective against extra-gastric *H. pylori* strains and no available measure has been proved to effectively eradicate *H. pylori* from the colon except the senna purge.[28,29,54-56] Accordingly; pregnant ladies who develop abnormal colonic *H. pylori* strains via an outside-home query meals would mostly remain dyspeptic and would become later in most instances the mothers of autistic children due to recurrence of a causative pathology which has triggered its effect during pregnancy and made the fetal brain already sensitive to the toxicity of ammonia earlier throughout the embryonic life.

As concerns revision of literature knowledge regarding existence of *H. pylori* in children, It is now recognized that *H. pylori* like most enteric infections is mainly acquired during childhood. The age at which children are most likely to become infected is still unclear but findings in a number of cross-sectional studies suggested that infection is acquired before the age of five.[57] Other studies suggested an earlier age before two years via trans-familial transmission from parents which is the time of weaning and it is at the same time the typical timing of developing autism.[28,58] Existence of *H. pylori* in children is community-related (less in developed and more in developing countries) and it has got a clear age-related prevalence; that is increasing with age.[59] All figures differ with life style changes, dependency on fast food meals and migration of food handlers from poor to rich countries. Children can contract *H. pylori* through poor hygiene, child care, or living with another person who has the bacteria. *H. pylori* is a common bacteria found in the stomachs of many children. In fact, some studies suggest that up to 50 percent of the world's population carries this bacteria. Children develop *H. pylori* by fecal-oral, gastric-oral, or oral-oral route. Risk factors for infection include poor socio-economic status, child care, close living quarters, poor hygiene and living with another person who has *H. pylori*. Asian Americans and African Americans get infected at about the same rate as children in developing countries.[58,60] The prevalence of infection is highest in children in the developing world where up to 75% of children may be infected by the age of 10, while in the developed world the prevalence of infection is noticeably increased among socially deprived children.[57]

Concerning prevalence of *H. pylori* among autistic children and their parents, it is worthy to mention that there is no available knowledge in literature about prevalence of *H. pylori* among children with autism; this might be a good point in favor of the value of this study as it might in this regard open a new field of study for researchers and investigators.

In addition to the toxic influence of ammonia, excess amounts of ammonia in the colon is smooth muscle spastic leading to multiple colonic spasms and a high rectal spasm which were demonstrated in *H. pylori*-dyspeptic adults by colonoscopy. These spasms interfere with the integral colonic function of forming the motion contents, instead it squeezes the colonic contents leading to constipation and formation of small pieces of dried stool.[50] Existence of *H. pylori* in the colon was confirmed by a specific test (*H. pylori* fecal antigen) which was found positive in all children and parents of this study. Constipation and passage of small pieces of dried stool are cardinal signs of colonic *H. pylori*-related dyspepsia;[50,51] these signs were found constant features in all children of the study.

The constant association of GI symptoms with autism to the extent that gluten-free diet and probiotics were employed to improve these symptoms could further support the possibility of the role of *H. pylori* behind pathogenesis of autism disorder. It has been furthermore suggested that strategies of probiotic supplements that can help to restore normal gut microbiota and reduce the gut production and absorption of toxins has been advised and employed not only to improve GI symptoms in autism, but also to improve the core deficits of the brain disorder.[32] The mucosal pathologic behavior of *H. pylori* abnormal strains includes apparent lymphoctic infiltration and lymphocytic mucosal inflammation;[61] small bowel enteropathy has been reported in literature among patients with autism that could be attributed to embedding of *H. pylori* colonization towards small intestinal mucosa which is a further unrecognized unusual behavior of *H. pylori*.[28,29,62] GI symptoms were frank and constant among patients of this study; minute-size continuous intestinal sounds were diffusely audible over the center of abdomen that had been related to small intestinal irritation. Small intestinal enteropathy could account for the observations of "No Appetite", "No Hunger" and "No Eat" symptoms among autistic children of the study as they would feel continuous abdominal discomfort. It was suggested that autonomic functions and GI problems in autistic children are linked together;[31] therefore, the quite passive peaceful attitude of some autistic children; "Non-Smiling", "Non-Reactive" was attributed in this study to a degree of parasympathetic activation caused by the minor dull somatic intestinal insult. The improvement of intestinal symptoms among children of this study upon intake of a warm mint drink, a soft caffeine drink or chocolate was attributed to improvement of this autonomic compromise. Constipation, weak appetite, passage of small pieces of dried stool or leaking small amount of soft retained/overflowing stool were encountered as constant features among children of this study.

Major colonization of abnormal-behavior *H. pylori* strains is necessary to induce symptoms and toxic complications. Spontaneous reduction below the pathologic level (50%) or even spontaneous elimination of *H. pylori* from the colon could occur due to variable reasons such as diarrhea or intake of foods containing bio-organic acid.[28,29,63] This could explain the wide variation in autistic features and the observation that some children develop some autistic symptoms then they skip the disease as they grow up.

This study included two children newly diagnosed for autism, one is two years old who started pronouncing some words and then he lost this skill. Immediate colon clear was employed for him and his parents within few days the clinical diagnosis was made up, that was followed by complete recovery of the child's skills. The other was three years old when diagnosed but he had lost the developed verbal skills one year earlier; he improved but did not recover completely after colon clear. The study also included a girl 11 months old; it is surprising to find a baby of that age who does not cry or even smile in response to her mother's plea, she was looking constantly to one direction and was never responsive or attentive towards her mother's voice. She was typically constipated and was crying only during passing the motion in the form of small pieces of dried hard stool. The father was having frank constipation and severe colonic dyspeptic symptoms due to frequent outside-home meals during his business lunch and dinner meetings. *H. pylori* fecal antigen test was strongly positive for the girl and the parents; definitely the bacteria travelled from husband to his wife who gave it to her kid possibly while preparing and tasting her feeds or kissing her baby on the lips. Unfortunately, this girl was seen few months after she developed these features; immediate colon clear with a calculated dose (45 CCs) of the senna leaves extract purge was employed for her followed by vinegar-mixed fruit yoghurt twice daily. The girl improved within few days but did not recover completely because of late discovery and management of her condition; her motion became easy without tragedy, the girl started to smile, look towards her mother, respond to her mother's voice and most importantly she learned to cry like any baby of her age when neglected for some time. *H. pylori* DNA extraction in the stool and *H. pylori* strain genotyping were done for the girl and parents; they were found having the same strain genotype with existence of cytotoxin-associated gene A (cagA) positive *H. pylori* strains. It was emphasized that cagA of *H. pylori* encodes a highly immunogenic and virulence-associated protein; the presence of this virulent gene in the body could affect the clinical out-come in many children.[64]

All living organisms produce ammonia as a byproduct of cellular metabolism, ammonia is the major end product of cellular amino acid metabolism. Ammonia is a highly toxic material in animals at even sub-millimolar concentrations. At high concentrations, ammonia is toxic and can cause adverse effects to the cell. Effects include disruption of cellular energy metabolism, mitochondrial dysfunction, modulation of inflammatory responses and neurotransmission in neurons. Existing evidences suggest that accumulation of ammonia in the brain affects neuronal function and may lead to several neurological abnormalities.[65-69] In mammalian brains, ammonia is derived mostly from protein metabolism. In the brain, ammonia is derived from two main pathways; endogenous and exogenous sources. Endogenous sources of brain ammonia involve hydrolysis of proteins and degradation of amino acids.[70-72] Exogenous sources produce large quantities of ammonia in the gastrointestinal tract resulting from bacterial splitting of urea and deamination of amino acids. Bacterial infections in the gut are major causes of accumulation of ammonia in the brain.[68,73] In addition to the fact that ammonia can diffuse blood-brain barriers (BBB) due to its small size and uncharged state leading to major toxic damage in the brain, elevated ammonia also could dissociate changes in BBB morphology and permeability allowing other toxins to diffuse with all expected bad sequels.[68,74,75] It was shown in individuals with hepatic encephalopathy that there is lack of balance between excitatory and inhibitory neurotransmission.[76]

In rat brain it has been shown that high ammonia concentrations markedly interact with mitochondrial function.[77] In most animal species, including mammals, the ammonia concentration of body fluids is typically low, high concentrations are usually toxic to mammalian cells.[69,78] In animals, high levels of ammonia can lead to disruption in the balance between mitochondrial fission and fusion, changes in mitochondria morphology, mitochondrial enzymatic failure, disruption of energy metabolism of mitochondria and a reduced rate of mitochondrial axonal transport.[79,80] The elevation of ammonia concentrations progressively leads to impaired mental status as concerns cognitive, learning, and memory functions. It has been shown that exposure of rat hippocampal slices to high ammonia concentrations compromised the neuro-receptors. It was found that elevated levels of ammonia impairs memory or conditioned learning in animals.[81,82]

In most species, including mammals, ammonia concentrations exceeding 1 mmol/L are usually toxic to mammalian cells. Because of its toxicity an effective ammonia detoxification or excretion system is crucial to maintain cellular and body fluid ammonia levels within a tolerable range to ensure normal systemic functions.[68,83,84] In this study, colon clear via employing the natural senna leaves extract purge was the method used for **H. pylori** eradication from the colon in order to clear the accumulated colonic ammonia.

Ammonia could have a biphasic effect on cerebral micro-capillary circulation, an early enhance due to endothelial-derived nitric oxide liberation via the effect of shear stress and a late harmful toxic effect. The possible mechanisms of the learning deficits produced by high levels of ammonia most likely involve a reduction of the neuronal glutamate-nitric oxide cyclic pathway.[69,78,83,84] This biphasic influence of ammonia on the cerebral micro-capillary function could account for the brilliant early skills or the high IQ scores of some autistic children which is followed by loss of already developed skills to the extent that the investigators of the study found some parents of autistic children believe that an evil eye has affected their children and they search spiritual therapies. Parents are looking everywhere for answers and best treatment even they are trying some traditional therapies including intensive behavioral approaches but with no "one-size-fits-all" treatment approach, parents often turn to diverse complementary and alternative therapies.[75] The investigators of this study noticed that people in some Middle East countries practice a lot of spiritual traditions and repeated sessions of bee bites therapy as an attempt for recovery of their children.

Permanent compromise of some areas of the brain among autistic children such as impairments of grey or white matter, decreased cortical thickness or cortical thinning leading to dysfunction of complex interactions in disadvantaged children was confirmed in literature;[13-15,22,24,26] possibly for this reason, most researchers were just able to achieve improvement through employing different measures but never complete cure of their autistic patients. The results of this study conform with the literature results in achieving incomplete cure of autistic features which could indicate that autism might not be a disease of definitive cure but it could be a typical disease of definite prevention via restriction of antibiotic use unless seriously indicated, extreme carefulness towards outside-home meals, colon care and colon clear on developing dyspeptic symptoms. If there is a chance for fundamental cure in autism, it might be via colon care and colon clear for both kids and parents. Early diagnosis and management are precious in this situation; recovery of the developed verbal skills for the two years old child of this study with the lucky advantage of early discovery of the onset of the disease upon losing the developed verbal words is an ideal example.

Prevention is always far better than treatment; scientific research efforts could not reach until to date an adequate cure of autism, while it could be greatly preventable by protecting children's brain from the bad sequels of the abnormal **H. pylori** strains of their dyspeptic mothers. Ladies should be extremely careful towards outside-home meals and strictly avoid un-necessary antibiotic use particularly before pregnancy. On developing any unusual or constant dyspepsia, parents should investigate for existence of colonic **H. pylori** strains and eradicate them if present by employing natural measures. Eradication of **H. pylori** from the colon can be done via employing the senna leaves purge as no other measure has been proved to be effective against colonic **H. pylori** strains; three times dilution of the natural senna leaves extract was found directly lethal to **H. pylori** on culture media. While antibiotics are seldom effective against extra-gastric **H. pylori** strains; on the contrary, it will force normal-behavior **H. pylori** to migrate to the colon.[28,54,56] During pregnancy, employing the senna leaves purge might not be confidently advisable as there is no available evidence against the possibility of development of sudden uterine contractions via a local axon reflex in response to the senna. In this situation, colon care can be employed by having a vinegar-mixed salad with food after any query meal to relief dyspeptic symptoms by buffering bacterial contents of the meal and to reduce colonic **H. pylori** strains below its pathologic level.[28,29,50,63] This could protect to a great extent the fetal blood and the embryonic brain from the toxic effect of the ammonia in maternal blood. After delivery, mothers must follow the same strict carefulness and measures particularly during the children's early critical ages of brain growth and development of skills. In addition, mothers should wash hands with white vinegar and water after washing with soap whenever using the bathroom or before preparing food for their children as soap does not kill *H. pylori*, while 20 times dilution of dietary white vinegar (acetic acid 6%) is directly lethal to *H. pylori*.[50,85]

The reason that there are some patients who developed autism before the last three decades which is the particular period of the abnormal-behavior *H. pylori* strains prevalence, is most probably due to chronic antibiotic exposure or recurrent antibiotic abuse that would force *H. pylori* to migrate to the colon; the suggestion of chronic antibiotic exposure in leading to autistic disorder has been suggested by some investigators.[1] The last three decades demonstrated flare up of abnormal-behavior *H. pylori* strains after the rediscovery of a bacterium surviving in the stomach by two Australian physicians and their strategic triple therapeutic violence against it with consequent flare up of medical challenges related to these drastic *H. pylori* strains. It might seem that the antibiotic violence has rendered a domestic bug to become wild in sequels instead of getting rid of it. The challenge of autism first appeared before the last three decades but it has mostly dominated during these last three decades.[1,28,29,86,87] The susceptibility or sensitivity of the brain to the undesired toxic effect of ammonia should differ from one child to another even they are all susceptible disadvantaged individuals; this could explain the apparent variable range of symptoms among autistic patients. It should be considered that those children who develop autism in relation to the toxic influence of the *H. pylori*-produced ammonia on the growing brain are susceptible predisposed individuals as exposure of some other children to the same circumstances was associated with different sequels such as toxic pancreatitis and development of childhood diabetes.[88]

The literature reports indicate increased risk and rising prevalence of identified ASD among U.S. children. An investigator with his 45 collaborators reported in 2009 that the increased prevalence of identified autism among U.S. children need to be regarded as an urgent public health concern.[4] The reason that autism prevails among U.S. children could be most probably related to the fact that U.S. is a typical country of fast food dependency and the food handlers are mostly poor people migrating from poor developing countries with inadequate health care standards carrying with them abnormal-behavior *H. pylori* strains; these abnormal strains travel from stomach to stomach via meals and remain in the gut with its abnormal behavior for life unless eradicated.[28,29] According to some personal communications; some mothers of autistic children indicated frankly that they love fast food to the extent that some particular fast food meals run in their blood while some mothers admitted that they are lazy to cook when they are pregnant and they depend on outside-home meals. Others mentioned that when they get pregnant while the previous baby is still between 2-3 years old, they depend mainly upon fast food delivery for themselves and their kids.

In Summary, realization of the real clue of a challenging illness constitutes the main success in its management; the hypothesis of the pathogenic influence of elevated serum ammonia in leading to the autistic behavioral disorder might remain just a hypothesis until approved or disapproved, but the unsolved puzzle of ASD has been considered as a "sequence" rather than a syndrome.[23] Apparently, the current available literature knowledge might seem articulating together to support a concept that the spread of the abnormal-behavior colonic *H. pylori* strains could lie behind the pathogenesis of a complex sequence of spectral events leading to the prevailing challenge known as the disorder of autistic spectrum. The following observational findings have been previously discussed: 1. Prevalence of the abnormal-behavior *H. pylori* strains followed the antibiotic violence towards it during the last three decades, 2. Flare up of medical challenges related to these *H. pylori* strains has started mainly during the last three decades, 3. Autistic behavioral syndrome appeared earlier but dominated during last three decades, 4. Antibiotic exposure was suggested as a factor leading to autistic disorder, 5. The association of GI troubles and autism is frank and constant in literature, 6. Development of autistic features or loss of developed skills occurs at the typical age where children could gain the abnormal *H. pylori* strains trans-familial from their parents, 7. *H. pylori* in the stomach was suggested to lead a behavior of natural bacteria while the role of microbiota and probiotics in autism is strongly suggested in literature, 8. The elevated serum level of ammonia among autistic children is constant in most scientific reports, 9. The toxic effect of **H. pylori**-produced ammonia on the whole brain conforms with the hypothesis of entire brain compromise suggested to explain inability of autistic children to perform complex interactions and 10. The concept of ammonia toxicity in leading to autistic sequels can still explain why many children with autism show early brilliance in developing skills which is followed by loss of already developed skills.

Accordingly, It seems that autism might not be a disease of definitive cure due to a permanent compromise of areas of the brain responsible for development of skills caused by a sustained toxic influence of ammonia throughout a critical period of brain growth during a child's early life. For this reason, scientific research efforts were just able to get improvement of autistic behavioral symptoms but did not achieve real or complete cure of autism. On the other hand, autism could be a typical disease of definite prevention via extreme carefulness towards outside-home meals, restriction of antibiotic use unless seriously indicated and colon care/colon clear for mothers who develop **H. pylori**-related dyspeptic symptoms before or during pregnancy or while nursing their kid's during the early critical ages of child's growth. Early diagnosis and management of autistic features in a child could greatly improve the out-coming results of treatment through colon clear for the kids themselves.

Conclusion: Until today, it seems that this research article may constitute the real fulfilled clue about autism sequences; autism might not be a disease of definitive cure due to permanent compromise of some areas of the brain responsible for development of skills during a critical period of a child's brain growth but it could be a typical disease of definite prevention via colon care and colon clear for parents employing natural measures for any developing **H. pylori**-related dyspepsia. If there is a chance for cure of autism, it might be via colon clear for kids in an early onset of developing autistic features. In spite of that; this research study invites and encourages all investigators to continue all persevere and enthusiastic efforts to approach a fundamental cure of autism.

REFERENCES:

1. **Li Q, Zhou JM.** The microbiota-gut-brain axis and its potential therapeutic role in autism spectrum disorder. *Neuroscience 2016 Jun 2; 324: 131-9.*

2. **Woolfenden S, Eapen V, Jalaludin B, et al. Prevalence and factors associated with parental concerns about development detected by the Parents' Evaluation of Developmental Status (PEDS) at 6-month, 12-month and 18-month well-child checks in a birth cohort.** *BMJ 2016 Sep 8; 6 (9): e012144.*

3. **Baio J. Prevalence of autism spectrum disorders - Autism and Developmental Disabilities Monitoring Network, United States, 2006.** *MMWR Surveill Summ 2009 Dec 18; 58 (10): 1-20.*

4. **Galichi F, Ghaemmaghami J, Malek A, et al. Effect of gluten free diet on gastrointestinal and behavioral indices for children with autism spectrum disorders: a randomized clinical trial.** *World J Pediatr 2016 Jun 10; 26(12): 1936-9. [Epub ahead of print]*

5. **Kiely B, Vettam S, Adesman A. Utilization of genetic testing among children with developmental disabilities in the United States.** *Appl Clin Genet 2016 Jul 11; 9: 93-100. eCollection 2016.*

6. **Allen DA. Autistic spectrum disorders: clinical presentation in preschool children.** *J Child Neurol 1988; 3Suppl: S48-56.*

7. **Emberti Gialloreti L, Benvenuto A, Battan B, et al. Can biological components predict short-term evolution in Autism Spectrum Disorders? A proof-of-concept study.** *Ital J Pediatr 2016 Jul 22; 42 (1): 70.*

8. Spjut Jansson B, Miniscalco C, Westerlund J, et al. Children who screen positive for autism at 2.5 years and receive early intervention: a prospective naturalistic 2-year outcome study. *Neuropsychiatr Dis Treat 2016 Sep 1; 12: 2255-63. eCollection 2016.*

9. Locke J, Williams J, Shih W, et al. Characteristics of socially successful elementary school-aged children with autism. *J Child Psychol Psychiatry 2016 Sep 13. doi: 10.1111/ jcpp.12636. [Epub ahead of print]*

10. Schwichtenberg AJ, Hensle T, Honaker S, et al. Sibling sleep-What can it tell us about parental sleep reports in the context of autism? *Clin Pract Pediatr Psychol 2016 Jun; 4 (2): 137-152.*

11. Donovan AP, Basson MA. The neuroanatomy of autism - a developmental perspective. *J Anat 2016 Sep 12. Doi: 10.1111/joa. 12542. [Epub ahead of print]*

12. Benitez-Burraco A, Lattanzi W, Murphy E. Language Impairments in ASD Resulting from a Failed Domestication of the Human Brain. *Front Neurosci 2016 Aug 29; 10: 373. eCollection 2016.*

13. Grecucci A, Rubicondo D, Siugzdaite R, et al. Uncovering the Social Deficits in the Autistic Brain. A Source-Based Morphometric Study. *Front Neurosci 2016 Aug 31; 10: 388. eCollection 2016.*

14. Richter J, Henze R, Vomstein K, et al. Reduced cortical thickness and its association with social reactivity in children with autismspectrum disorder. *Psychiatry Res 2015 Oct 30; 234 (1): 15-24. Epub 2015 Aug 22.*

15. Blanken LM, Mous SE, Ghassabian A, et al. Cortical morphology in 6- to 10-year old children with autistic traits: a population-based neuroimaging study. *Am J Psychiatry 2015 May; 172 (5): 479-86. Epub 2015 Jan 13.*

16. Blatt GJ, Fatemi SH. Alterations in GABAergic biomarkers in the autism brain: research findings and clinical implications. *Anat Rec (Hoboken) 2011 Oct; 294 (10): 1646-52. Epub 2011 Sep 8.*

17. Jou RJ, Mateljevic N, Kaisern MD, et al. Structural neural phenotype of autism: preliminary evidence from a diffusion tensor imaging study using tract-based spatial statistics. *AJNR Am J Neuroradiol 2011 Oct; 32 (9): 1607-13. Epub 2011 Jul 28.*

18. Jaber M. The cerebellum as a major player in motor disturbances related to Autistic Syndrome Disorders. *Encephale 2016 Sep 8. doi: 10.1016/1. encep.2016.03.018. [Epub ahead of print]*

19. Sperdin HF, Schaer M. Aberrant Development of Speech Processing in Young Children with Autism: New Insights from Neuroimaging Biomarkers. *Front Neurosci 2016 Aug 25; 10: 393. eCollection 2016.*

20. Happe F, Conway JR. Recent progress in understanding skills and impairments in social cognition. *Curr Opin Pediatr 2016 Sep 6. [Epub ahead of print]*

21. Dinan TG, Cryan JF. Gut Instincts: microbiota as a key regulator of brain development, ageing and neurodegeneration. *J Physiol 2016 Sep 19. Doi: 10.1113/JP273106. [Epub ahead of print]*

22. **Peeva MG, Tourville JA, Agam Y, et al. White matter impairment in the speech network of individuals with autism spectrum disorder.** *Neuroimage 2013 Aug 28; 3: 234-41. eCollection 2013.*

23. **Casanova MF, El-Baz AS, Kamat SS, et al. Focal cortical dysplasias in autism spectrum disorders.** *Acta Neuropathol Commun 2013 Oct 11; 1: 67. Doi: 10.1186/2051.5960.1.67.*

24. **Misaki M, Wallace GL, Dankner N, et al. Characteristic cortical thickness patterns in adolescents with autism spectrum disorders: interactions with age and intellectual ability revealed by canonical correlation analysis.** *Neuroimage 2012 Apr 15; 60 (3): 1890-901. Epub 2012 Feb 3.*

25. **Randolph-Gips M, Srinivasan P. Modeling autism: a systems biology approach.** *J Clin Bioinforma 2012 Oct 8; 2 (1): 17. Doi: 10.1186/2043.9113.2.17.*

26. **Chiang HL, Chen YJ, Lin HY, et al. Disorder-Specific Alteration in White Matter Structural Property in Adults With AutismSpectrum Disorder Relative to Adults With A DHD and Adult Controls.** *Hum Brain Mapp 2016 Sep 15y. doi: 10.1002/ hbm.23367. [Epub ahead of print]*

27. **Chang J, Gilman SR, Chiang AH, et al. Genotype to phenotype relationships in autism spectrum disorders.** *Nat Neurosci 2015 Feb; 18 (2): 191-8. Epub 2014 Dec 22.*

28. **Farinha P, Gascoyne RD. Helicobacter pylori and MALT Lymphoma.** *Gastroenterology 2005 May; 128 (6): 1579-605.*

29. **Nasrat AM, Nasrat SAM, Nasrat RM, et al. Misconception and misbehavior towards Helicobacter pylori is leading to major spread of illness.** *Gen Med 2015; S1: 002.* **[Open Access]**

30. **Horvath K, Peman JA. Autism and gastrointestinal symptoms.** *Curr Gastroenterol Res 2002 Jun; 4 (3): 251-8.*

31. **Ferguson BJ, Marler S, Altstein LL, et al. Psychophysiological associations with gastrointestinal symptomatology in Autism Spectrum Disorder.** *Autism Res 2016 Jun 20. doi: 10. 1002/aur. 1646. [Epub ahead of print]*

32. **Santocchi E, Guiducci L, Fulceri F, et al. Gut to brain interaction in Autism Spectrum Disorders: a randomized controlled trial on the role of probiotics on clinical, biochemical and neurophysiological parameters.** *BMC Psychiatry 2016 Jun 4; 16: 183.*

33. **Marler S, Ferguson BJ, Lee EB, et al. Brief Report: Whole blood serotonin levels and gastrointestinal symptoms in Autism Spectrum Disorder.** *J Autism Dev Diord 2016 Mar; 46 (3): 1124-30.*

34. **Fulceri F, Morelli M, Santocchi E, et al. Gastrointestinal symptoms and behavioral problems in preschoolers with Autism Spectrum Disorder.** *Dig Liver Dis 2016 Mar; 48 (3): 248-54.*

35. **Kushak RI, Buie TM, Murray KF, et al. Evaluation of intestinal function in children with Autism and gastrointestinal symptoms.** *J Pediatr Gastroenterol Nutr 2016 May; 62 (5): 687-91.*

36. **Inoue R, Sakaue, Sawai C. A preliminary investigation on the relationship between gut microbiota and gene expressions in peripheral mononuclear cells of infants with autism spectrum disorders.** *Biosci Biotechnol Biochem 2016 Sep 1: 1-9. [Epub ahead of print]*

37. **Ge Z. Potential of fumarate reductase as a novel therapeutic target in Helicobacter pylori infection.** *Expert Opin Ther Targets 2002 Apr; 6(2): 135-46.*

38. **Nasrat SAM, Nasrat RM, Nasrat MN, et al. The dramatic spread of diabetes mellitus worldwide and influence of Helicobacter pylori.** *General Med. 2015; 3 (1): 159-62.*

39. **Kiykim E, Zeybek CA, Zubarioglu T, et al. Inherited metabolic disorders in Turkish patients with autism spectrum disorders.** *Autism Res 2016 Feb; 9 (2): 217-23. Epub 2015 Jun 7.*

40. **Burrus CJ. A biochemical rationale for the interaction between gastrointestinal yeast and autism.** *Med Hypotheses 2012 Dec; 79 (6): 784-5. Epub 2012 Sep 26.*

41. **Abu Shmais GA, Al-Ayadhi LY, Al-Dbass AM, et al. Mechanism of nitrogen metabolism-related parameters and enzyme activities in the pathophysiology of autism.** *J Neurodev Disord 2012 Feb 13; 4 (1): 4. doi: 10.1186/1866.1955.4.4.*

42. **Wang L, Christophersen CT, Sorich MJ, et al. Elevated fecal short chain fatty acid and ammonia concentrations in children with autism spectrum disorder.** *Dig Dis Sci 2012 Aug; 57 (8): 2096-102. Epub 2012 Apr 26.*

43. **Good P. Do salt cravings in children with autistic disorders reveal low blood sodium depleting brain taurine and glutamine?** *Med Hypotheses 2011 Dec; 77 (6): 1015-21. Epub 2011 Sep 16.*

44. **Cohen BI. Ammonia (NH3), nitric oxide (NO) and nitrous oxide (N2O)--the connection with infantile autism.** *Autism 2006 Mar; 10 (2): 221-3.*

45. **Corker I, Tuzun U. Autistic-like findings associated with a urea cycle disorder in a 4-year-old girl.** *J Psychiatry Nerosci 2005 Mar; 30 (2): 133-5.*

46. **Filipek PA, Juranek J, Naguyen MT, et al. Relative carnitine deficiency in autism.** *J Autism Dev Disord 2004 Dec; 34 (6): 615-23.*

47. **Fallon J. Could one of the most widely prescribed antibiotics amoxicillin/clavulanate "augmentin" be a risk factor for autism?** *Med Hypotheses 2005; 64 (2): 312-5.*

48. **Clark-Taylor T, Clark-Taylor BE. Is autism a disorder of fatty acid metabolism? Possible dysfunction of mitochondrial beta-oxidation by long chain acyl-CoA dehydrogenase.** *Med Hypotheses 2004; 62 (6): 970-5.*

49. **Cohen BI. The significance of ammonia/gamma-aminobutyric acid (GABA) ratio for normality and liver disorders.** *Med Hypotheses 2002 Dec; 59 (6): 757-8.*

50. **Nasrat AM, Nasrat SAM, Nasrat RM, et al. An alternate natural remedy for symptomatic relief of Helicobacter pylori dyspepsia.** *Gen Med 2015; 3: 4.* **[Open Access]**

51. Nasrat AM, Nasrat SAM, Nasrat RM, et al. **Characteristics of Helicobacter pylori-related dysglycemia.** *Gen Med 2015; S1 (4).* [Open Access]

52. Nasrat AM. **Functional dyspepsia.** *Gen Med 2015; 3: 3. doi: org/10.4172/2327-5146.1000192.*

53. Blatt GJ. **The neuropathology of autism.** *Scientifica (Cairo) 2012; 2012: 703675. Epub 2012 Dec 19.*

54. Grünberger B, Wöhrer S, Streubel B, et al. **Antibiotic treatment is not effective in patients infected with Helicobacter pylori suffering from extragastric MALT lymphoma.** *J Clin Oncol 2006 Mar 20; 24 (9): 1370-5.*

55. Nasrat AM, Nasrat SAM, Nasrat RM, et al. **A comparative study of natural eradication of Helicobacter pylori vs. antibiotics.** *Gen Med 2015; S1:1.* [Open Access]

56. Nasrat AM, Nasrat SAM, Nasrat RM, et al. **The definitive eradication of Helicobacter pylori from the colon.** *Gen Med 2015; S1:1.* [Open Access]

57. Rowland M, Imrie Bourke B, et al. **How should Helicobacter pylori infected children be managed?** *Gut 1999; 45 (1): 136-9.*

58. Nasrat AM, Nasrat SAM, Nasrat RM, et al. **An alternate natural remedy for symptomatic relief of Helicobacter pylori dyspepsi.** *Gen Med 2015; 3: 4. doi: org/10.4172/2327-5146.1000200.*

59. Asaka M. **Epidemiology of Helicobacter pylori infection in Japan.** *Nihon Rinsho 2003; 61: 19-24.*

60. Thomas DW, Greer FR. **Probiotics and prebiotics in pediatrics.** *Pediatrics 2010 Dec; 126 (6): 1217-31.*

61. Copie-Bergman C, Locher C, Levy M, et al. **Metachronous gastric MALT lymphoma and early gastric cancer: is residual lymphoma a risk factor for the development of gastric carcinoma?** *Ann Oncol 2005 Aug; 16 (8): 1232-6. Epub 2005 May 12.*

62. Torrente F, Anthony A, Heuschkel RB, et al. **Focal-enhanced gastritis in regressive autism with features distinct from Crohn's and Helicobacter pylori gastritis.** *Am J Gastroenterol 2004 Apr; 99 (4): 598-605.*

63. Zentilin P, Iiritano E, Vingale C, et al. **Helicobacter pylori infection is not involved in the pathogenesis of either erosive or non-erosive gastro-oesophageal reflux disease.** *Aliment Pharmacol Ther 2003 Apr; 17 (8): 1057-64.*

64. Bulut Y, Agacayak A, Karlidag D, et al. **Association of CagA+ Helicobacter pylori with adenotonsillar hypertrophy.** *Tohoku J Exp Med 2006 Jul; 209 (3): 1057-64.*

65. Wright PA. **Nitrogen excretion: three end products, many physiological roles.** *J Exp Biol 1995; 198 (2): 273-281.*

66. Marcaida G, Felipo V, Hermenegildo C, et al. **Acute ammonia toxicity is mediated by the NMDA type of glutamate receptors.** *FEBS Lett 1992 Jan 13; 296 (1): 67-8.*

67. Britto DT, Kronzucker HJ. **NH4+ toxicity in higher plants: a critical review.** *J Plant Physiol 2002; 159 (6): 567-584.*

68. 68. Adlimoghaddam A, Sabbir MG, Albensi BC. Ammonia as a Potential Neurotoxic Factor in Alzheimer's Disease. *Front Mol Neurosci 2016 Aug 8; 9: 57. doi: 10.3389/fnmol.2016.00057.*

69. Cooper AJ, Plum F. Biochemistry and physiology of brain ammonia. *Physiol Rev 1987; 67: 440-519.*

70. Seiler N. Is ammonia a pathogenetic factor in Alzheimer's disease? *Neurochem Res 1993; 18: 235-245.*

71. Seiler N. Ammonia and Alzheimer's disease. *Neurochem Int 2002; 41: 189-207.*

72. Seglen PO. Inhibitors of lysosomal function. *Meth Enzymol 1983; 96: 737-764.*

73. Marcaggi P, Coles JA. Ammonium in nervous tissue: transport across cell membranes, fluxes from neurons to glial cells, and role in signalling. *Prog Neurobiol 2001; 64: 157-183.*

74. Laursen , Diemer NH. Morphometric studies of rat glial cell ultrastructure after urease-induced hyperammonaemia. *Neuropathol Appl Neurobiol 1979; 5: 345-362.*

75. Fiorentino M, Sapone A, Senger S, et al. Blood-brain barrier and intestinal epithelial barrier alterations in autism spectrum disorders. *Mol Autism 2016 Nov 29; 7: 49. eCollection 2016.*

76. Albrecht J, Jones EA. Hepatic encephalopathy: molecular mechanisms underlying the clinical syndrome. *J Neurol Sci 1999; 170: 138-146.*

77. Veauvy CM, Wang Y, Walsh PJ, et al. Comparison of the effects of ammonia on brain mitochondrial function in rats and gulf toadfish. *Am J Physiol Regul Integr Comp Physiol 2002; 283: 598-603.*

78. Hrnjez BJ, Song JC, Prasad M, et al. Ammonia blockade of intestinal epithelial K+ conductance. *Am J Physiol 1999; 277 (3): 521-532.*

79. Zhu X, Perry G, Smith MA, et al. Abnormal mitochondrial dynamics in the pathogenesis of Alzheimer's disease. *J Alzheimers Dis 2013; 33 (1): 253-262.*

80. Cadonic C, Sabbir MG, Albensi BC. Mechanisms of mitochondrial dysfunction in Alzheimer's disease. *Mol Neurobiol 2016 Nov; 53 (9): 6078-6090.*

81. Albert MS. Cognitive and neurobiologic markers of early Alzheimer disease. *Proc Natl Acad Sci U S A 1996 Nov 26; 93 (24): 13547-51.*

82. Aguilar MA, Minarro J, Felipo V. Chronic moderate hyperammonemia impairs active and passive avoidance behavior and conditional discrimination learning in rats. *Exp Neurol 2000; 161: 704-713.*

83. Sumii T, Nakano Y, Abe T, et al. The Effect of Nitric Oxide on Ammonia Decomposition in Co-cultures of Hepatocytes and Hepatic Stellate Cells. *In Vitro Cell Dev Biol Anim 2016 Jun; 52 (6): 625-31.*

84. Kosenko EA, Solomadin IN, Tikhonova LA, et al. Pathogenesis of Alzheimer disease: role of oxidative stress, amyloid-beta peptides, systemic ammonia and erythrocyte energy metabolism. *CNS Neurol Disord Drug Targets 2014; 13: 112-119.*

85. Debevere J, Devlieghere F, van Sprundel P, et al. Influence of acetate and CO2 on the TMAO – reduction reaction by Shewanella baltica. *Int J Food Microbiol 2001 Aug 15; 68 (1-2): 115-23.*

86. Aksoy H, Sebin SO. H. pylori and cardiovascular diseases. *Gen Med 2015; S1: 1.* [Open Access]

87. Jaber M. The cerebellum as a major player in motor disturbances related to Autistic Syndrome Disorders. *Encephale 2016 Sep 8. doi: 10.1016/j. encep.2016.03.018. [Epub ahead of print]*

88. Nasrat AM, Nasrat SAM, Nasrat RM, et al. The challenge of childhood diabetes. *Gen Med 2015; 3: 4. doi: org/10.4172/2327-5146.1000193.*

ALZHEIMER AND HELICOBACTER PYLORI; SHOULD WE FIGHT AND KILL OR SAVE H. PYLORI!! WE SHOULD SAVE H. PYLORI

*Alzheimer Could be Readily Delayed until End of Life of a Person*SCIENTIFIC EVIDENCES ON THE INFLUENCE OF HELICOBACTER PYLORI IN ALZHEIMER DISEASE

Alzheimer and Helicobacter Pylori; Should We Fight and Kill or Save H. Pylori!! We Should Save H. Pylori; Review Article: Published in the American Journal of Medicine and Medical Sciences; 2017; 7 (5): 221-228. Nasrat et al. Alzheimer and Helicobacter pylori; should we fight and kill or save H. pylori!! We should save H. pylori. *Am J Med Med Sci 2017; 7 (5): 221-228.* [doi: 10.5923/j.ajmms.20170705.03]

Abstract: This review study aimed at assessment of the bacterium **Helicobacter pylori** whether it is guilty, not guilty or innocent towards the brain and Alzheimer disease (AD).

AD is a chronic age-related degenerative disease characterized by loss of cognitive and memory functions. A genetic theory was suggested while the amyloid hypothesis is the most accepted. There are many medical pathologies that could contribute to Alzheimer such as diabetes, hypertension and dyslipidemia. Other factors like toxic elements, air pollution and nutrition are also under consideration.

A lot of controversy entails the influence of systemic ammonia and the endothelial-liberated nitric oxide (NO) on the pathogenesis of the amyloid disease and in turn on the onset and progress of Alzheimer disease. Elevated levels of ammonia is toxic and is associated with progress of the amyloid disease and dementia symptoms. Excess NO is involved in nitro-oxidative stress sequels resulting in endothelial and neuronal degeneration. Meanwhile, the normal level of ammonia could help to maintain the neuro-protective function of NO via its endothelial liberation due to the effect of shear stress. Accordingly, the normal-behavior **H. pylori** strains in the stomach could be biologic and healthy towards Alzheimer and the brain while the colonic **H. pylori** strains could be considered pathologic and toxic to the brain and dementia symptoms.

AD remains a disease without real cure or prevention because of permanent degeneration of some areas of the brain; therefore, attempts to delay the onset and symptoms of Alzheimer constitute intelligent and practical strategies. Eradication of colonic **H. pylori** strains via natural colon clear might be the most effective measure among these strategies as it eliminates the main pathologic source with its greater toxic influence in addition to amelioration of other factors contributing to AD such as diabetes, hypertension and dyslipidemia.

On conclusion, ***H. pylori***-produced ammonia in accordance could constitute at the mean time a cure and a poison towards Alzheimer while the natural existence of the bacterium ***H. pylori*** is biologic and protective; hence, it should be saved not killed.

Key words: Alzheimer, dementia, Helicobacter pylori, senna purge, vinegar.

Introduction: Alzheimer is a chronic, progressive and prevalent neuro-degenerative disease characterized by loss of higher cognitive functions with an associated memory loss. Alzheimer is the most common age-related degenerative disease. It should be admittedly that a lot is not known about Alzheimer's. More than 100 years after its discovery, it is still not exactly known what causes this neuro-degenerative disease and an exact cure is still not known. However, it is important not to lose sight of how far what has been achieved since the unique symptoms of the disease were first noticed; the interest and hope in realizing fundamental cure should not be lost. AD was first described in 1906 in a female patient who experienced memory loss, paranoia and psychological changes. Autopsy revealed shrinkage in and around nerve cells in her brain. Cognitive measurement scales were created in 1968 which allowed researchers to investigate degree of impairment and estimate the volume of damaged brain tissue. A National Alzheimer's Disease Genetic Study started in 2003 to hopefully identify risk genes for the disease. In 2010, Alzheimer's was considered the sixth leading cause of death in the United States.[1,2] There still a lot of work ahead is needed to find a cure or at least control of the challenge of Alzheimer's.

Dementia is defined as a clinical syndrome characterized by variety of symptoms and signs manifested by difficulties in memory or memory loss, disturbances in language and cognitive functions, changes in behaviors and impairments in activities of daily life. AD is the most common cause of dementia accounting for up to 75 % of dementia cases, AD is a progressive and challenging neuro-degenerative disorder. During the last few decades, epidemiological study of the disease has noticed tremendous progress in its researches and marked increase in the disease incidence.[3]

Alzheimer's disease represents an increasing challenge to public health and the health care system which has had tremendous impact on both the individual and societal levels. Epidemiologic researches have provided sufficient evidence that vascular risk factors in middle-aged and older adults play a significant role in the development and progression of dementia and AD whereas extensive social network and active engagement in mental, social, and physical activities may postpone the onset of dementia. Multi-domain community intervention trials are warranted to determine to what extent preventive strategies toward optimal control of multiple vascular factors and disorders as well as the maintenance of an active lifestyle are effective against dementia and AD.[1,3]

Population aging has become a worldwide universal phenomenon. The number of older people (65+ years) in the world is expected to increase with the proportion of older people being increased from 7% to 12%. Developing countries will see the largest increase in absolute numbers of older persons. As the occurrence of AD is strongly associated with increasing age, it is anticipated that the disorders of dementia will pose huge challenges to public health and elderly care systems in all countries all over the world.[3]

Concerning prevalence, the pooled data of population-based studies in Europe suggests that the age-standardized prevalence in people 65+ years old is 6.4 % for dementia and 4.4 % for AD. In the US, the study of a national representative sample of people aged >70 years yielded a prevalence for AD of 9.7 %. Worldwide, the global prevalence of dementia was estimated to be 3.9 % in people aged 60+ years. More than 25 million people in the world who are currently affected by dementia are mostly suffering from AD with around 5 million new cases occurring every year. The number of people with dementia is anticipated to double every 20 years. The age-specific prevalence of AD almost doubles every 5 years after the age of 65.[1,2,4-6]

The pooled incidence rate of AD among people 65+ years of age in Europe was 19.4 per 1000 person-years. The pooled incidence of population aged 65+ years in US yielded an incidence rate for AD of 13.0 in males and 16.9 in females per 1000 person-years. The incidence rate of AD increases almost exponentially with increasing age until 85 years of age.[7-9]

Alzheimer's dementia is a multi-factorial disease in which old age is the strongest risk factor suggesting that the aging-related biological processes may be implicated in the pathogenesis of the disease. Furthermore, the strong association of AD with increasing age may partially reflect the cumulative effect of different risk and protective factors over the lifespan including the effect of complex interactions of genetic susceptibility, psycho-social factors, biological factors and environmental exposures over the life. Various etiologic hypothetical studies support the role of genetic, vascular, and psycho-social factors in the development of AD whereas evidence for the etiologic role of other factors such as dietary or nutritional factors, occupational exposures and inflammation is insufficient.[10]

AD significantly shortens life expectancy and is one of the principal causes of physical disability and impaired quality of life. Epidemiologic studies have confirmed that AD is associated with increased risk of death for older people in a similar extent to that of malignant tumors. Several follow-up studies showed that AD was associated with a two to five-fold increased risk of death. The years of survival for people with newly diagnosed AD ranges from 3 to 6 years.[11,12]

Objective: The aim of this review study of the literature is attempting to approach a conclusion whether the bacterium *Helicobacter pylori* is healthy or toxic to the brain and whether it is biologic or pathologic as concerns the onset and progress of Alzheimer disease (AD) in addition to assessing the observational findings concerning the association between the colonic *H. pylori* strains and the frequency of Alzheimer during late decades.

Review: The genetic hypothesis of the disease which accounts for only about 2 to 5 % of all Alzheimer patients emphasizes that early-onset familial AD is often caused by autosomal dominant mutations such as mutations in amyloid precursor protein.[13] According to the vascular hypothesis moderate to strong evidence from multidisciplinary research works has emerged supporting the concept that vascular risk factors such as smoking, alcohol consumption, obesity and high total cholesterol together with vascular morbidity factors such as hypertension, diabetes, silent brain infarcts and white matter lesions are associated with an increased impact on the risk of dementia including AD.[14-26]

Silent strokes or small spots of dead brain cells were found linked to memory loss in the elderly people in a rate about one out of four. Both hippocampal volume and brain infarcts independently contribute to low memory performance in elderly individuals. A group of 658 people aged 65 and older were studied by MRI for silent strokes and hippocampal shrinkage; 174 of them were found having silent strokes and they scored worse on memory tests. A small hippocampus, which is the memory center of the brain, related to silent strokes was considered a new clue as regards why some older people lose their memory leading to the development of a new intervention for prevention of Alzheimer via stroke prevention as a mean for staving off memory problems.[27]

Air pollution may contribute to white matter loss in the brain; long-term exposure to air pollution may pose risk to brain structure and cognitive functions among middle-aged and older adults. It was found that air pollution over long periods could have impact on brain shrinkage with time and other risks including stroke and dementia. On the other way, having a purpose in life, physical or simple modified aerobic activities and mental activities might improve health of aging brain.[28-31]

Other factors that could have an impact on the development of Alzheimer's include nutritional or dietary pattern, educational and economic status, social engagement, physical or mental activity and traumatic head injury. Further important factors include inflammation, toxic exposure and pathogens.[31]

The emerging roles of pathogens in leading to Alzheimer via causing slowly progressive dementia, cortical atrophy and amyloid deposition have supported a hypothetical research concept that dementia might be prevented by the combined effect of antibiotic, antiviral and anti-inflammatory therapies. A possible link of the influence of the abnormal-behavior *H. pylori* strains in AD has been documented in literature. An association was found between *H. pylori* and AD but the contribution of *H. pylori* in the neuro-inflammatory process in Alzheimer was not confirmed or denied.[32] AD is associated with amyloid beta peptide deposition that could lead ultimately to neuro-degeneration. An infectious hypothesis is suggesting an alteration of the blood-brain barriers (BBB) and activation of a neuro-inflammation in the brain which could play a role in AD especially in the presence of decreased amyloid beta peptide clearance. Several viral or bacterial agents have been incriminated including *H.*

pylori; *H. pylori* can induce systemic inflammation and increase homocysteine levels contributing to worsen AD.[33,34] Homocysteine levels and amyloid beta peptide levels were found elevated in association with Alzheimer and *H. pylori*. AD patients associated with existence of *H. pylori* tend to show more cognitive impairment.[35,36]

As concerns the role of *H. pylori* in neurological diseases such as Alzheimer's, since the latest decade several studies have reported on the link between chronic *H. pylori* infection and a variety of extra-gastric manifestations including dementia. A recent longitudinal population-based cohort study found that after 20 years of follow-up, 28.9% of *H. pylori*-positive versus 21.1% of *H. pylori*-negative subjects developed dementia. Existence of *H. pylori* usually persists throughout life resulting in a chronic inflammatory response with local secretion of numerous inflammatory mediators including chemokines such as interleukin and cytokines such as tumor necrosis factor and interferon which can pass into the circulation and have a systemic effect. The persistence of detectable systemic and local concentrations of inflammatory mediators is likely to alter the outcome of neurological diseases. These pro-inflammatory factors can induce brain inflammation, death of neurons and could eventually be involved in the development of AD. Although most neurological diseases are the result of a combination of multiple factors, yet the systemic inflammatory response is a common component and determinant in the onset, evolution, and outcome of diseases in general. However, a sufficient understanding of the mechanism by which the inflammatory response generated by *H. pylori* affects neurological diseases is still required.[37-39]

The pathologic behavior of the abnormal-attitude *H. pylori* strains includes its migration or being forced to migrate to the colon under the influence of antibiotic violence. *H. pylori* in the colon will continue producing ammonia for a reason or no reason, unopposed or buffered by any acidity, leading to accumulation of profuse toxic amounts of ammonia, ammonia is neuro-toxic and toxic to the brain; hepatic ammonia encephalopathy is a frank example. The elevation of ammonia concentrations progressively leads to impaired mental status as concerns cognitive and memory functions. It has been also shown that exposure of rat hippocampal slices to high ammonia concentrations compromised the neuro-receptors. It was found that elevated levels of ammonia impairs memory and cognition in animals.[40-44]

The amyloid hypothesis is the classical theory explaining AD pathogenesis and hence is currently targeted for drug development; Alzheimer's is marked by progressive accumulation of beta amyloid peptide which appears to trigger neuro-toxic and inflammatory sequels. The hypothesis signifies that certain cellular proteins which are normally soluble in the living organisms, under certain conditions change behavior to form aggregates with a specific structure called beta amyloid. These intra or extra-cellular insoluble aggregates whether fibers or plaques constitute marks of many neuro-degenerative pathologies including AD. Amyloidoses are widespread disorders in the elderly human population showing rapid demographic expand in many global population. Increasing age is the most significant risk for these degenerative diseases associated with amyloid deposition. Role of amyloidosis in the pathogenesis of AD and dementia development has been significantly and adequately confirmed in literature.[45-47] Beta amyloid peptides exert pro-oxidant or anti-oxidant effects based on the metal ion concentrations that it sequesters, at low metal ion concentrations it is an anti-oxidant whereas at relatively higher concentration it is a pro-oxidant. Therefore; increased oxidative stress in the human brain includes accumulating evidences that could be a key causative factor for AD and treatment strategies could be hence largely based on beta amyloid clearance.[48]

Does ammonia play an essential role in amyloid disease of the CNS!! The excessive formation of ammonia in the brain of AD patients has been demonstrated and it has been also shown that AD patients exhibit elevated serum ammonia levels. The formation of amyloid plaques is currently considered as the key event of AD. The histological hallmarks of the disease include formation of fibrillary tangles and astrocytosis in some cortical areas of the brain. Among the toxic factors which have been considered to contribute to the symptoms and progression of AD, ammonia deserves special interest for many reasons; 1. Ammonia is formed in nearly all tissues and organs of the vertebrates and it is the most common endogenous neuro-toxic compound, 2. Several symptoms and histological sequels of hepatic ammonia encephalopathy caused by impairment of ammonia detoxification resemble those of AD, 3. Ammonia is the most important natural modulator of lysosomal protein processing and there are sufficient evidences for the involvement of aberrant lysosomal processing of beta-amyloid precursor protein in the formation of amyloid deposits, 4. Ammonia is able to affect the characteristic functions of microglia such as endocytosis and cytokine production whereas inflammatory processes and activation of microglia are widely believed to be implicated in the pathology of AD. It has been further reported that elevated level of serum ammonia causes biochemical and cellular dysfunctions in the brain which can be found in the brain of dementia and AD patients. Experimental attempts were made to demonstrate evidences in favor of the idea that ammonia plays a definite role in dementia of the Alzheimer type. Astrocytosis and impairment of neuro-transmission with net increase in excitability and glutamate release were considered among these evidences. Derangement of lysosomal processing of proteins is another potential site of ammonia action which is especially important in view of the growing evidence for the role of the endosomal-lysosomal system in the formation of amyloidogenic fragments from beta-amyloid precursor protein. Based on these facts, an ammonia hypothesis of AD has been first suggested in 1993 which is in support of the findings that ammonia is a factor able to produce symptoms of AD and to affect the progression of the disease.[48-50]

All living organisms produce ammonia as a by-product of cellular metabolism, ammonia is the major end product of cellular amino acid metabolism. Ammonia is a highly toxic material in animals at even sub-millimolar concentrations. At high concentrations, ammonia is toxic and can cause adverse effects to the cell. Effects include disruption of cellular energy metabolism, mitochondrial dysfunction, modulation of inflammatory responses and neuro-transmission in neurons. Existing evidences suggest that accumulation of ammonia in the brain affects neuronal function and may lead to several neurological abnormalities.[51-55] In mammalian brains, ammonia is derived mostly from protein metabolism. In the brain, ammonia is derived from two main pathways; endogenous and exogenous sources. Endogenous sources of brain ammonia involve hydrolysis of proteins and degradation of amino acids.[49,50,56] Exogenous sources produce large quantities of ammonia in the gastro-intestinal tract resulting from bacterial splitting of urea and de-amination of amino acids. Bacterial infections in the gut are major causes of accumulation of ammonia in the brain.[54,57] In addition to the fact that ammonia can diffuse BBB due to its small size and uncharged state leading to major toxic damage in the brain. Elevated ammonia could also dissociate changes in BBB morphology and permeability allowing other toxins to diffuse with all expected bad sequels.[54,58,59] In most animal species, including mammals, the ammonia concentration of body fluids is typically low, high concentrations are usually toxic to mammalian cells.[55,60] The elevation of ammonia concentrations progressively leads to impaired mental status as concerns cognitive, learning, and memory functions. It has been shown that exposure of rat hippocampal slices to high ammonia concentrations compromised the neuro-receptors. It was found that elevated levels of ammonia impairs memory or conditioned learning in animals.[43,44] In most species, including mammals, ammonia concentrations exceeding 1 mmol/L are usually toxic to mammalian cells. Because of its toxicity an effective ammonia detoxification or excretion system is crucial to maintain cellular and body fluid ammonia levels within a tolerable range to ensure normal systemic functions.[48,54,61]

Nitric oxide (NO) is an intelligent molecule produced by neurons and endothelial cells in the brain. The endothelial NO is essential for the integrity of the micro-capillary vasculature and it acts in the neurons as a neuro-transmitter. It is consistent that NO has got a significant neuro-protective role. NO is a specific micro-capillary vasodilator, the challenge and intelligence in NO is its specific production in response to particular requirements and its approach to a specific targeted pathological site such as in Alzheimer's. Unlike medicinal preparations like Viagra, NO could include toxic side-effects on the heart, blood pressure or the retina because of lack of specificity.[48,62,63] NO deficiency is associated with progression of AD and abscence of NO synthase 3 increases beta amyloid disease pathology in mice; it has been reported that fibrillary beta-amyloid deposits are closely associated with atrophic nitric oxide synthase.[63-65] Whereas NO can be scavenged in a rapid reaction with superoxide (O_2-) to generate peroxynitrite (ONOO-) which is a potent oxidant and the primary component of nitro-oxidative stress. At high concentrations ONOO- can undergo homolytic or heterolytic cleavage to produce highly reactive oxidative components and secondary components of nitro-oxidative stress. This high nitro-oxidative stress can initiate a cascade of reactions that can trigger and evoke neuronal and endothelial degeneration similar to what is observed in AD. The role of oxidative stress and nitro-oxidative stress associated with increased systemic ammonia in AD has been sufficiently emphasized in literature. The vast accumulating evidences that increased oxidative stress in the human brain is a key causative factor for Alzheimer have attracted the treatment strategies towards this field.[48,63] Accordingly, NO could constitute a cure and a poison at the mean time in AD.

The natural biological behavior of the bacterium *H. pylori* includes its existence under the shelter of the gastric mucus layer. *H. pylori* colonized the stomach since an immemorial time as if both the gastric wall and the bacterium used to live together in peace harmless to each other. The bacterium does not exist in the gastric lumen during presence of food where it stays settling on the gastric mucosa protected from any acidity reaching adjacent to the gastric wall by the ammonia produced at its immediate vicinity, protecting in turn the gastric mucosa from its acid if it goes in excess. The bacterium gains nutrition from food remnants after travel of the meal from the stomach and drop of the acid to a minimum in a blink-like momentum protected by a shield of ammonia and leaving some scattered ammonia after it in the gastric lumen. This scattered ammonia excites the gastric wall to secrete its acid to buffer the ammonia; *H. pylori* in this way protects from absence of the defensive role of the gastric acid during absence of food.[41,42,66] Hence; this biological balance between ammonia of *H. pylori* and gastric acid is constant life-long round the clock ensuring a residual level of ammonia that could further account for a constant systemic serum ammonia level. Systemic ammonia derived from the natural biological behavior of *H. pylori* could therefore have a healthy effect on the cerebral micro-capillary circulation via ensuring an endothelial-derived NO liberation due to the effect of shear stress.[48,60,61,67] NO is neuro-protective; hence, normal levels of serum ammonia could be protective towards the brain and Alzheimer. According to a population based study, it has been reported that eradication of *H. pylori* was associated with progression of dementia.[68] Whereas excess systemic ammonia constitutes a potential neuro-toxic factor in AD.[69] Similarly then, ammonia is a cure and a poison at the mean time in AD; as if ammonia or NO or both of them function as a cure and a poison at the same situation in Dementia and Alzheimer's.

Motive of the Review: As Alzheimer is a degenerative disease, treatment and prevention remain until current time a great challenge. Delaying the onset of Alzheimer could be a logic attempt. Many investigators have followed the policy of delaying the symptoms or onset of the disease relying mainly on early detection of symptoms because if not early detected, improvement might not be expected.[1,3] Revision of the records of the research investigators of this review study since 2011 revealed the medical information of eleven elderly patients with newly-discovered symptoms of dementia of Alzheimer who have undergone follow up for the purpose of evaluating the role of colon clear in delaying the symptoms of the disease. Those patients were actually referred by their relatives to do blood-let out cupping therapy for them in order to improve memory functions. Cupping therapy was not done for them but they were investigated for existence of colonic *H. pylori* strains and tested for serum ammonia level. Age of patients ranged between 71 and 99 years, they were seven males and four females. All patients were positive for existence of colonic *H. pylori* strains according to a specific test (*H. pylori* fecal antigen test).[40] Serum ammonia was elevated in all patients which ranged between 113-147 umol/L. All patients underwent colon clear employing the natural senna leaves extract purge for eradication of colonic *H. pylori* strains. After colon clear, they followed a vinegar therapy in the form of a vinegar-mixed salad amidst of principal meals once or twice daily, 3-5 days/week for six months. Vinegar therapy should be given in the middle of a meal in order to fight the abnormal-behavior *H. pylori* strains only that exist in the gastric lumen while presence of food whereas the normal-behavior strains are sheltered under the gastric mucus layer during presence of food where no violence can defeat them even the strongest antibiotics except forcing them to migrate to the colon particularly those antibiotics given in excess mal-use on empty stomach with consequent loss of the protective function of *H. pylori* at least in the stomach.[41,66] Colon clear was repeated after further one month and after two months later if required. Patients were followed up for every 3 years survival with adequate observation of recurrence of dementia symptoms throughout the life of the patient. Three patients showed mild improvement and four patients showed moderate improvement of memory functions after undergoing colon clear three times whereas two patients showed marked recovery of memory after the first colon clear and two patients did not show any improvement in spite of revision of colon clear two times. Five patients developed recurrence of dementia symptoms after 1-3 years but they recovered their previous memory level after colon clear while six patients died after 2-2.5 years in peace for a reason un-related to Alzheimer without developing any recurrent symptoms of dementia. The case of one female patient was amazingly interesting, she was seen in year 2011 for early dementia symptoms, she was from Yemen living in Gizan in the Southern region of Saudi Arabia, her age that time was 96 years, she improved completely after colon clear, three years later (in 2014) at age of 99 she developed marked loss of memory to the extent that she could not recognize her sons and daughters or distinguish her grand kids, suddenly she went into coma and developed diabetes, she was severely constipated, *H. pylori* fecal antigen test was strongly positive, level of serum ammonia was 146 umol/L, random blood sugar was 334 mg/dL and she was put on insulin therapy, she recovered completely from coma after colon clear, her diabetic condition was also corrected and insulin therapy was discontinued, most importantly she recovered her memory even relatives were astonished that she was able to recognize and distinguish perfectly her sons, daughters and grand kids again after recovery from coma, she died two years later in year 2016 without developing any dementia symptoms. Her coma and memory loss were attributed to the toxic effect of ammonia on the brain while her diabetic condition was considered a potential condition of toxic pancreatitis due to a biological toxic stress caused by accumulation of profuse toxic amounts of ammonia in the colon.[66,70] The sequence of events of this patient was actually the motive for the research team to review the influence of *H. pylori*-produced ammonia on cognitive and memory functions.

Ammonia is not considered the only primary factor of the AD. However, since elevated levels of serum ammonia and the release of ammonia from the brains of AD patients is well supported by observational findings, ammonia could be taken into account as a factor that contributes to manifestations and the progression of AD.[50] Therefore; traditional therapeutic strategies that can help elimination of excess ammonia such as colon clear can lead to the amelioration of symptoms and progression of AD. The abnormal-behavior colonic *H. pylori* strains contribute also in different ways in leading to some medical problems that could further contribute in the pathogenesis of AD such as diabetes mellitus, hypertension and dyslipidemia.[10,40,41,70-72] Hence, elimination of these colonic *H. pylori* strains via colon clear employing natural measures (the senna leaves extract purge) could constitute the most effective strategy to improve or improve and delay the symptoms of Alzheimer when newly detected.

Accordingly, a normal-behavior of *H. pylori* seems to be useful to the cerebral micro-capillary circulation as it is responsible for maintaining a normal residual systemic ammonia level which contributes to ensure the endothelial-derived NO liberation via the effect of shear stress; NO is an intelligent neuro-protective and an essential element to maintain the integrity of the cerebral micro-capillary circulation. While the abnormal colonic *H. pylori* strains are the reason for accumulation of profuse toxic amounts of ammonia in the colon which is leading to increased systemic serum ammonia level with consequent ammonia toxicity and NO toxicity in turn; elevated systemic ammonia is a major reason in the pathogenesis and progression of amyloid disease of the brain whereas high nitro-oxidative stress can evoke cytotoxic effects in neuronal and endothelial degeneration observed in Alzheimer.[48,62,67-69] Therefore; it might be safely suggested that both ammonia and NO resemble a cure and a poison at the same time for Alzheimer and dementia.

Summary: In Summary, It seems that the strategy of delaying the onset and symptoms of Alzheimer constitutes a practical solution for a medical challenge that does not currently have any fundamental treatment or prevention. It might be also considered that elimination of the potential source of excess toxic amounts of ammonia via natural eradication of the abnormal colonic *H. pylori* stains is the most effective measure among these strategies in order to delay or postpone symptoms and the onset of AD.[43,44,48,50] In spite of that all scientific efforts should continue persevere attempts to achieve real cure or prevention of Alzheimer by means of investigating all fields and factors contributing to the disease.

Conclusion: The natural structure and existence of the normal-behavior ***H. pylori*** strains contributing to maintain a normal residual systemic ammonia level is healthy to the brain as it supports the endothelial-derived NO liberation which is a neuro-protective element via maintaining the integrity of the cerebral micro-capillary circulation. Preservation of the natural structure and existence of the normal behavior-***H. pylori*** strains could delay the onset of Alzheimer and dementia symptoms. Therefore; we should not fight and kill but we should save ***H. pylori*** for the sake of brain health and for delaying the onset and symptoms of Alzheimer disease for many elderly people.

Alzheimer's is still until now a non-curable/non-preventable degenerative disease; hence, attempts to delay the onset of the disease upon early detection of symptoms constitute an effective practical strategy. Accordingly, elimination of the abnormal colonic ***H. pylori*** strains responsible for the profuse colonic ammonia toxicity might be the most effective measure among these strategies. In addition, observational findings indicating that eradication of the colonic ***H. pylori*** strains could help improving other factors contributing to Alzheimer such as diabetes, hypertension and dyslipidemia may further support the natural strategy of ***H. pylori*** eradication as a measure to delay Alzheimer and dementia symptoms.

REFERENCES:

1. **Lobo A, Launer LJ, Fratiglioni L, et al.** Prevalence of dementia and major subtypes in Europe: A collaborative study of population-based cohorts. *Neurology 2000; 54: S4-S9.*

2. **Plassman BL, Langa KM, Fisher GG, et al. Prevalence of dementia in the United States: the aging, demographics, and memory study.** *Neuroepidemiology 2007; 29: 125-132.*

3. **Kalaria RN., Maestre GE., Arizaga R., et al. Alzheimer's disease and vascular dementia in developing countries: prevalence, management, and risk factors.** *Lancet Neurol 2008; 7: 812-826.*

4. **Ferri CP, Prince M, Brayne C, et al. Global prevalence of dementia: a Delphi consensus study.** *Lancet 2005; 366: 2112-2117.*

5. **Wimo A, Winblad B, Agüero-Torres H, et al. The magnitude of dementia occurrence in the world.** *Alzheimer Dis Assoc Disord 2003; 17: 63-67.*

6. **Brookmeyer R, Johnson E, Ziegler-Graham K, et al. Forecasting the global burden of Alzheimer's disease.** *Alzheimers Dement 2007; 3: 186-191.*

7. **Fratiglioni L, Launer LJ, Andersen K, et al. Incidence of dementia and major subtypes in Europe: a collaborative study of population-based cohorts.** *Neurology 2000; 54: S10-S15.*

8. **Kawas C, Gray S, Brookmeyer R, et al. Age-specific incidence rates of Alzheimer's disease: the Baltimore Longitudinal Study of Aging.** *Neurology 2000; 54: 2072-2077.*

9. **Kukull WA, Higdon R, Bowen JD, et al. Dementia and Alzheimer disease incidence: a prospective cohort study.** *Arch Neurol 2002; 59: 1737-1746.*

10. **Blennow K, de Leon MJ, Zetterberg H. Alzheimer's disease.** *Lancet 2006; 368: 387-403.*

11. **Helzner EP, Scarmeas N, Cosentino S, et al. Survival in Alzheimer disease: a multiethnic, population-based study of incident cases.** *Neurology 2008; 71: 1489-1495.*

12. **Mehta KM, Yaffe K, Pérez-Stable EJ, et al. Race/ethnic differences in AD survival in US Alzheimer's Disease Centers.** *Neurology 2008; 70: 1163-1170.*

13. Blennow K, de Leon MJ, Zetterberg H. Alzheimer's disease. *Lancet 2006; 368: 387–403.*

14. Aggarwal NT, Bienias JL, Bennett DA, et al. The relation of cigarette smoking to incident Alzheimer's disease in a biracial urban community population. *Neuroepidemiology 2006; 26: 140–146.*

15. Anstey KJ, von Sanden C, Salim A, et al. Smoking as a risk factor for dementia and cognitive decline: a meta-analysis of prospective studies. *Am J Epidemiol 2007; 166: 367–378.*

16. Ding J, Eigenbrodt ML, Mosley T H Jr, et al. Alcohol intake and cerebral abnormalities on magnetic resonance imaging in a community-based population of middle-aged adults: the Atherosclerosis Risk in Communities (ARIC) study. *Stroke 2004; 35: 16–21.*

17. Paul CA, Au R, Fredman L, et al. Association of alcohol consumption with brain volume in the Framingham study. *Arch Neurol 2008; 65: 1363–1367.*

18. Rosengren A, Skoog I, Gustafson D, et al. Body mass index, other cardiovascular risk factors, and hospitalization for dementia. *Arch Intern Med 2005; 165: 321–326.*

19. Fitzpatrick AL, Kuller LH, Lopez OL, et al. Midlife and late-life obesity and the risk of dementia: cardiovascular health study. *Arch Neurol 2009; 66: 336–342.*

20. Kivipelto M, Helkala EL, Laakso MP, et al. Apolipoprotein E Â4 allele, elevated midlife total cholesterol level, and high midlife systolic blood pressure are independent risk factors for late-life Alzheimer disease. *Ann Intern Med 2002; 137: 149–155.*

21. Launer LJ, Ross GW, Petrovitch H, et al. Midlife blood pressure and dementia: the Honolulu-Asia aging study. *Neurobiol Aging. 2000; 21: 49–55.*

22. Kivipelto M, Helkala EL, Laakso MP, et al. Midlife vascular risk factors and Alzheimer's disease in later life: longitudinal, population based study. *BMJ 2001; 322: 1447–1451.*

23. Arvanitakis Z, Wilson RS, Bienias JL, et al. Diabetes mellitus and risk of Alzheimer disease and decline in cognitive function. *Arch Neurol 2004; 61: 661–666.*

24. Irie F, Fitzpatrick AL, Lopez OL, et al. Enhanced risk for Alzheimer disease in persons with type 2 diabetes and APOE e4: the Cardiovascular Health Study Cognition Study. *.Arch Neurol. 2008; 65: 89–93.*

25. Vermeer SE, Prins ND, den Heijer T, et al. Silent brain infarcts and the risk of dementia and cognitive decline. *N Engl J Med 2003; 348: 1215–1222.*

26. Honig LS, Tang MX, Albert S, et al. Stroke and the risk of Alzheimer disease. *Arch Neurol 2003; 60: 1707–1712.*

27. Blum S, Luchsinger JA, Manly JJ, et al. Memory after silent stroke: hippocampus and infarcts both matter. *Neurology 2012 Jan 3; 78 (1): 38-46.*

28. WU YC, Lin YC, YU HL, et al. Association between air pollutants and dementia risk in the elderly. *Alzheimers Dement (Amst) 2015 May 14; 1 (2): 220-8.*

29. Calderón-Garcidueñas L, Calderón-Garcidueñas A, Torres-Jardón R, et al. Air pollution and your brain: what do you need to know right now. *Prim Health Care Res Dev 2015 Jul; 16 (4): 329-45.*

30. Weuve J. Invited commentary: how exposure to air pollution may shape dementia risk, and what epidemiology can say about it. *Am J Epidemiol 2014 Aug 15; 180 (4): 367-71.*

31. Qiu C, Kivipelto M, von Strauss E. Epidemiology of Alzheimer's disease: occurrence, determinants, and strategies toward intervention. *Dialogues Clin Neurosci 2009; 11 (2): 111-28. Review.*

32. Miklossy J. Emerging roles of pathogens in Alzheimer disease. *Expert Rev Mol Med 2011 Sep 20; 13: e30. doi: 10.1017/S1462399411002006.*

33. Malaguarnera M, Bella R, Alagona G, et al. Helicobacter pylori and Alzheimer's disease: a possible link. *Eur J Int Med 2004 Oct; 15 (6): 381-386.*

34. Roubaud Baudron C, Varon C, Mégraud F, et al. Alzheimer's disease and Helicobacter pylori infection: a possible link? *Geriatr Psychol Neuropsychiatr Vieil 2016 Mar; 14 (1): 86-94.*

35. Roubaud Baudron C, Krolak-Salmon P, Quadrio I, et al. Impact of chronic Helicobacter pylori infection on Alzheimer's disease: preliminary results. *Neurobiol Aging 2012 May; 33 (5): 1009. e11-9.* doi: 10.1016/j.neurobiolaging.2011.10.021. Epub 2011 Dec 1.

36. Roubaud Baudron C, Varon C, Mégraud F, et al. Alzheimer's disease: the infectious hypothesis. *Geriatr Psychol Neuropsychiatr Vieil 2015 Dec; 13 (4): 418-24.*

37. Adriani A, Fagoonee S, De Angelis C, et al. Helicobacter pylori infection and dementia: can actual data reinforce the hypothesis of a causal association? *Panminerva Med 2014 Sep; 56 (3): 195-9.*

38. Roubaud Baudron C, Letenneur L, Langlais A, et al. Does Helicobacter pylori infection increase incidence of dementia? The Personnes Agées QUID Study. *J Am Geriatr Soc 2013 Jan; 61 (1): 74-8.*

39. Alvarez-Arellano L, Maldonado-Bernal C. Helicobacter pylori and neurological diseases: Married by the laws of inflammation. *World J Gastrointest Pathophysiol 2014 Nov 15; 5 (4): 400-4.*

40. Farinha P, Gascoyne RD. Helicobacter pylori and MALT Lymphoma. *Gastroenterology 2005 May; 128 (6): 1579-605.*

41. Nasrat AM, Nasrat SAM, Nasrat RM, et al. Misconception and misbehavior towards Helicobacter pylori is leading to major spread of illness. *GM 2015; S1: 002.* [Open Access]

42. Butterworth RF. Pathophysiology of hepatic encephalopathy: a new look at ammonia. *Metab Brain Dis 2002 Dec; 17 (4): 221-7.*

43. Albert MS. Cognitive and neurobiologic markers of early Alzheimer disease. *Proc Natl Acad Sci U S A 1996 Nov 26; 93 (24): 13547-51.*

44. Aguilar MA, Minarro J, Felipo V. Chronic moderate hyperammonemia impairs active and passive avoidance behavior and conditional discrimination learning in rats. *Exp Neurol 2000; 161: 704-713.*

45. **Shukla M, Boontem P, Reiter RJ, et al. Mechanisms of melatonin in alleviating Alzheimer's disease.** *Curr Neuropharmacol 2017 Mar 13.* **doi: 10.2174/1570159X15666170313123454. [Epub ahead of print]**

46. **Andreeva TV, Lukiw WJ, Rogaev EI. Biological Basis for Amyloidogenesis in Alzheimer's Disease.** *Biochemistry (Mosc) 2017 Feb; 82 (2): 122-139.*

47. **Cahill MK, Huang EJ. Testing the Amyloid Hypothesis with a Humanized AD Mouse Model.** *Neuron 2017 Mar 8; 93 (5): 987-989.*

48. **Kosenko EA, Solomadin IN, Tikhonova LA, et al. Pathogenesis of Alzheimer disease: role of oxidative stress, amyloid-β peptides, systemicammonia and erythrocyte energy metabolism.** *CNS Neurol Disord Drug Targets 2014 Feb; 13 (1): 112-9.*

49. **Seiler N. Ammonia and Alzheimer's disease.** *Neurochem Int 2002 Aug-Sep; 41 (2-3): 189-207.*

50. **Seiler N. Is ammonia a pathogenetic factor in Alzheimer's disease?** *Neurochem Res 1993 Mar; 18 (3): 235-45.*

51. **Wright PA. Nitrogen excretion: three end products, many physiological roles.** *J Exp Biol 1995; 198 (2): 273-281.*

52. **Marcaida G, Felipo V, Hermenegildo C, et al. Acute ammonia toxicity is mediated by the NMDA type of glutamate receptors.** *FEBS Lett 1992 Jan 13; 296 (1): 67-8.*

53. **Britto DT, Kronzucker HJ. NH4+ toxicity in higher plants: a critical review. J** *Plant Physiol 2002; 159 (6): 567-584.*

54. **Adlimoghaddam A, Sabbir MG, Albensi BC. Ammonia as a Potential Neurotoxic Factor in Alzheimer's Disease.** *Front Mol Neurosci 2016 Aug 8; 9: 57. doi: 10.3389/fnmol.2016.00057.*

55. **Cooper AJ, Plum F. Biochemistry and physiology of brain ammonia.** *Physiol Rev 1987; 67: 440-519.*

56. **Seglen PO. Inhibitors of lysosomal function.** *Meth Enzymol 1983; 96: 737-764.*

57. **Marcaggi P, Coles JA. Ammonium in nervous tissue: transport across cell membranes, fluxes from neurons to glial cells, and role in signalling.** *Prog Neurobiol 2001; 64: 157-183.*

58. **Laursen H, Diemer NH. Morphometric studies of rat glial cell ultrastructure after urease-induced hyperammonaemia.** *Neuropathol Appl Neurobiol 1979; 5: 345-362.*

59. **Fiorentino M, Sapone A, Senger S, et al. Blood-brain barrier and intestinal epithelial barrier alterations in autism spectrum disorders.** *Mol Autism 2016 Nov 29; 7: 49. eCollection 2016.*

60. **Hrnjez BJ, Song JC, Prasad M, et al. Ammonia blockade of intestinal epithelial K+ conductance.** *Am J Physiol 1999; 277 (3): 521-532.*

61. **Sumii T, Nakano Y, Abe T, et al. The Effect of Nitric Oxide on Ammonia Decomposition**

in Co-cultures of Hepatocytes and Hepatic Stellate Cells. *In Vitro Cell Dev Biol Anim 2016 Jun; 52 (6): 625-31.*

62. Nasrat AM, El-Sayed SM, Shabaka AA, et al. Male pelvic congestion and erectile dysfunction; obscure reasons for an obvious phenomenon among the young. *GM 2016; S1 (1).* [Open Access]

63. Malinski T. Nitric oxide and nitroxidative stress in Alzheimer's disease. *J Alzheimers Dis 2007 May; 11 (2): 207-18.*

64. Hartlage-Rübsamen M, Apelt J, Schliebs R. Fibrillary beta-amyloid deposits are closely associated with atrophic nitric oxide synthase (NOS)-expressing neurons but do not upregulate the inducible NOS in transgenic Tg2576 mouse brain with Alzheimer pathology. *Neurosci Lett 2001 Apr 20; 302 (2-3): 73-6.*

65. Hu ZI, Kotarba AM, Van Nostrand WE. Absence of Nitric Oxide Synthase 3 Increases Amyloid ⬚Protein Pathology in Tg-5xFAD Mice. *Neurosci Med 2013 Jun; 4 (2): 84-91.*

66. Nasrat AM. The world misconception and misbehavior towards Helicobacter pylori is leading to major spread of illness. *The 7th Anti-Aging Medicine World Congress, Monte-Carlo, Monaco, 2009 Mar.* Available from URL, *www.euromedicom.com*

67. Cooper AJ, Plum F. Biochemistry and physiology of brain ammonia. *Physiol Rev 1987; 67: 440-519.*

68. Chang YP, Chiu GF, Kuo FC, et al. Eradication of Helicobacter pylori is associated with the progression of dementia: A population-based study. *Gastroenterol Res Pract 2013; 2013: 175729.* doi: org/10.1155/2013/175729. Epub 2013 Nov 25.

69. Adlimoghaddam A, Sabbir MG, Albensi BC. Ammonia as a potential neurotoxic factor in Alzheimer's disease. *Front Mol Neurosci 2016 Aug 8; 9: 57.* doi: 10.3389/fnmol.2016.00057. eCollection 2016.

70. Nasrat SAM, Nasrat RM, Nasrat MN, et al. The dramatic spread of diabetes mellitus worldwide and influence of Helicobacter pylori. *General Med 2015; 3 (1): 159-62.*

71. Nasrat SAM, Nasrat AM. An alternative approach for the rising challenge of hypertensive illness via Helicobacter pylori eradication. *Cardiol Res 2015; 6 (1): 221-225.* [Open Access] doi: org/10.14740/cr382e

72. Aksoy H, Sebin SO. H. pylori and cardiovascular diseases. *General Med 2015; S1: 1.* [Open Access] doi: org/10.4172/2327-5146.1000S1-007

AUTISM AND ALZHEIMER; THE ETIOPATHOLOGIC TWINS
SCIENTIFIC EVIDENCES ON THE TWIN LINK BETWEEN AUTISM AND ALZHEIMER

*A*utism *and Alzheimer; the etio-pathologic twins; Review Article:* Published in the American Journal of Medicine and Medical Sciences; 2017; 7 (6): 277-280. Nasrat et al. Autism and Alzheimer; the etio-pathologic twins. *Am J Med Med Sci* 2017; 7 (6): 277-280. [doi: 10.5923/j.ajmms.20170706.07]

Abstract: This short review aims at demonstration of the aspects of similarity in etiology and pathology between autism and Alzheimer.

An etio-pathologic similarity exists between autism and Alzheimer's disease; both disorders include obscure etiology and indefinite cure. The toxic influence of abnormal profuse amounts of *Helicobacter pylori*-produced colonic ammonia and the elevated serum ammonia level are constant in both disorders. *H. pylori*, ammonia and nitric oxide constitute a cure and a poison at the same time in both diseases. Colon care/colon clear could be a good clinical measure to avoid development of autism among disadvantaged kids and to delay onset of Alzheimer in susceptible elderly people. It could be considered that autism is the Alzheimer's of kids and Alzheimer is the autism of elderly people.

Key Words: Alzheimer, ammonia, autism, Helicobacter pylori, nitric oxide, senna.

Introduction: Autism is a brain disorder that limits a person's ability to communicate, correlate and relate to other people. It is a series of neuro-developmental disorders that are characterized by deficits in both social and cognitive functions.[1] It first appears in young children who fall along a spectrum from mild to severe presentation. Autism spectrum disorders (ASD) affect about one child in 68, striking nearly five times as many boys as girls.[2,3] While Alzheimer disease (AD) is a chronic, progressive and prevalent neuro-degenerative disease characterized by loss of higher cognitive functions with an associated memory loss. Alzheimer is the most common age-related degenerative disease.[4,5]

It was concluded that genetic and environmental factors could be both responsible for the etiology of ASD. Although epidemiological studies have been conducted to clarify these factors but this conclusion remains unclear.[6,7] Rather similarly, a lot is not well known about Alzheimer's; more than 100 years after its discovery it is still not exactly known what causes this neuro-degenerative disease and an exact cure is still not known.[4,5]

A child with autism remains detached showing loss of the already developed language skills while AD is associated with memory loss.[4,5,8,9] Children with more autistic disorder showed widespread areas of decreased gyrification of the brain.[10,11] White matter impairment, dysplasia with abnormal cortical thinning or decreased cortical thickness have been identified among children with autism.[12-15] Investigator considered that the increased prevalence of identified cases of autism among U.S. children need to be regarded as an urgent public health concern.[6] While on the other way round, AD was first described in a female patient who experienced memory loss, paranoia and psychological changes. Autopsy revealed shrinkage in and around nerve cells in her brain. Cognitive measurement scales allowed to investigate the degree of impairment and estimate the volume of the damaged brain tissue. A National Alzheimer's Disease Genetic Study started in 2003 to hopefully identify risk genes for the disease. In 2010, Alzheimer's was considered the sixth leading cause of death in the United States.[4,5]

The healthy effect of residual ammonia in the gut that is remaining after the protective biological functions of ***Helicobacter pylori***-produced ammonia close to the gut mucosa which is also sharing to maintain a constant systemic serum ammonia level has been emphasized as concerns the integrity of the micro-capillary circulation among all ages including children and elderly people via ensuring the endothelial-derived nitric oxide (NO) liberation according to the effect of shear stress.[16,17] Migration of ***H. pylori*** to the colon under the influence of antibiotics will lead to continuous production of ammonia for a reason or no reason, un-opposed or buffered by any acidity, leading to accumulation of profuse toxic amounts of ammonia and NO toxicity in turn that could lead to adverse toxic effects in the body;[17-19] The healthy value of residual ammonia will turn accordingly into a toxin and the cure becomes a poison.

The symphony of cure and poison played by the bacterium ***H. pylori***, ammonia of ***H. pylori*** and NO of micro-capillary endothelium is being clearly manifested in both autism and Alzheimer; when it deviates towards the toxic poison side because of the antibiotic violence it is standing most probably behind the permanent compromise of some areas of the brain leading to cognitive dysfunction, loss of already developed skills or memory loss.[18,19]

Objective: The aim of this mini review is demonstration of the aspects of similarity in both etiology and pathology between autistic disorder and Alzheimer's disease.

Review: The similarity in etiology and pathogenesis between autism and Alzheimer disease seems rather evidently obvious. Autism is a neuro-developmental disorder with unknown etiology and treatment is obscure until recently. Similarly, Alzheimer disease is a neuro-degenerative disorder with indefinite etiology and all efforts of treatment are only successful in attempting to postpone or delay the symptoms and onset of the disease.[1-7,20,21] Autism is characterized by deficits in social and cognitive functions with loss of already developed skills while AD is a progressive disease characterized by cognitive disorders associated with memory loss.[4,5]

The toxic influence of colonic ammonia produced by the abnormal existence/behavior of colonic ***H. pylori*** strains is the most reasonable pathogenesis behind both autism and Alzheimer as serum ammonia level was found elevated among patients of both disorders to the extent that preservation of the natural structure and existence of ***H. pylori*** was suggested as a good preventive measure towards development of autism and colon clear was found an effective measure to delay the symptoms and onset of Alzheimer if employed at the proper timing.[16,17] The amyloid theory in Alzheimer's disease is greatly accepted but the toxic influence of ammonia in the amyloid disorder is still greatly valid.[22]

Both disorders, ASD and AD, remained for long time without a definite etiology but the ammonia hypothesis is adequately accepted. Autism once established is not a curable disorder or is not a disease of definitive cure due to permanent compromise of the centers of the brain responsible for development of skills but it is a typical disease of definite prevention via natural elimination of the abnormal colonic ***H. pylori*** stains for the mother and the kid particularly at the critical time of child weaning (18-24 month of age) and the strict sanitary measures during serving food to the kid. Prevention is always far better than treatment; accordingly, the challenge of autism could be greatly controlled. Alzheimer in the same way once established is difficult to cure or improve but so long colon clear employing natural measures namely the senna leaves extract purge was found an effective method to postpone or delay the symptoms and onset of the disease particularly if employed at the early critical timing of development of symptoms; accordingly the disease could be readily controlled or prevented by watching the colonic condition and supporting the structure of natural microbiota.[16,17,19] Hence, the symptoms of Alzheimer and dementia should not be considered un-avoidable so long an effective measure to delay the onset and symptoms is becoming available that could in such way render the disease possibly prevented or at least readily controlled.

The concept of cure and poison of *H. pylori*, residual *H. pylori*-produced ammonia close to the gut mucosa and the endothelial-derived NO liberation induced via the effect of shear stress caused by systemic ammonia is perfectly applicable in both disorders; *H. pylori*, ammonia and NO within natural limits constitute cure and protection while beyond natural parameters become poisonous and toxic.[16,17]

Summary: In Summary, the etiopathologic similarity in autism and Alzheimer includes the following characteristics:

1. **Both disorders were leading sufficient time with obscure etiology and indefinite cure.**

2. **Residual levels of ammonia could be healthy towards both conditions.**

3. **The toxic influence of ammonia and its elevated serum level are constant findings in both disorders.**

4. **The influence of the abnormal-behavior/existence colonic *H. pylori* strains is valid in both disorders and is mostly due to antibiotic abuse.**

5. **Both disorders when established could have no chance of cure.**

6. **Both disorders could be typically preventable via employing colon care and colon clear at proper timing.**

Twin similarity between autism and Alzheimer disease does not mean that it is an identical twin similarity as there should be essential differences between them. Autism as example is more prevalent in boys than girls while Alzheimer is more frequent in females than males. According to observational findings that autism could be *H. pylori*-related, it was found in some studies that *H. pylori* in children prevails significantly among boys more than girls which could contribute for explanation of the frequency of autism among boys.[23-25] On the other way, the rate of Alzheimer disease is more in females as elderly females dissociate from the society earlier than males who could maintain a degree of association and socialization for an older age than females, this could constitute a sort of cognitive rehabilitation which could contribute for explanation of the frequency of Alzheimer in females more than males.

Furthermore, autistic disorder could have a fast onset to develop while Alzheimer could take some years to establish; autism is a neuro-developmental disorder occupying the critical timing of development of centers responsible for skills during early chilhood,[16] toxins could compromise these developing centers in a short duration and hence affecting their development faster. While Alzheimer is a neuro-degenerative disease affecting already developed brain centers among adults,[17] degeneration of these centers is a slower process needing therefore some years to establish.

Conclusion: The twin similarity between autism and Alzheimer in etiology and pathology is clearly obvious; both of them are of indefinite etiology and cure. Both disorders are ideal examples for the concept of cure when it turns a poison to be applied for them; namely *H. pylori*, ammonia and NO. It might be accordingly considered that autism is the Alzheimer's of kids and Alzheimer is the autism of elderly people.

REFERENCES:

1. **Li Q, Zhou JM.** The microbiota-gut-brain axis and its potential therapeutic role in autism spectrum disorder. *Neuroscience 2016 Jun 2; 324: 131-9.*

2. **Woolfenden S, Eapen V, Jalaludin B, et al. Prevalence and factors associated with parental concerns about development detected by the Parents' Evaluation of**

Developmental Status (PEDS) at 6-month, 12-month and 18-month well-child checks in a birth cohort. *BMJ 2016 Sep 8; 6 (9): e012144.*

3. Baio J. Prevalence of autism spectrum disorders - Autism and Developmental Disabilities Monitoring Network, United States, 2006. *MMWR Surveill Summ 2009 Dec 18; 58 (10): 1-20.*

4. Lobo A, Launer LJ, Fratiglioni L, et al. Prevalence of dementia and major subtypes in Europe: A collaborative study of population-based cohorts. *Neurology 2000; 54: S4-S9.*

5. Plassman BL, Langa KM, Fisher GG, et al. Prevalence of dementia in the United States: the aging, demographics, and memory study. *Neuroepidemiology 2007; 29: 125-132.*

6. Galichi F, Ghaemmaghami J, Malek A, et al. Effect of gluten free diet on gastrointestinal and behavioral indices for children with autism spectrum disorders: a randomized clinical trial. *World J Pediatr 2016 Jun 10; 26 (12): 1936-9. [Epub ahead of print]*

7. Kiely B, Vettam S, Adesman A. Utilization of genetic testing among children with developmental disabilities in the United States. *Appl Clin Genet 2016 Jul 11; 9: 93-100. eCollection 2016.*

8. Allen DA. Autistic spectrum disorders: clinical presentation in preschool children. *J Child Neurol 1988; 3Suppl: S48-56.*

9. Emberti Gialloreti L, Benvenuto A, Battan B, et al. Can biological components predict short-term evolution in Autism Spectrum Disorders? A proof-of-concept study. *Ital J Pediatr 2016 Jul 22; 42 (1): 70.*

10. Richter J, Henze R, Vomstein K, et al. Reduced cortical thickness and its association with social reactivity in children with autismspectrum disorder. *Psychiatry Res 2015 Oct 30; 234 (1): 15-24. Epub 2015 Aug 22.*

11. Blanken LM, Mous SE, Ghassabian A, et al. Cortical morphology in 6- to 10-year old children with autistic traits: a population-based neuroimaging study. *Am J Psychiatry 2015 May; 172 (5): 479-86. Epub 2015 Jan 13.*

12. Peeva MG, Tourville JA, Agam Y, et al. White matter impairment in the speech network of individuals with autism spectrum disorder. *Neuroimage 2013 Aug 28; 3: 234-41. eCollection 2013.*

13. Casanova MF, El-Baz AS, Kamat SS, et al. Focal cortical dysplasias in autism spectrum disorders. *Acta Neuropathol Commun 2013 Oct 11; 1: 67. Doi: 10.1186/2051.5960.1.67.*

14. Misaki M, Wallace GL, Dankner N, et al. Characteristic cortical thickness patterns in adolescents with autism spectrum disorders: interactions with age and intellectual ability revealed by canonical correlation analysis. *Neuroimage 2012 Apr 15; 60 (3): 1890-901. Epub 2012 Feb 3.*

15. Chiang HL, Chen YJ, Lin HY, et al. Disorder-Specific Alteration in White Matter Structural Property in Adults With Autism Spectrum Disorder Relative to Adults With A DHD and Adult Controls. *Hum Brain Mapp 2016 Sep 15y. doi: 10.1002/hbm.23367. [Epub ahead of print]*

16. **Nasrat AM, Nasrat RM, Nasrat MM. Autism; an approach for definite etiology and definitive etiologic management.** *Am J Med Med Sci 2017; 7 (3): 108-118.* **[Open Access]**

17. **Nasrat AM, Nasrat RM, Nasrat MM. Alzheimer and Helicobacter pylori; should we fight and kill or save H. pylori!! We should save H. pylori.** *Am J Med Med Sci 2017; 7 (5): 221-228.* **[Open Access]**

18. **Farinha P, Gascoyne RD. Helicobacter pylori and MALT Lymphoma.** *Gastroenterology 2005 May; 128 (6): 1579-605.*

19. **Nasrat AM, Nasrat SAM, Nasrat RM, et al. Misconception and misbehavior towards Helicobacter pylori is leading to major spread of illness.** *GM 2015; S1: 002.* **[Open Access]**

20. **Aguilar MA, Minarro J, Felipo V. Chronic moderate hyperammonemia impairs active and passive avoidance behavior and conditional discrimination learning in rats.** *Exp Neurol 2000; 161: 704-713.*

21. **Seiler N. Is ammonia a pathogenetic factor in Alzheimer's disease?** *Neurochem Res 1993 Mar; 18 (3): 235-45.*

22. **Kosenko EA, Solomadin IN, Tikhonova LA, et al. Pathogenesis of Alzheimer disease: role of oxidative stress, amyloid-☒ peptides, systemic ammonia and erythrocyte energy metabolism.** *CNS Neurol Disord Drug Targets 2014 Feb; 13 (1): 112-9.*

23. **Hestvik E, Tylleskar T, Kaddu-Mulindwa DH, et al. Helicobacter pylori in apparently healthy children aged 0-12 years in urban Kampala, Uganda: a community-based cross sectional survey.** *BMC Gastroenterol 2010 Jun 16; 10 (62).* **doi: 10.1186/1471-230X-10-62.**

24. **Leandro Liberato SV, Hernández Galindo M, Torroba Alvarez L, et al. Helicobacter pylori infection in the child population in Spain: prevalence, related factors and influence on growth.** *Ann Pediatr (Barc) 2005 Dec; 63 (6): 489-94.* **[Open Access]**

25. **Ndip RN, Malange AE, Akoachere JF, et al. Helicobacter pylori antigens in the faeces of asymptomatic children in the Buea and Limbe health districts of Cameroon: a pilot study.** *Trop Med Int Health 2004; 9 (9): 1036-1040.*

FREQUENCY OF LEUKEMIA DURING LATE DECADES MAY INDICATE THAT THE ANTI-HELICOBACTER PYLORI ANTIBIOTIC STRATEGY WAS A THERPEUTIC MISTAKE

Does Leukemia in Late Decades Constitute an Influenza!!

Itroduction: While cancer has been long recognized as a disease of the genome, the importance of epigenetic mechanisms in neoplasms was acknowledged more recently. Leukemia was first described in 1827, a more detailed description was given by a pathologist in 1845. Around ten years after, it was concluded that a bone marrow problem was responsible for the abnormal blood of leukemia patients.[1-4]

By year 1900, leukemia was considered as a family of diseases not a single disease. The cause for most cases of leukemia is unknown; different types of leukemia likely do have different causes. Both inherited and environmental (non-inherited) factors are believed to be involved.[1,2,5,6]

In 2012, leukemia developed in 352.000 people globally and caused 265.000 deaths. It is the most common type of cancer in children, with three quarters of leukemia cases in children being the acute lymphoblastic type. However, about 90% of all leukemias are diagnosed in adults, with acute myeloid leukemia and chronic lymphocytic leukemia being most common in adults. It occurs more commonly in the developed world.[1,2,7]

Prognosis and success of treatment depend on type of leukemia and age of the patient; outcomes of treatment have improved in the developed world while the five-years survival rate is variable in different countries.[2,8,9]

Near 1947, it was believed that a folic acid mimic could potentially cure leukemia in children. The majority of children with acute lymphoblastic leukemia showed signs of improvement in their bone marrow, but none of them was actually cured. In 1962, a combination chemotherapy was tested to attempt leukemia cure, the tests were successful with some patients surviving long after the tests;[10,11]

Helicobacter pylori could migrate or get forced to migrate to the colon under the influence of antibiotic violence where it will continue producing ammonia for a reason or no reason, unopposed or buffered by any acidity leading to accumulation of profuse toxic amounts of ammonia in the colon;[12,13] these excess amounts of ammonia could lead to adverse toxic effects in the body.

The motive of this study was a striking observation which attracted the attention of the research investigators of the study. In addition to the prevalence of the abnormal-behavior ***H. pylori*** stains and their direct relation to many medical challenges, it was observed that two cases of leukemia which were proved by blood count and bone marrow biopsy, have been cured spontaneously simply due to movement to a different environment for just three weeks; true leukemia is not known to improve fast as such even under medications.

<u>*REFERENCES:*</u>

1. **McGuire S.** World Cancer Report 2014. Geneva, Switzerland: World Health Organization, International Agency for Research on Cancer, WHO Press, 2015. *Adv Nutr 2016 Mar 15; 7 (2): 418-9.*

2. **Reddy A, Vidal M, de la Cruz M, et al. Snapshot of an acute palliative care unit in a tertiary cancer hospital.** *Palliat Support Care 2014 Aug; 12 (4): 331-7.*

3. **Tzelepis F, Rose SK, Sanson-Fisher RW, et al. Are we missing the Institute of Medicine's mark? A systematic review of patient-reported outcome measures assessing quality of patient-centred cancer care.** *BMC Cancer 2014 Jan 25; 14: 41. doi: 10.1186/1471.2407.14.41.*

4. **Kazandjian D. Multiple myeloma epidemiology and survival: A unique malignancy.** *Semin Oncol 2016 Dec; 43 (6): 676-681.*

5. **Ross JA, Kasum CM, Davies SM, et al. Diet and risk of leukemia in the Iowa Women's Health Study.** *Cancer Epidemiol Biomarkers Prev 2002 Aug; 11 (8): 777-81.*

6. **Boniol M, Koechlin A, Sorahan T, et al. Cancer incidence in cohorts of workers in the rubber manufacturing industry first employed since 1975 in the UK and Sweden.** *Occup Environ Med 2017 Jan 6. doi: 10.1136/oemed.2016.103989. [Epub ahead of print]*

7. **Arun AK, Senthamizhselvi A, Mani S, et al. Frequency of rare BCR-ABL1 fusion transcripts in chronic myeloid leukemia patients.** *Int J Lab Hematol 2016 Dec 29. Doi: 10.1111/ijlh.12616. [Epub ahead of print]*

8. **Kang MH, Smith MA, Morton CL, et al. National Cancer Institute pediatric preclinical testing program: model description for in vitro cytotoxicity testing.** *Pediatr Blood Cancer 2011 Feb; 56 (2): 239-49.*

9. **Weiss NS. Use of acetaminophen in relation to the occurrence of cancer: a review of epidemiologic studies.** *Cancer Causes Control 2016 Dec; 27 (12): 1411-1418. Epub 2016 Nov 10.*

10. **Patlak M.** *Targeting leukemia: From bench to bedside.* *FASEB J 2002 Mar; 16 (3): 273.*

11. **Navada SC, Silverman LR. Safety and efficacy of azacitidine in elderly patients with intermediate to high-risk myelodysplastic syndromes.** *Ther Adv Hematol 2005 May; 128 (6): 1579-605.*

12. **Farinha P, Gascoyne RD. Helicobacter pylori and MALT Lymphoma.** *Gastroenterology 2005 May; 128 (6): 1579-605.*

13. **Nasrat AM, Nasrat SAM, Nasrat RM, et al. Misconception and misbehavior towards Helicobacter pylori is leading to major spread of illness.** *Gen Med 2015; S1: 002.* **[Open Access]**

SCIENTIFIC EVIDENCES ON THE RISK CAUSED BY THE ANTI-HELICOBACTER PYLORI ANTIBIOTICS ON THE FREQUENCY OF LEUKEMIA DURING LATE DECADES

Frequency of Leukemia May Indicate that the Anti-Helicobacter Pylori Antibiotic Strategy was a Therapeutic Mistake. Published in the American Journal of Medicine and Medical Sciences; 2017; 7 (3): 103-107. Nasrat et al. Frequency of leukemia during late decades may indicate that the anti-Helicobacter pylori antibiotic strategy was a therapeutic mistake. *Am J Med Med Sci 2017; 7 (3): 103-107.* *[doi: 10.5923/j.ajmms.20170703.03]*

Background: Leukemia is considered as a family of diseases not a single disease. The cause for most types of leukemia is unknown; different types of leukemia are likely to have different causes. It is the most common type of cancer in children; however, about 90% of all leukemias are diagnosed in adults. Prognosis and success of treatment depend on type of leukemia and age of the patient; outcomes of treatment have improved in the developed world while the five-years survival rate is variable in different countries.[1-7]

In 2012, leukemia developed in 352.000 people globally and caused 265.000 deaths. It is the most common type of cancer in children, with three quarters of leukemia cases in children being the acute lymphoblastic type. However, about 90% of all leukemias are diagnosed in adults, with acute myeloid leukemia and chronic lymphocytic leukemia being most common in adults. It occurs more commonly in the developed world.[8-11]

Helicobacter pylori could migrate or get forced to migrate to the colon under the influence of antibiotics where it will continue producing ammonia for a reason or no reason, unopposed or buffered by any acidity leading to accumulation of profuse toxic amounts of ammonia in the colon with consequent initiation of a biological toxic stress to the body. This toxic stress condition could be expressed by the bone marrow as a toxic invasion to the body exciting the bone marrow to produce excess defensive white cells and hence, the development of a potential picture of leukemia.[12-13]

Objective: Demonstration of ***H. pylori*** as a recent pathological reason behind the rising figures of leukemia in developing countries during last three decades.

Design & Setting: A Multiple-case clinical study which has been done in Jeddah/Saudi Arabia between May 2014 and October 2015.

Patients & Methods: The study included seven patients with frank long history of dyspepsia at different stages of different types of leukemia (two myeloid, four lymphoblastic and one lymphocytic). Those patients were actually seeking a second opinion consultation of an alternative therapy for their condition after the diagnosis and strategy of treatment was already established. They were males with age range between 23-33 years except one female patient aged 70 years. Two male patients were suffering acute myeloid leukemia with leucocytic count range of 42.000-44.000/Cmm at inclusion of the study. Four male patients were suffering lymphoblstic leukemia with total leucocytic count ranging between 45.000-88.000/Cmm on admission in a healthcare center or at inclusion of the study. The female patient was suffering a neglected case of lymphocytic leukemia with leucocytic count of 120.000/Cmm, her hemoglobin was 9 gm/dl and platelet count was 6.000/Cmm with many bleeding incidents. Patients were mostly under care of skilled qualified healthcare centers. They were investigated for existence of colonic **H. pylori** strains by a specific test (**H. pylori** fecal antigen test). Colon clear using the natural senna leaves extract purge was advised for natural eradication of **H. pylori** from the colon for patients with positive fecal antigen test.[12,13] Patients were advised to follow up strictly with their treating oncologists.

Results: All patients were found positive for existence of colonic **H. pylori** strains; it was strongly positive in four patients (three males and the female patient), colon clear was done for them. There was no chance or no need to employ colon clear for the other three male patients whose fecal antigen test was found weakly positive; spontaneous elimination of toxins from the colon has possibly occurred due to moving to the healthy hospital atmosphere with consequent avoidance of the bad habit of misbehavior in outside-home meals.

Two males with myeloid leukemia achieved normal leucocytic count without myeloid cells after colon clear; one has reached a leucocytic count of 3.800/Cmm in three weeks after colon clear while the other has reached 5.400/Cmm in two weeks after colon clear. One male patient with lymphoblastic leukemia (45.000/Cmm) has reached a normal leucocytic count of 6.700/Cmm without lymphoblasts in two weeks after colon clear. The total leucocytic count of the female patient dropped from 120.000/Cmm to 90.000/Cmm just in two days after colon clear before she died one day later because of deterioration of her general condition.

The leucocytic count of the other three males with lymphoblastic leukemia reached a normal level after two-three weeks of observation in hospital and intake of a single dose of combination therapy without employing colon clear possibly because of spontaneous clearance of the colonic toxins upon moving to the healthy hospital atmosphere and intake of healthy meals. In one of them, the leucocytic count dropped from 66.000/Cmm to 1.800/Cmm in three weeks following intake of a single dose of combination therapy taken near end of the third week of hospital stay, while the second patient with total leucocytic count 88.000/Cmm on admission has reached a leucocytic count of 7.200/Cmm just in two weeks with intake of a single dose of combination therapy shortly after admission. The third patient with leucocytic count of 76.000/Cmm on admission in hospital reached a count of 5.800/Cmm after three weeks of hospital stay and one dose of combination therapy taken few days after admission.

Patients were followed up for their colonic condition and recurrence of leukemia around 12-16 months. They were also advised to follow up strictly with their treating oncologists during the same period. Patients included in this study were not selected cases; they were just the seven consecutive patients during a particular period who have requested a second opinion of an alternative therapy for their illness.

Recurrence was not shown during the first six months after recovery as concerns the six male patients; serious carefulness towards their meals was of course expected. Recurrence occurred once or twice between the ninth and eleventh month for the six male patients possibly because of negligence towards their meals and their colonic condition. All recurrences were mild and improved smoothly within 1-2 weeks after colon clear.

The individual analysis of patients and their results might be useful as being illustrative and it is as follows:

First patient was a young male 23 years old with frank history of dyspepsia due to frequent outside-home meals. He was diagnosed as acute myeloid leukemia with leucocytic count of 55.000/Cmm, he was under combination therapy by a National Guard healthcare center. His leucocytic count became 52.000/Cmm at end of first week of therapy, 49.000/Cmm at end of second week, 47.000/Cmm at the end of third week and 44.000/Cmm at the end of the fourth week. He was confirmed positive for colonic **H. pylori** strains and colon clear was done for him in the middle of the fifth week of therapy. Leucoctyic count dropped from 44.000/Cmm to 21.000/Cmm in three days after colon clear, the leucocytic count further dropped to 7.000/Cmm with residual myeloid cells one week after, and the leucocytic count became just 3.800/Cmm without myeloid cells after further two weeks.

Second patient was a young male 25 years old, military soldier having most of his meals according to the kitchen routine of the military unit. He was diagnosed as lymphoblastic leukemia with leucocytic count 66.000/Cmm and he was in care of a National Guard hospital. He was under careful observation in the hospital for three weeks after bone marrow confirmation of his diagnosis then he was given a first dose of combination therapy where his leucocytic count dropped suddenly to 1.800/Cmm. Medications were ceased, patient was isolated from reasons of cross infection, while repeat bone marrow examination revealed a normal picture. Colon clear was not needed for this patient.

Third patient was a young male 30 years old with frank history of dyspepsia due to frequent fast food meals, he was diagnosed by a specialized research and healthcare center as lymphoblastic leukemia with leucocytic count 88.000/Cmm.

He was staying in the hospital for observation as the leucocytic count was dropping after a single dose of combination therapy; his leucocytic count reached a normal figure (7.200/Cmm without lymphoblastic cells) in two weeks. Colon clear was not employed for this patient.

Fourth patient was a young male 28 years old with frank history of dyspepsia due to frequent outside-home meals, he was diagnosed as acute myeloid leukemia with leucocytic count of 49.000/Cmm and he was under combination therapy by a national guard hospital. His leucocytic count dropped to 42.000/Cmm after three weeks of therapy.

After colon clear which was done in the beginning of the fourth week, the leucocytic count became normal in two weeks (5.400/Cmm without myeloid cells).

Fifth patient was a young male 27 years old, military soldier having most of his meals in the military unit. He was diagnosed as lymphoblastic leukemia with total leucocytic count of 45.000/Cmm, he was under care of a military hospital and he was scheduled for observation and follow up for two weeks as an outpatient before admission for commencing therapy.

Colon Clear was employed for him with dramatic improvement of his blood count as repeat blood count on admission two weeks after colon clear revealed a normal picture (leucocytic count 6.700/Cmm without lymphoblastic cells), revision of bone marrow biopsy confirmed recovery of his condition.

Sixth patient was a young male 33 years old with frank history of dyspepsia due to frequent fast food meals, he was diagnosed by a specialized research and healthcare center as having lymphoblastic leukemia with leucocytic count 76.000/Cmm.

He has been kept in hospital under watchful waiting for three weeks after the first dose of therapy according to the policy of the healthcare center. It was noticed that his leucocytic count was dropping until it reached 5.800/Cmm without any further medications. Colon clear was not done for this patient.

Seventh patient was a female aged 70 years with a neglected condition of lymphocytic leukemia, at inclusion in the study her leucocytic count was 120.000/Cmm, hemoglobin was 9 gm/dl, platelet count was 6.000/Cmm with many bleeding incidents. She was under care of a private general hospital for enough time then she was discharged because of inability to afford the hospital bill and she was scheduled next day for admission in a university hospital for blood and platelet transfusion before starting chemotherapy.

She was receiving quite inadequate medications because of financial reasons. Colon clear was done for her immediately before admission in the university hospital, the blood count done two days later showed drop of total leucocytic count to 90.000/Cmm. Sadly, this poor patient died on the third day in hospital due to heart failure secondary to bleeding events and severe anemia.

Ethical Considerations: An informed signed consent was taken from all patients, they were made aware about safety of the natural colon clear; they were free to quit participation in the study whenever they like. Patients were advised to follow strictly their own medications according to the strategy of their healthcare providers. Patients were allowed to follow their own style of life if they are outpatients except restriction of outside-home meals or the routine of hospital ward if they are inpatients. The research proposal was approved and the study followed the rules of the Research Ethics Committee.

Discussion: There is no single known cause for the different types of leukemia; the few known causes which are not generally factors account for few cases. Leukemia, like any other cancer can result from mutations in the DNA. Certain mutations can trigger leukemia by activating oncogenes or deactivating tumour suppressor genes hence, disrupting the regulation of cell death, cell differentiation or division. These mutations may occur spontaneously or because of exposure to radiation or carcinogenic substances. Diet has got very limited or no effect, although eating more vegetables may confer a small protective benefit.[5,14] Different risk factors could further include smoking, ionizing radiation, direct chemical exposure and prior chemotherapy.[1,15,16]

Clinical symptoms may include fever, easy fatigue, bruising problems and bleeding. Diagnosis is usually based on clinical symptoms, repeated blood counts and bone marrow biopsy, lymph node biopsy could be performed to diagnose certain types of leukemia in some situations. There are four main types of leukemia; acute lymphoblastic leukemia, acute myeloid leukemia, chronic lymphocytic leukemia and chronic myeloid leukemia in addition to a number of less common types. Three quarters of leukemia cases in children are being the acute lymphoblastic type while acute myeloid leukemia and chronic lymphocytic leukemia are being the most common in adults. Despite diagnostic methods many people may not be diagnosed as many symptoms could be vague, non-specific or misleading to other diseases. For this reason, one-fifth of the people with leukemia may remain undiagnosed for sometime as blood tests occasionally may not show that a person has leukemia specially in the early stages of the disease or during remission.[1,2,17]

Treatment of leukemia may involve combination of chemotherapy, radiation therapy and bone marrow transplant in addition to supportive and palliative care. Outcomes of treatment depend on whether leukemia is acute which is generally more severe versus chronic, the specific abnormal white cell type, stage of progression of the disease, the grade of tissue abnormality, the presence of metastasis, lymph node involvement, bone marrow infiltration and the skills of the healthcare team. The average five-year survival is 57% in the United States; in children under 15, the five-year survival is greater than 60-85% depending on the type of leukemia. Children with acute leukemia who are cancer-free after five years, cancer is unlikely to return.[1,2,8,18-23]

Migration of ***H. pylori*** to the colon might cause accumulation of profuse toxic amounts of ammonia in the colon leading to a biological toxic stress to the body;[13,24-26] this toxic influence could be either directly expressed by the bone marrow or translated by the defensive mechanisms as a toxic invasion to the body exciting the bone marrow to produce excess defensive white cells and hence, the developing picture of leukemia in such situation should not be considered an established chronic illness but could be carefully watched and treated as a potential condition related to a temporary underlying pathologic reason. The exaggerated compensatory defensive behavior of the bone marrow could be therefore absolutely corrected by elimination of the underlying pathology as verified by the results of this study.

The fast improvement after colon clear compared to the slow response to the combination therapy was attributed in this study to elimination of the potential toxins from the colon. While the drop of the leucocytic count of the patients who did not employ the senna purge was explained in the study by the patient's movement to the healthy hospital environment and intake of healthy meals allowing spontaneous elimination of most of the colonic toxins below its pathologic level. This suggested spontaneous clearance of the colon from its toxins due to moving to a healthy atmosphere with healthy dieting might support a concept of colonic toxins-induced onset of leukemia among disadvantaged population. The miserable female patient, in spite of her deteriorated general condition, her circulation got rid of 30.000 bad white cells/Cmm without real therapy in just two days after colon clear; a matter that could support the concept of the influence of accumulated ***H. pylori***-produced colonic toxins in inducing leukemia in susceptible predisposed individuals and the role of the natural senna purge in the management of the resulting potential leukemic condition through elimination of colonic toxins.

Leukemia as many diseases could be falsely misdiagnosed or undiagnosed and although observation and watchful waiting is one of the early lines of certain types of newly discovered leukemia therapy,[1] but an established leukemia with confirmed diagnosis after repeated blood count and bone marrow biopsy is not expected to vanish spontaneously in such a short period of time. In accordance, the leukemic patients encountered in this study were considered to suffer a potential condition induced by a temporary toxic influence; otherwise they would not improve simply after moving to a healthier environment or following elimination of the colonic toxins via natural colon clear.

Conclusion: Colonic ***H. pylori*** strains could be responsible for a considerable figure of leukemia spread among developing countries during last three decades which could be considered a compensatory response to the biological toxic influence related to ***H. pylori***-produced ammonia in excess amounts in the colon. ***H. pylori*** antibiotic eradication therapies might require detailed revision and further accurate re-determination. Newly discovered leukemia patients with frank ***H. pylori*** dyspepsia could be given a chance of adequate close observation until spontaneous cure is achieved via colon clear employing natural measures. Those patients with colonic ***H. pylori***-induced leukemia should be considered susceptible predisposed disadvantaged individuals liable for recurrence; hence, they should watch their meals and colonic condition.

Conflict of Interest: There is no conflict of interest existing.

REFERENCES:

1. **McGuire S.** World Cancer Report 2014. Geneva, Switzerland: World Health Organization, International Agency for Research on Cancer, WHO Press, 2015. *Adv Nutr 2016 Mar 15; 7 (2): 418-9.*

2. **Reddy A, Vidal M, de la Cruz M, et al. Snapshot of an acute palliative care unit in a tertiary cancer hospital.** *Palliat Support Care 2014 Aug; 12 (4): 331-7.*

3. **Tzelepis F, Rose SK, Sanson-Fisher RW, et al. Are we missing the Institute of Medicine's mark? A systematic review of patient-reported outcome measures assessing quality of patient-centred cancer care.** *BMC Cancer 2014 Jan 25; 14: 41. doi: 10.1186/1471.2407.14.41.*

4. **Kazandjian D. Multiple myeloma epidemiology and survival: A unique malignancy.** *Semin Oncol 2016 Dec; 43 (6): 676-681.*

5. **Ross JA, Kasum CM, Davies SM, et al. Diet and risk of leukemia in the Iowa Women's Health Study.** *Cancer Epidemiol Biomarkers Prev 2002 Aug; 11 (8): 777-81.*

6. **Boniol M, Koechlin A, Sorahan T, et al. Cancer incidence in cohorts of workers in the rubber manufacturing industry first employed since 1975 in the UK and Sweden.** *Occup Environ Med 2017 Jan 6. doi: 10.1136/oemed.2016.103989. [Epub ahead of print]*

7. **Arun AK, Senthamizhselvi A, Mani S, et al. Frequency of rare BCR-ABL1 fusion transcripts in chronic myeloid leukemia patients.** *Int J Lab Hematol 2016 Dec 29. Doi: 10.1111/ijlh.12616. [Epub ahead of print]*

8. **8. Kang MH, Smith MA, Morton CL, et al. National Cancer Institute pediatric preclinical testing program: model description for in vitro cytotoxicity testing.** *Pediatr Blood Cancer 2011 Feb; 56 (2): 239-49.*

9. **Weiss NS. Use of acetaminophen in relation to the occurrence of cancer: a review of epidemiologic studies.** *Cancer Causes Control 2016 Dec; 27 (12): 1411-1418. Epub 2016 Nov 10.*

10. **Patlak M.** *Targeting leukemia: From bench to bedside. FASEB J 2002 Mar; 16 (3): 273.*

11. **Navada SC, Silverman LR. Safety and efficacy of azacitidine in elderly patients with intermediate to high-risk myelodysplastic syndromes.** *Ther Adv Hematol 2005 May; 128 (6): 1579-605.*

12. **Farinha P, Gascoyne RD. Helicobacter pylori and MALT Lymphoma.** *Gastroenterology 2005 May; 128 (6): 1579-605.*

13. **Nasrat AM, Nasrat SAM, Nasrat RM, et al. Misconception and misbehavior towards Helicobacter pylori is leading to major spread of illness.** *Gen Med 2015; S1: 002.* **[Open Access]**

14. **Radivoyevitch T, Sachs RK, Gale RP, et al. Defining AML and MDS second cancer risk dynamics after diagnoses of first cancers treated or not with radiation.** *Leukemia 2016 Feb; 30 (2): 285-94. doi: 10.1038/leu.2015.258. Epub 2015 Sep 22.*

15. **Hutter JJ. Childhood leukemia.** *Pediatr Rev 2010 Jun; 31 (6): 234-41. doi: 10.1542/ pir.31.6.234*

16. **Ganguly BB, Dolai TK, De R, et al. Spectrum of complex chromosomal aberrations in a myelodysplastic syndrome and a brief review.** *J Cancer Res Ther 2016 Jul-Sep; 12 (3): 1203-1206. doi: 10.4103/0973.1482.197563.*

17. **Faderl S, O'Brien S, Pui CH, et al. Adult acute lymphoblastic leukemia: concepts and strategies.** *Cancer 2010 Mar 1; 116 (5): 1165-76. doi: 10.1002/cancr.24862.*

18. **Zaorsky NG, Williams GR, Barta SK, et al. Splenic irradiation for splenomegaly: A systematic review.** *Cancer Treat Rev 2016 Dec 22; 53: 47-52. [Epub ahead of print]*

19. **van Dalen EC, Raphael MF, Caron HN, et al. Treatment including anthracyclines versus treatment not including anthracyclines for childhood cancer.** *Cochrane Datbase Syst Rev 2014 Sep 4; (9): CD006647. doi: 10.1002/14651858.CD006647.pub4.*

20. **Bak M, Ibfelt EH, Stauffer Larsen T, et al. The Danish National Chronic Myeloid Neoplasia Registry.** *Clin Epidemiol 2016 Oct 25; 8: 567-572. eCollection 2016.*

21. **da Cunha-Bang C, Geisler CH, Enggaard L, et al. The Danish National Chronic Lymphocytic Leukemia Registry.** *Clin Epidemiol 2016 Oct 25; 8: 561-565. eCollection 2016.*

22. **Østgard LS, Nørgaard JM, Raschou-Jensen KK, et al. The Danish National Acute Leukemia Registry.** *Clin Epidemiol 2016 Oct 25; 8: 553-560. eCollection 2016.*

23. **Schrøder H, Rechnitzer C, Wehner PS, et al. Danish Childhood Cancer Registry.** *Clin Epidemiol 2016 Oct 25; 8: 461-464. eCollection 2016.*

24. **Nasrat SAM, Nasrat RM, Nasrat MN, et al. The dramatic spread of diabetes mellitus worldwide and influence of Helicobacter pylori.** *General Med. 2015; 3 (1): 159-62.*

25. **Nasrat RM, Nasrat MM, Nasrat AM, et al. Improvement of idiopathic cardiomyopathy after colon clear.** *J Cardiol Res 2015 Apr; 6 (2): 249-254. doi: org/10.14740/cr398c.* **[Open Access]**

26. **Nasrat AM, Nasrat SAM, Nasrat RM, et al. The challenge of childhood diabetes.** *Gen Med 2015; 3: 4. doi: org/10.4172/2327-5146.1000193.*

A PATHOLOGIC ETIOLOGY FOR THE RISING WORLD CHALLENGE OF OBESITY AND DYSLIPIDEMIA DURING LATEST THREE DECADES
Dyslipidemia was the Fake of Last Century

Introduction: Obesity constitutes a serious global health concern reaching pandemic prevalence rates. Obesity is a quite significant major risk factor for many diseases and is considered an economic complicating factor, it is becoming a common health problem in the United States. Obesity has got its impact on the short/long-term survival and major adverse cardiovascular events; obese patients have lower free survival because of increased incidence of congestive heart failure.[1-3] Childhood obesity prevalence has tripled over the last three decades. Pediatric obesity has got important implications on both child and adult health. It is an economic burden in the United States as well. Professionals should find ways to involve children in various sports settings and policies as well as helping obese children to engage more in sports.[4,5]

Cardiovascular disease (CVD) has become a concerning health problem because of its increasing prevalence. CVD remains the most common health problem in developed countries and the residual risk after implementing all the current therapies is still high. Changing demographics and lifestyles over the past few decades have resulted in an epidemic of the atherogenic dyslipidemia complex.[6,7] In most clinical trials it was found that the reduction of LDL-cholesterol (LDL-C) reduces the incidence of cardiovascular events by approximately one third meaning that a sizeable "residual risk" remains. In the last decade, the importance of HDL-cholesterol (HDL-C) was overvalued while the importance of triglycerides (TG) has been underestimated.[8]

REFERENCES:

1. **Sakellariou P, Valente A, Carrillo AE, et al.** Chronic l-menthol-induced browning of white adipose tissue hypothesis: A putative therapeutic regime for combating obesity and improving metabolic health. *Med Hypotheses 2016 Aug; 93: 21-6.*

2. **Moretti E, Gonnelli S, Campagna M, et al. Influence of Helicobacter pylori infection on metabolic parameters and body composition of dyslipidemic patients.** *Intern Emerg Med. 2014 Oct; 9 (7): 767-72.*

3. **Aksoy H, Sebin SO. H. pylori and cardiovascular disease.** *Gen Med 2015; S1: 1.* **[Open Access]**

4. **Parikh Y, Mason M, Williams K. Researchers' perspectives pediatric obesity research participant recruitment.** *Clin Transl Med 2016 Dec; 5 (1): 20. Epub 2016 Jun 23.*

5. **Lee JE, Pope Z, Gao Z. The Role of Youth Sports in Promoting Children's Physical Activity and Preventing Pediatric Obesity: A Systematic Review.** *Behav Med 2016 Jun 23: 0. [Epub ahead of print]*

6. **Jolfaie NR, Rouhani MH, Surkan PJ, et al. Rice Bran Oil Decreases Total and LDL Cholesterol in Humans: A Systematic Review and Meta-Analysis of Randomized Controlled Clinical Trials.** *Horm Metab Res 2016 Jun 16. [Epub ahead of print]*

7. **Xiao C, Dash S, Morgantini C, et al. Pharmacological Targeting of the Atherogenic Dyslipidemia Complex: The Next Frontier in CVD Prevention Beyond Lowering LDL Cholesterol.** *Diabetes 2016 Jul; 65 (7): 1767-78.*

8. **Grammer T, Kleber M, Silbernagel G, et al. Residual risk: The roles of triglycerides and high density lipoproteins.** *Dutsch Med Wochenschr 2016 Jun; 141 (12): 870-7.*

SCIENTIFIC EVIDENCES ON THE PATHOLOGIC ETIOLOGY FOR THE RISING WORLD CHALLENGE OF OBESITY AND DYSLIPIDEMIA DURING LATEST THREE DECADES

Pathologic Etiology for the Rising World Challenge of Obesity and Dyslipidemia during Latest Three Decades: Published in the American Journal of Medicine and Medical Sciences; 2017; 7 (8): 318-322. Nasrat et al. A pathologic etiology for the rising world challenge of obesity and dyslipidemia during latest three decades. *Am J Med Med Sci 2017; 7 (8): 318-322. [doi: 10.5923/j.ajmms.20170708.03]*

Background: Prevalence of obesity and dyslipidemia constitutes a world health challenge. The latest decades demonstrated flare up of abnormal-existence/behavior colonic ***Helicobacter pylori pylori*** strains and rising figures of disease spread related to these colonic ***H. pylori*** strains. The association of overweight/obesity with ***H. pylori*** is controversial in different studies while it has been confirmed that colonic ***H. pylori*** strains could interfere with fat turnover and lipid-lipoprotein metabolism. ***H. pylori*** was found significantly associated with dyslipidemia; ***H. pylori*** can induce dyslipidemia by means of increasing triglyceride and decreasing HDL-cholesterol (HDL-C), hence; increasing the risk of atherosclerosis.[1-8]

Objective: Demonstration of the existence frequency of the colonic strains of the bacterium ***H. pylori*** among an overweight/obese and dyslipidemic sample of population and illustration of the pathologic role of these colonic ***H. pylori*** strains in leading to obesity and dyslipidemia.

Design& Setting: A Prospective clinical study done in Jeddah/Saudi Arabia between May 2014 and October 2015.

Patients& MethodS: A group of 100 overweight/obese individuals who were equally distributed between males and females within the age range of 30-45 years were investigated for the existence of colonic ***H. pylori*** strains employing ***H. pylori*** fecal antigen test.[9] The ***H. pylori*** fecal antigen test was obtained from Acon Laboratory, USA, Batch No. HP8040008. They were also investigated for serum levels of cholesterol and TG. A group of 30 volunteers with dyslipidemia and positive for colonic ***H. poylri*** strains were selected from the first group so that males are equal to females. They followed a natural measure for eradication of ***H. pylori*** from the colon which consisted of the senna leaves extract purge and vinegar therapy. The senna purge was employed every month for three successive times to ensure eradication of the colonic ***H. pylori*** strains while vinegar therapy was used to protect from recurrence of the abnormal-behavior ***H. pylori*** strains via buffering the bacterium ingested with any query meal. Vinegar therapy consisted of a vinegar-mixed salad with principal meals, once or twice daily/five days every week continued for five months or until a satisfactory target as concerns overweight/obesity and dyslipidemia is achieved; vinegar is dietary white vinegar 6%. Patients were advised to refrain from any gastric sedative medications particularly those including anti-urease activity in order to avoid forcing normal-behavior ***H. pylori*** strains to escape to the colon.[10] Patients were not following any particular diet regimen or slimming measures and they were allowed to follow their own style of life except absolute restriction of outside-home meals to avoid recurrence of colonic *H. pylori* strains.

Results: 93 patients (93%), 52 males and 41 females, were found positive for colonic *H. pylori* strains. The weight of the 30 patients selected to follow the natural therapy was ranging between 105-123 KG with body mass index (BMI) above 25. The level of their serum TG ranged between 171-199 mg/dl, total serum cholesterol range was between 221-268 mg/dl, serum HDL-C ranged between 41-44mg/dl and LDL-cholesterol (LDL-C) was ranging between 180-224 mg/dl. All patients became negative for colonic *H. pylori* strains after the senna purge as confirmed by the *H. pylori* fecal antigen test. Marked slimming was demonstrated in 27 patients (90%) within 3-5 months with improvement of their BMI and a range of body weight of 83-92 KG. Slimming was frankly characterized by stretched skin without any redundancy as the loss of weight occurred just gradual. Serum TG dropped to a normal range between 106-144 mg/dl. Total serum cholesterol improved to a range of 154-176 mg/dl with HDL-C ranging between 56-61 mg/dl and a range of LDL-C between 98-115 mg/dl.

Ethical considerations An informed signed consent was taken from all patients, they were made aware about safety of the natural vinegar therapy and senna extract purge, they were free to quit the study whenever they like. The research proposal was approved and the study followed the rules of the Research Ethics Committee.

Discussion: The latest reports in literature demonstrated a definite flare up of many medical challenges in a dramatic way through different reasons. Some of these diseases such as diabetes and hypertension which were once considered diseases of the developed world have become a worldwide pandemic resembling an ocean wave flooding the whole world with its two thirds occupying the developing side of the globe. Diabetes and hypertension, diseases of rich, are now flaring up as a challenge among poor population. Some reports consider disease spread in developing countries a consequence of progress and lifestyle change.[9,11-15] In spite of that, traditional risk rules do not appear fully sufficient to explain the rising figures of spread of chronic illness in those countries. Prevalence of the challenge of obesity and dyslipidemia has been demonstrated worldwide during the latest few decades.[4,7,8] Obesity and diabetes in the developing world constitute an actual growing challenge.[16]

The latest three decades confirm the prevalence of abnormal-existence/behavior colonic *H. pylori* strains with flare up of a lot of medical challenges related to these strains through immune, inflammatory, toxic or different unknown reasons.[9,10] Obesity has got an epidemic growth but the association of overweight/obesity with *H. pylori* is controversial in different studies, some studies have reported that *H. pylori* is not associated with overweight/obesity while other studies emphasized that this association is undefined or there is inverse correlation between *H. pylori* colonization and overweight.[17-19] Whereas some studies have considered that *H. pylori* increases the prevalence of metabolic syndrome and mentioned that existence of *H. pylori* and vitamin D deficiency could be predictors of metabolic syndrome.[20,21] Surgeons doing gastric interventions for treatment of obesity has found positive existence of *H. pylori* in more than 50% of their patients and they advised that *H. pylori* should be eradicated in order to achieve successful reduction of weight after surgery.[22,23]

Although epidemiologic and clinical data suggest that *H. pylori* is a contributing factor in the progression of atherosclerosis, specific CVD risk factors which could be associated with *H. pylori* remain

unclear. However, *H. pylori* was found significantly and independently associated with dyslipidemia. *H. pylori* has been also found associated significantly with low serum levels of HDL-C. It has been reported that *H. pylori* can induce dyslipidemia which may result in the development of coronary heart disease by increasing TG and decreasing HDL-C, accordingly increasing the risk of atherosclerosis.[24-26]

H. pylori colonized the stomach since an immemorial time as if both the stomach wall and the bacterium used to live together in peace harmless to each other. *H. pylori* could migrate or get forced to migrate to the colon under the influence of antibiotic violence to become foreign structure to the tissues beyond the stomach as the bacterium is recognized only to the gastric wall tissues. *H. pylori* outside the stomach is rendered a poison itself by inducing auto-immunity and also a source of poison by leading to inflammatory reactions and tissue pathology. Colonic *H. pylori* strains will continue producing ammonia for a reason or no reason, un-opposed or buffered by any acidity, leading to accumulation of profuse toxic amounts of ammonia that might cause different adverse toxic sequels in the body.[9,10] Different reports in literature have confirmed the association of cytotoxin-associated gene A (cagA) with colonic *H. pylori* strains and emphasized that cagA of *H. pylori* encodes a highly immunogenic and virulence-associated protein; the presence of this virulent gene in the body could affect the clinical outcome in many patients.[27,28]

It has been confirmed that colonic *H. pylori* strains could interfere with lipid and glucose metabolism. The most plausible hypothesis is emphasizing that alterations in fat turnover, interference with lipid-lipoprotein metabolism and glucose metabolism may exist due to low-grade systemic inflammatory situations causing increased insulin resistance. In spite of a century old hypothesis that infection is a known cause for atherosclerosis, this is an issue which is still debatable. *H. pylori* can induce dyslipidemia by increasing TG and decreasing HDL-C, accordingly increasing the risk for developing atherosclerosis. While *H. pylori* does not essentially enter the circulation, these remote manifestations beyond the stomach are probably mediated by the cytokines and acute phase proteins produced by the inflamed mucosa. The role of extra-gastric *H. pylori* cytotoxins and associated chronic inflammatory situations with consequent increase of insulin resistance creating atherogenic lipid profile and increased body mass index have been confirmed in further studies.[26,29-31]

The association of overweight/obesity and dyslipidemia with colonic *H. pylori* strains in this study constituted a considerable figure (93%). The reason that some studies did not report a similar association was due to the finding that these studies were only searching for the existence of the gastric *H. pylori* strains employing urea breath test or endoscopic gastro-duodenal biopsy missing to assess the percentage of *H. pylori* in the colon.[17-19,32,33] Gastric *H. pylori* strains, so long within the stomach, do not induce antigenicity as the bacterium is being recognized to the stomach wall tissues. More-over, these gastric strains of the bacterium even including abnormal behavior within the stomach do not lead to accumulation of toxic amounts of ammonia and therefore are not supposed to cause systemic inflammatory sequels beyond the stomach.[9,10] Whereas existence of *H. pylori* strains in the colon among patients of this study was confirmed by the *H. pylori* fecal antigen test and it is further confirmed by the stool picture. The stool was in the form of solid hard dried small pieces in 87 patients (87%) denoting presence of multiple colonic spasms while it was small amount soft in 13 patients (13%) which is the picture of retention with overflow indicating a loaded colon due to a high rectal severe spasm caused by the excess ammonia as ammonia is smooth muscle tonic but its accumulation is spastic for the colon.[27] The multiple colonic spasms were demonstrated by colonoscopy while the high rectal spasm was detected by sigmoidoscopy.

The principle of employing the senna extract purge in the current study is eradication of the colonic *H. pylori* strains which are the suggested main pathogenesis of compromising the lipid metabolism among patients of the study. The senna leaves extract purge was demonstrated as the typical natural measure for definitive eradication of *H. pylori* from the colon. Three-time dilution of the standard senna leaves extract was found directly lethal to *H. pylori* strains on culture media.[34-36] Whereas employment of the vinegar therapy was meant to protect from recurrence of any abnormal-behavior *H. pylori* strains via buffering any query food intake. The complex nutritional requirements of *H. pylori* are achieved via its unique energy metabolism as the major routes of generation of energy for *H. pylori* are via pyruvate while the activity of the pyruvate dehydrogenase complex is controlled by the rules of product inhibition and feedback regulation.[37,38] As acetate is demonstrated as an end product among the metabolic pathway of **H. pylori**;[39,40] therefore, addition of acetic acid to the atmosphere around **H. pylori** could compromise the energy metabolism of **H. pylori** or interfere with the organism's respiratory chain metabolism. So long the matter includes interference with the energy metabolism and respiratory chain metabolism of **H. pylori**, an immediate dramatic lethal effect on the bacterium should be considered. Twenty times-dilution of dietary white vinegar 6% was found directly lethal to **H. pylori** strains on culture media.[35]

Revision of the clinical records of the research team of this study in order to compare different ways for management of overweight/obesity and dyslipidemia associated with colonic **H. pylori** strains, it revealed that combination of the senna extract purge and vinegar therapy was superior to employment of the senna purge alone or the vinegar therapy alone. The purge regimen needs seven months to approach the target results as concerns cure of obesity and dyslipidemia while the vinegar therapy requires nine months to reach the same target whereas combination of the senna purge monthly for three successive months together with vinegar therapy for five months from the start of the combination therapy is sufficient to achieve ideal results.

Further revision of several series for the research team of this study which were done for the purpose of demonstrating the existence of **H. pylori** in the colon among dyslipidemic slim individuals. It was revealed that existence of colonic **H. pylori** strains was associated with dyslipidemia even among slim individuals in a frequency of 82-90% which confirms the role **H. pylori** in leading to dyslipidemia regardless of the body weight of the person. Some investigators confirmed the influence of **H. pylori** in leading to atherosclerosis and CVD via different mechanisms including interference with fat turnover, lipid-lipoprotein metabolism, glucose metabolism and increased insulin resistance,[3,26,29,31] while other workers faced controversy or uncertainty as regards the influence of **H. pylori** in CVD as they did not find improvement of the atherogenic lipid profile after eradication of **H. pylori**.[24,32,41] The reason for that controversy could be most probably due to the employment of antibiotics for **H. pylori** eradication instead of natural measures, this would further force the bacterium for migration towards the colon. Accordingly, dyslipidemia is not expected to improve, on the contrary it might even go worse.

Conclusion colonic **H. pylori** strains could be significantly responsible for the spreading phenomena of obesity and dyslipidemia during latest decades. Eradication of the abnormal-existence colonic **H. pylori** strains could be a definitive and effective measure for controlling the phenomena of overweight/obesity and dyslipidemia worldwide.

Conflict of Interest There is no conflict of interest existing.

REFERENCES:

1. **Sakellariou P, Valente A, Carrillo AE, et al.** Chronic l-menthol-induced browning of white adipose tissue hypothesis: A putative therapeutic regime for combating obesity and improving metabolic health. *Med Hypotheses 2016 Aug; 93: 21-6.*

2. **Moretti E, Gonnelli S, Campagna M, et al. Influence of Helicobacter pylori infection on metabolic parameters and body composition of dyslipidemic patients.** *Intern Emerg Med. 2014 Oct; 9 (7): 767-72.*

3. **Aksoy H, Sebin SO. H. pylori and cardiovascular disease. Gen Med 2015**; *S1: 1.* **[Open Access]**

4. **Parikh Y, Mason M, Williams K. Researchers' perspectives pediatric obesity research participant recruitment.** *Clin Transl Med 2016 Dec; 5 (1): 20. Epub 2016 Jun 23.*

5. **Lee JE, Pope Z, Gao Z. The Role of Youth Sports in Promoting Children's Physical Activity and Preventing Pediatric Obesity: A Systematic Review.** *Behav Med 2016 Jun 23: 0. [Epub ahead of print]*

6. Jolfaie NR, Rouhani MH, Surkan PJ, et al. Rice Bran Oil Decreases Total and LDL Cholesterol in Humans: A Systematic Review and Meta-Analysis of Randomized Controlled Clinical Trials. *Horm Metab Res 2016 Jun 16. [Epub ahead of print]*

7. Xiao C, Dash S, Morgantini C, et al. Pharmacological Targeting of the Atherogenic Dyslipidemia Complex: The Next Frontier in CVD Prevention Beyond Lowering LDL Cholesterol. *Diabetes 2016 Jul; 65 (7): 1767-78.*

8. Grammer T, Kleber M, Silbernagel G, et al. Residual risk: The roles of triglycerides and high density lipoproteins. *Dutsch Med Wochenschr 2016 Jun; 141 (12): 870-7.*

9. Farinha P, Gascoyne RD. Helicobacter pylori and MALT Lymphoma. *Gastroenterology 2005 May; 128 (6): 1579-605.*

10. Nasrat AM, Nasrat SAM, Nasrat RM, et al. Misconception and misbehavior towards Helicobacter pylori is leading to major spread of illness. *Gen Med 2015; S1: 002.* [Open Access]

11. Katulanda P, Sheriff MH, Matthews DR. The diabetes epidemic in Sri Lanka-a growing problem. *Ceylon Med J 2006 Mar; 51 (1): 26-8.*

12. Wissow LS. Diabetes, poverty and Latin America. *Patient Educ Couns 2006 May; 61 (2): 169-70. Epub 2006 Apr 18.*

13. Einecke D. Like a tsunami: diabetes wave floods the whole world. *MMC 2006 Apr 6; 148 (14): 4-6.*

14. Yach D, Stuckler D, Brownell KD. Epidemiologic and economic consequences of the global epidemics of obesity and diabetes. *N Med 2006 Jan; 12 (1): 62-6.*

15. Reddy KS, Naik N, Prabhakaran D. Hypertension in developing world: a consequence of progress. *Curr Cardiol Rep 2006; 8 (6): 399-404.*

16. Hossain P, Kawar B, El Nahas M. Obesity and diabetes in developing world-a growing challenge. *N Engl J Med 2007 Jan 18; 356 (3): 213-5.*

17. Xu MY, Liu L, Yuan BS, et al. Association of obesity with Helicobacter pylori infection: A retrospective study. *World J Gastroenterol 2017 Apr 21; 23 (15): 2750-2756.*

18. Abadi ATB. Obesity and Helicobacter pylori: An undefined association. *Obesity (Silver Spring) 2017 Jun; 25 (6): 981. Epub 2017 May 5.*

19. Moran-Lev H, Lubetzky R, Mandel D, et al. Inverse Correlation between Helicobacter pylori Colonization and Pediatric Overweight: A Preliminary Study. *Child Obes 2017 May 1. doi: 10.1089/chi.2016.0275. [Epub ahead of print]*

20. Vafaeimanesh J, Bagherzadeh M, Mirzaei A, et al. Effect of Helicobacter pylori on metabolic syndrome parameters in diabetic patients. *Gastroenterol Hepatol Bed Bench 2016 Dec; 9 (Suppl 1): S36-S41.*

21. Chen LW, Chien CY, Hsieh CW, et al. The Associations between Helicobacter pylori Infection, Serum Vitamin D, and Metabolic Syndrome: A Community-Based Study. *Medicine (Baltimore) 2016 May; 95 (18): e3616. doi: 10.1097/MD. 0000000003616.*

22. Kassir R, Lointier P, Phelip JM, et al Barrett's Oesophagus and Oesophageal Carcinogenesis Following Obesity Surgery: Helicobacter Pylori Must Be Eradicated?. *Obes Surg 2017 Jun 28. doi: 10.1007/s11695-017-2785-4. [Epub ahead of print]*

23. Danciu M, Simion L, Poroch V. The role of histological evaluation of Helicobacter pylori infection in obese patients referred to laparoscopic sleeve gastrectomy. *Rom J Morphol Embryol 2016; 57 (4): 1303-1311.*

24. Kim TJ, Lee H, Kang M, et al. Helicobacter pylori is associated with dyslipidemia but not with other risk factors of cardiovascular disease. *Sci Rep 2016 Nov 28; 6: 38015. doi: 10.1038/srep38015.*

25. Pohjanen VM, Koivurova OP, Niemelä SE, et al. Role of Helicobacter pylori and interleukin 6 -174 gene polymorphism in dyslipidemia: a case-control study. *BMJ Open 2016 Jan 18; 6 (1): e009987. doi: 10.1136/bmjopen-2015-009987.*

26. Chen Z, Xu C, Luo L, et al. Helicobacter pylori infection and gastric mucosa change and blood-lipid in people undergoing the physical examination in Changsha. *Zhong Nan Da Xue Xue Bao Yi Xue Ban 2014 Mar; 39 (3): 265-9.*

27. Nasrat SAM, Nasrat RM, Nasrat MN, et al. The dramatic spread of diabetes mellitus worldwide and influence of Helicobacter pylori. *General Med. 2015; 3 (1): 159-62.*

28. Bulut Y, Agacayak A, Karlidag D, et al. Association of CagA+ Helicobacter pylori with adenotonsillar hypertrophy. *Tohoku J Exp Med. 2006 Jul; 209 (3): 229-33.*

29. Vijayvergiya R, Vadivelu R. Role of Helicobacter pylori infection in pathogenesis of atherosclerosis. *World J Cardiol 2015 Mar 26; 7 (3): 134-43.*

30. Buzás GM. Metabolic consequences of Helicobacter pylori infection and eradication. *World J Gastroenterol 2014 May 14; 20 (18): 5226-34.*

31. Sharma V, Aggarwal A. Helicobacter pylori: Does it add to risk of coronary artery disease. *World J Cardiol 2015 Jan 26; 7 (1): 19-25.*

32. Rogha M, Dadkhah D, Pourmoghaddas Z, et al. Association of Helicobacter pylori infection with severity of coronary heart disease. *ARYA Atheroscler 2012 winter; 7 (4): 138-41.*

33. Rogha M, Nikvarz M, Pourmoghaddas Z. Is Helicobacter pylori infection a risk factor for coronary heart disease?. *ARYA Atheroscler 2012 spring; 8 (1): 5-8.*

34. Nasrat AM, Nasrat SAM, Nasrat RM, et al. The definitive eradication of Helicobacter pylori from the colon. Gen Med 2015*; S1: 1.* [Open Access]

35. Nasrat RM, Nasrat MM, Nasrat AM, et al. Improvement of idiopathic cardiomyopathy after colon clear. *J Cardiol Res 2015 Apr; 6 (2): 249-254.* [Open Access]

36. Nasrat AM, Nasrat RM, Nasrat MM. Frequency of leukemia during late decades may indicate that the anti-Helicobacter pylori antibiotic strategy was a therapeutic mistake. *Am J Med Med Sci 2017; 7 (3): 103-107.* [Open Access]

37. Hughes NJ, Clayton CL, Chalk PA, et al. Helicobacter pylori porCDAB oorDABC genes encode distinct pyruvate: flavodoxin and 2-oxoglutarate: acceptor oxidoreductases which mediate electron transport to NADP. *J Bacteriol 1998 Mar; 180 (5): 1119-28.*

38. Berg JM, Tymoczko JL, Stryer L. Biochemistry. *WH Freeman and Company. 2002; 5ᵗʰ Ed: 480.*

39. Mendz GL, Hazell SL. Fumarate catabolism in Helicobacter pylori. *Biochem Mol Biol Int. 1993 Oct; 31 (2): 325-32.*

40. **Mendz GL, Hazell SL, van Gorkom L. Pyruvate metabolism in Helicobacter pylori.** *Arch Microbiol. 1994; 162(3):187-92.*

41. **Jang SH, Lee H, Kim JS, et al. Association between Helicobacter pylori Infection and Cerebral Small Vessel Disease.** *Korean J Fam Med 2015 Sep; 36 (5): 227-32.*

THE HIDDEN TRUTH BEHIND OSTEOPOROSIS AND VITAMIN D DEFICIENCY
Why Osteoporosis and Vitamin D Deficiency are Lately Running among People like Common Cold!!

Introduction: Osteoporosis is an almost increasing public health problem worldwide. Osteoporosis is one of the most prevalent forms of age-related bone diseases, increased bone loss with advancing age has become a grave public health concern. Osteoporosis results from imbalance between bone resorption and bone formation; reduction in the quantity of bone tissue with deterioration of the bone micro-structure leads to general loss in bone strength and greater fracture risk. While it is part of the natural aging process, osteoporosis does not affect everyone to the same degree.[1-3]

Genetic factors are considered major contributors to the pathogenesis of osteoporosis while menopause constitutes a major health risk as concerns osteoporosis because it is characterized by decreased bone density and increased fracture risk due to over-activation of osteoclastogenesis. Patients with organ transplantation are at further orthopedic risk as they require life-long immune-suppressive therapy to minimize the risk of immune-mediated graft rejection; complications of the immune-suppressive therapy such as impaired bone strength and increased fracture risk are common among those patients leading to increased morbidity and mortality rates.[1,4,5]

Osteoporosis is diagnosed primarily by measurement of bone mineral density and several advanced techniques are available while treatment relies upon encouraging osteogenesis or inhibition of osteoclastogenesis.[4,6,7]

Vitamin D has been appreciated for its role in bone health since its identification in 1921, it is important for non-skeletal health as much as for skeletal health. Vitamin D deficiency is a major association with the phenomena of osteoporosis due to lack of proper function of vitamin D in both calcium and phosphorus homeostasis in the bones. Vitamin D deficiency is recently a common health problem worldwide, it is more common than previously thought; more people have been found severely deficient in vitamin D. Sun exposure is considered the single most important source of vitamin D which is obtained primarily from skin exposure to ultraviolet radiation in sunlight. Hypovitaminosis D resulting from lack of ultraviolet rays exposure is not easily corrected by dietary intake alone in the absence of supplements.[8-12]

The association between *Helicobacter pylori* and serum vitamin D level was found controversial by some investigators.[13] Previous studies have also reported conflicting results on the association between *H. pylori* and osteoporosis as the development of osteoporosis is complex and multi-factorial but recent reports have emphasized that early eradication could reduce the influence of *H. pylori* on osteoporosis.[14-16] It was collectively reported that advanced age, low body mass index and *H. pylori* positivity were the main risk factors for osteoporosis; however, the success of antibiotic *H. pylori* eradication was not shown to decrease the risk for osteoporosis.[17]

REFERENCES:

1. Wang H, Gong C, Liu X, et al. Genetic interaction of purinergic P2X7 receptor and ER-α polymorphisms in susceptibility to osteoporosis in Chinese postmenopausal women. *J Bone Miner Metab 2017 Sep 7. doi: 10.1007/s00774-017-0862-3. [Epub ahead of print]*

2. Antika LD, Lee EJ, Kim YH, etal. Dietary phlorizin enhances osteoblastogenic bone formation through enhancing β-catenin activity via GSK-3β inhibition in a model of senile osteoporosis. *J Nutr Biochem 2017 Jul 28; 49: 42-52.*

3. Zhao XL, Chen JJ, Zhang GN, et al. Small molecule T63 suppresses osteoporosis by modulating osteoblast differentiation via BMP and WNT signaling pathways. *Sci Rep 2017 Sep 4; 7 (1): 10397. doi: 10.1038/s41598-017-10929-3.*

4. Chen X, Zhi X, Cao L, et al. Matrine derivate MASM uncovers a novel function for ribosomal protein S5 in osteoclastogenesis and postmenopausal osteoporosis. *Cell Death Dis 2017 Sep 7; 8 (9): e3037. doi: 10.1038/cddis.2017.394.*

5. Löfdahl E, Rådegran G. Osteoporosis following heart transplantation and immunosuppressive therapy. *Transplant Rev (Orlando) 2017 Aug 12. pii: S0955-470X (17)30039-3. doi: 10.1016/j.trre.2017.08.002. [Epub ahead of print]*

6. Kemp JP, Morris JA, Medina-Gomez C, et al. Identification of 153 new loci associated with heel bone mineral density and functional involvement of GPC6 in osteoporosis. *Nat Genet 2017 Sep 4. doi: 10.1038/ng.3949. [Epub ahead of print]*

7. Meier C, Uebelhart B, Aubry-Rozier B, et al. Osteoporosis drug treatment: duration and management after discontinuation. A position statement from the SVGO/ASCO. *Swiss Med Wkly 2017 Sep 5; 147:w14484. doi: smw.2017.14484. eCollection 2017 Sep 5*

8. Holick MF. Vitamin D deficiency. *N Engl J Med 2007 Jul 19; 357 (3): 266-81.*

9. Kizilgul M, Kan S, Ozcelik O, et al. Vitamin D replacement improves tear osmolarity in patients with vitamin D deficiency. *Semin Ophthalmol 2017 Sep 6: 1-6. doi: 10.1080/08820538.2017.1358752. [Epub ahead of print]*

10. Pilecka I, Sandin S, Reichenberg A, et al. Sun exposure and psychotic experiences. *Front Psychiatry 2017 Jun 19; 8: 107. doi: 10.3389/fpsyt.2017.00107. eCollection 2017.*

11. Rolvien T, Krause M, Jeschke A, et al. Vitamin D regulates osteocyte survival and perilacunar remodeling in human and murine bone. *Bone 2017 Jun 27; 103: 78-87.*

12. Iqbal AM, Dahl AR, Lteif A, et al. Vitamin D deficiency: A potential modifiable risk factor for cardiovascular disease in children with severe obesity. *Children (Basel) 2017 Aug 28; 4 (9). pii: E80. doi: 10.3390/children4090080.*

13. Chen LW, Chien CY, Hsieh CW, et al. The associations between Helicobacter pylori infection, serum vitamin D, and metabolic syndrome: A Community-Based Study. *Medicine (Baltimore) 2016 May; 95 (18): e3616. doi: 10.1097/ MD.0000000000003616.*

14. Shih HM, Hsu TY, Chen CY, et al. Analysis of patients with Helicobacter pylori infection and the subsequent risk of developing osteoporosis after eradication therapy: A nationwide population-based cohort study. *PLoS One 2016 Sep 14; 11 (9): e0162645*. doi: *10.1371/journal.pone.0162645. eCollection 2016.*

15. Chung YH, Gwak JS, Hong SW, et al. Helicobacter pylori: A possible risk factor for bone health. *Korean J Fam Med 2015 Sep; 36 (5): 239-44.*

16. Fotouk-Kiai M, Hoseini SR, Meftah N, et al. Relationship between Helicobacter pylori infection (HP) and bone mineral density (BMD) in elderly people. *Caspian J Intern Med 2015 spring; 6 (2): 62-6.*

17. Asaoka D, Nagahara A, Shimada Y, et al. Risk factors for osteoporosis in Japan: is it associated with Helicobacter pylori? *Ther Clin Risk Manag 2015 Mar 6; 11: 381-91.*

SCIENTIFIC EVIDENCES ON THE HIDDEN TRUTH BEHIND OSTEOPOROSIS AND VITAMIN D DEFICIENCY

The Hidden Truth behind Osteoporosis and Vitamin D Deficiency: Published in the American Journal of Medicine and Medical Sciences; 2017; 7 (11):369-377. Nasrat et al. The hidden truth behind osteoporosis and vitamin D deficiency. *Am J Med Med Sci 2017; 7 (11):369-377. [10.5923/j.ajmms.20170711.02]*

Background: Osteoporosis is one of the most prevalent forms of age-related bone diseases, increased bone loss with advancing age has become a grave public health concern. While it is part of the natural aging process, osteoporosis does not affect everyone to the same degree.[1-3] Genetic factors are considered major contributors to the pathogenesis of osteoporosis while menopause constitutes a major health risk as concerns osteoporosis. Complications of the immune-suppressive therapy such as impaired bone strength and increased fracture risk are common.[4-7]

Vitamin D has been appreciated for its role in bone health since its identification in 1921, it is important for non-skeletal health as much as for skeletal health. Vitamin D deficiency is a major association with the phenomena of osteoporosis.[8-12]

Prevalence of osteopenia/osteoporosis and vitamin D deficiency constitutes a world health challenge. The latest decades demonstrated flare up of abnormal-existence/behavior colonic ***Helicobacter pylori*** strains and rising figures of disease spread related to these strains. The association of vitamin D deficiency with ***H. pylori*** is controversial in literature whereas it has been confirmed that colonic ***H. pylori*** strains could lead to abnormal lipid metabolism interfering with absorption of the fat-soluble vitamin D. ***H. pylori*** was found significantly associated with osteoporosis; ***H. pylori*** can influence osteoporosis directly by increasing the release of toxic inflammatory mediators and through the developed ***H. pylori*** related-vitamin D deficiency.[13-17]

Motive of Study: The marked prevalence of vitamin D deficiency during latest decades as if every living individual should have a degree of vitamin D deficiency and the common medical attitude that lack of sun exposure is the main reason behind this spreading and challenging frequency of vitamin D deficiency to the extent that a national survey in a sunny country like Saudi Arabia including 5000 individuals of all age groups of school students, boys and girls, and their male and female teachers has revealed prevalence of some degree of vitamin D deficiency among most of them which was attributed mainly to lack of sun exposure and next to bad nutritional habits.[18,19] Exposure to the sun and lack of exposure to the sun should not vary very much during these latest decades from the decades before them and in spite of the fact that lack of sun exposure is the common traditional factor for vitamin D deficiency, it is still insufficient alone to explain the dramatic frequency of vitamin D deficiency during latest decades like a worldwide spreading influenza. These conflicting conceptions have attracted the attention of the research team and constituted part of the motive for this study.

Revision of the clinical records of the research team of this study revealed the findings of 5 groups of patients with vitamin D deficiency as 10 patients per each group. These groups resembled civil service workers, traffic police officers, real estate professionals, golf players and owners of private boats for fishing and sailing. All these subjects showed moderate to severe vitamin D deficiency although they are candidates of sufficient sun exposure and the last three groups are supposed to be well to do having good nutrition advantages. In addition, frank colonic upsets were common features in all of them; that was exactly the main and real motive of this study. A general impression has developed that an environmental error could be there most probably in the colon as most population stepping on the earth are suffering colonic troubles. Lack of proper sun exposure is an integral reason for vitamin D deficiency but it seems that it is not the only or at least it is not the main factor responsible for the dramatic challenge of osteopenia/osteoporosis and vitamin D deficiency during latest decades as traditional risk rules such as age and gender are still insufficient alone to explain the flare up of osteoporosis/vitamin D deficiency during these decades. Therefore; efforts had been raised to search for a hidden reason apart of lack of exposure to the sun together with investigation of a colonic pathology that could have an influence on vitamin D uptake by the body, the blame was almost pointing towards existence of colonic *H. pylori* strains.

Objective: Demonstration of the possibility of an existing hidden underlying environmental error behind the spreading challenge of the increased frequency of osteopenia/osteoporosis and vitamin D deficiency during latest decades.

Design& Settung: A prospective clinical study done in Jeddah/Saudi Arabia between October 2015 and May 2017.

Patients& Methods: The study included four groups of patients with different grades of moderate low bone density (LBD) due to vitamin D deficiency. The first group included 100 patients equally distributed between males and females known with different grades of LBD/vitamin D deficiency and colonic upsets having an age range of 45-59 years, they were randomly included in the study without any selection. The purpose of this group was to investigate the association of LBD/vitamin D deficiency with existence of the colonic *H. pylori* strains using a specific test (*H. pylori* fecal antigen test).[20] The second group consisted of 19 patients (8 males and 11 females) with Osteopenia/osteoporosis due to moderate to severe grades of vitamin D deficiency, their age ranged between 47-56 years. They were referred from a nutritional center for an alternative therapy for their resistant colonic upsets in spite of adequate medications, their response to vitamin D replacement therapy was also not satisfactory but they were not referred for this purpose. *H. pylori* fecal antigen test was employed for them and the patients who proved to be positive for colonic *H. pylori* strains followed natural measures for *H. pylori* eradication from the colon that was consisting of the senna leaves extract purge and vinegar therapy. The senna purge was used for eradication of *H. pylori* from the colon done once monthly for consequent three months to ensure eradication of the bacterium whereas vinegar therapy consisted of a vinegar-mixed salad with principal meals, once or twice daily/3-5days a week, in order to protect from the recurrence of any abnormal behavior *H. pylori* strains via food intake.[21] This group has been employed to demonstrate the effect of eradication of *H. pylori* from the colon via natural measures on the recovery of vitamin D serum level without further vitamin D supplements. As regards the third group, patients were selected from the first group including 20 patients equally distributed between males and females with an age range of 48-57 years, positive for colonic *H. pylori* strains and having minor or tolerable colonic troubles that were not in need of symptomatic or therapeutic medications, they were having rather a similar grade of vitamin D deficiency as that of the second group and they were receiving standard vitamin D supplement therapy. The purpose of the third group was comparative with patients of the second group as concerns the effect of *H. pylori* eradication on improvement of vitamin D serum level. A fourth group of patients who were selected also from the first group including 20 patients equally distributed between males and females with an age range of 46-56 years, positive for colonic *H. pylori* strains and having colonic troubles that were in need of natural therapy (senna leaves purge colon clear and vinegar therapy), patients of this group received standard vitamin D supplements for comparative reasons. All patients were of average body built or well-built. An additional fifth group to illustrate the effect of anti-**H. pylori** antibiotic therapy on the response of the body to vitamin D supplement therapy was not included for ethical reasons as **H. pylori** antibiotic eradication therapies demonstrate a lot of controversy.[20] Patients were followed up for 16-18 months.

Results: The vast majority, 96 patients, of the first group (96%) were found positive for colonic **H. pylori** strains while all patients of the second group were positive for these colonic strains. Serum vitamin D level of the second group patients was ranging between 27-33 nmol/L and the range in the third group was 26-31 nmol/L while in the fourth group it was 29-37 nmol/L. Serum calcium and phosphorus were also compromised in all patients, that was at the lowest range of the normal average (Serum calcium 9.4-9.7 mg/dL and phosphorus 2.7-3.1 mg/dL). Serum vitamin D level of the second group (the group of colon clear/no vitamin D supplement) improved to 78-91 nmol/L after 12-14 weeks of colon clear and eradication of colonic **H. pylori** strains without any further vitamin D supplement therapy whereas it did not improve among the third group patients (vitamin D supplement/no colon clear) except to a range of 67-72 nmol/L after 16-20 weeks in spite of an adequate vitamin D supplement therapy. Serum vitamin D level of the fourth group (the colon clear/vitamin D supplement group) improved to 89-99 nmol/L after 8-9 weeks of colon clear and supplement therapy. The nutritional center has given a feedback comment that their referred patients (the second group) who followed the colon clear measures without vitamin D supplement therapy have shown relief of their colonic troubles and demonstrated stop in the progress of osteoporosis for 12 months follow up. Recurrence of vitamin D deficiency did not occur in the second group (colon clear/no vitamin D supplement) except in 4 patients due to recurrence of colonic **H. pylori** strains via query meals which has been corrected in few months after revision of colon clear. Recurrence of vitamin D deficiency occurred in most patients of the third group (vitamin D supplement/ no colon clear), 17 patients (85%), within few months (3-5 months) after discontinuation of the supplement therapy. The fourth group of patients demonstrated good recovery of vitamin D serum level in shorter duration while showing no recurrence of vitamin D deficiency until 12 months follow up.

The table demonstrates the serum vitamin D of the second, third and fourth groups before and after therapy together with calcium and phosphorus levels upon start of the study.

Group	Vit. D (Before)	Vit. D (After)	Ca	P
Second	27-33 nmol/L	78-91 nmol/L		
Third	26-31 nmol/L	67-72 nmol/L	9.4-9.7 mg/dL	2.7-3.1 mg/dL
Fourth	29-37 nmol/L	89-99 nmol/L		

The table illustrates comparative aspects of the second, third and fourth groups as regards employment of colon clear, intake of vitamin D supplements, rate of recovery of vitamin D serum level and incidence of vitamin D deficiency recurrence.

Group	Description	Vitamin D Recovery	Vitamin D Deficiency Recurrence
Second	Colon Clear/No vitamin D Supplement	After 3-3.5 Months	Present (+)
Third	Vitamin D Supplement/ No Colon Clear	After 4-5 Months	Present (+++)
Fourth	Colon Clear/Vitamin D Supplement	After 2 Months	Not Present

Ethical Cconsiderations: An informed signed consent was taken from all patients, they were made aware about safety of the natural vinegar therapy and senna extract purge, they were free to quit the study whenever they like. The research proposal was approved and the study followed the rules of the Research Ethics Committee.

Discussion: The most important risk factors for developing osteoporosis are advanced age in both men and women, female sex and estrogen deficiency. Osteoporosis can be present without any symptoms for decades because osteoporosis does not cause symptoms until bone breaks. Therefore; patients may not be aware of their osteoporosis until they suffer a painful fracture.[1,7,8]

The association between *H. pylori* existence and serum vitamin D deficiency was found controversial in the literature whereas conflicting results were reported on the association between *H. pylori* and osteoporosis.[13,14] *H. pylori* may cause systemic inflammation and increase the production of tumor necrosis factors and interleukins; bone mineral density could be accordingly affected by these cytokines.[15,16] Further studies investigating the risk factors for osteoporosis and whether the existence or eradication of *H. pylori* is associated with osteoporosis have reached a conclusion that *H. pylori* positivity is considered a risk factor for osteoporosis whereas the success of *H. pylori* eradication was not demonstrated to improve osteoporosis risk.[17]

H. pylori existence as determined by serum antibodies and atrophic gastritis diagnosed on the basis of serum pepsinogen was found to significantly increase the risk of low trabecular bone density; accordingly it was emphasized that serological diagnosis of *H. pylori* existence and atrophic gastritis, which is usually utilized for risk assessment of gastric cancer, could be suggested as useful risk assessment for osteoporosis.[22-24] This matter has been attributed to the fact that *H. pylori* was linked to extra-digestive conditions and lifestyle-related diseases like osteoporosis as it could elicit a chronic cellular inflammatory response not only in the gastric mucosa but also in the extra-digestive organs particularly when cytotoxin-associated gene A (cagA) positive cytotoxic *H. pylori* strains are present.[25]

The latest reports in the literature demonstrated a definite flare up of many medical challenges in a dramatic way through different reasons.[20] Traditional risk rules do not appear fully sufficient to explain the rising figures of the world's spread of chronic illness. The latest three decades confirm the prevalence of abnormal-existence/behavior colonic *H. pylori* strains with flare up of a lot of medical challenges related to these abnormal strains through immune, inflammatory, toxic or different unknown reasons.[20,21]

H. pylori colonized the stomach since an immemorial time as if both the stomach wall and the bacterium used to live together in peace harmless to each other. *H. pylori* could migrate or get forced to migrate to the colon under the influence of antibiotic violence to become foreign structure to the tissues beyond the stomach as the bacterium is recognized only to the gastric wall tissues. *H. pylori* outside the stomach is therefore rendered a poison itself by inducing auto-immunity and a source of poison by leading to inflammatory reactions and local tissue pathology. Colonic *H. pylori* strains will continue producing ammonia for a reason or no reason, un-opposed or buffered by any acidity, leading to accumulation of profuse toxic amounts of ammonia that might cause different adverse toxic sequels inside the body.[20,21] Different reports in literature have confirmed the association of cagA with colonic *H. pylori* strains and emphasized that cagA of *H. pylori* encodes a highly immunogenic and virulence-associated protein; the presence of this virulent gene in the body could affect the clinical outcome in many patients.[26,27]

Although vitamin D deficiency is common and prevalent, measurement of serum vitamin D level is expensive and universal screening is not supported.[8,10] The association of overweight/obesity and dyslipidemia with existence of the colonic *H. pylori* strains has been emphasized and confirmed in literature. Obesity is found to be associated with abnormal lipid metabolism and as vitamin D is a fat soluble vitamin, hence obesity could be a logic risk factor for vitamin D deficiency.[12,28-33]

As long it was emphasized that the risk of developing osteoporosis is increased with the association of extra-gastric cagA positive *H. pylori* strains; early eradication of *H. pylori* was suggested in order to reduce the influence of *H. pylori* on osteoporosis via reducing the incidence of systemic inflammation and lowering cytokines production.[14-16,22,23] Accordingly; existence of the colonic *H. pylori* strains could have double influence in predisposing to osteoporosis; a direct influence through the release of pro-inflammatory mediators and indirect influence via predisposing to vitamin D deficiency due to impairment of lipid metabolism.[12,28]

The principle of employing the senna extract purge in the current study is eradication of the colonic *H. pylori* strains which are suggested to be the main pathogenesis leading to osteoporosis and vitamin D deficiency among the patients of this study. The senna leaves extract purge was demonstrated as the typical natural measure for definitive eradication of *H. pylori* from the colon. Three times dilution of the standard senna leaves extract was found directly lethal to *H. pylori* strains on culture media.[33-35] Whereas employment of the vinegar therapy was meant to protect from recurrence of any abnormal-behavior *H. pylori* strains via buffering any query food intake. The complex nutritional requirements of *H. pylori* are achieved via its unique energy metabolism as the major routes of generation of energy for *H. pylori* are via pyruvate while the activity of the pyruvate dehydrogenase complex is controlled by the rules of product inhibition and feedback regulation.[36,37] As acetate is demonstrated as an end product among the metabolic pathway of *H. pylori*;[38,39] therefore, addition of acetic acid to the atmosphere around *H. pylori* could compromise the energy metabolism of *H. pylori* or interfere with the organism's respiratory chain metabolism. So long the matter includes interference with the energy metabolism and respiratory chain metabolism of *H. pylori*, an immediate dramatic lethal effect on the bacterium could be considered. Twenty times-dilution of dietary white vinegar 6% was found instantly lethal to *H. pylori* strains on culture media.[34]

Most of the miscorrelation as concerns the reported association between *H. pylori* and osteoporosis/vitamin D deficiency in literature is the result of missing the fact that colonic *H. pylori* strains could lead to pathologic sequels because of its abnormal existence while gastric *H. pylori* strains even with abnormal behavior do not induce inflammatory or toxic sequels beyond the stomach, most of the workers were searching only for the gastric but not for the colonic strains. The association of cagA with colonic *H. pylori* strains is confirmed in literature and it is emphasized that cagA of *H. pylori* encodes a highly immunogenic and virulence-associated protein.[40,41] This matter is peculiar to extra-gastric *H. pylori* strains in general or most commonly to colonic *H. pylori* strains in particular while gastric *H. pylori* strains so long confined within the stomach seem to be innocent as concerns inducing immunogenicity as the bacterium is being recognized to the stomach wall tissues. More-over, these gastric strains even including abnormal behavior within the stomach do not lead to accumulation of toxic amounts of ammonia because of the buffering effect of gastric acid and therefore are not supposed to cause systemic inflammatory or toxic sequels beyond the stomach.[20,21,42] Most researches working on osteoporosis were looking for *H. pylori* in the stomach employing serological and urea breath tests or upper endoscopy,[16,17] while *H. pylori* serum anti-body test is extremely non-specific,[20,21] this could be most probably the reason for the resulting miscorrelation as colonic *H. pylori* strains could be co-existing and could be the reason behind the recorded bad sequels not the gastric strains.

The association of *H. pylori* with osteoporosis is controversial in literature; different reports in literature have given conflicting results about the association between *H. pylori* and osteoporosis. Few studies have discussed the influence of *H. pylori* eradication therapy on bone mineral density. Some investigators reported that existence of *H. pylori* might be associated with an increased risk of developing osteoporosis but they did not demonstrate value of *H. pylori* eradication on osteoporosis risk. They emphasized that early eradication could reduce the influence of *H. pylori* on osteoporosis when the follow-up is greater than 5 years;[14] which is rather a long period to confirm exclusion of other related factors or ruling out other variables. The reason for this controversy is most probably because investigators were employing antibiotics for *H. pylori* eradication forcing more *H. pylori* strains to migrate to the colon,[20,21,34] which is unfortunate for the progress of osteoporosis. Antibiotic eradication therapies seem to have no effect on gastric *H. pylori* strains except forcing them to migrate from the stomach as evidenced by the observational finding of development of new symptoms and new sequels.[20,34] This suggestion is supported by the findings that pseudo-membranous toxic colitis and toxic megacolon have developed after eradication of *H. pylori* by antibiotic therapy,[43,44] whereas antibiotics are seldom effective against extra-gastric *H. pylori* strains.[45]

Although osteoporosis is expected after the age of 50 years, physicians usually look for it at older age. The prominent observation in the current study is presentation of osteoporosis in rather lower age range without association of frank risk factors for developing osteoporosis in addition of finding osteoporosis among men rather similar as in females, therefore; this study might gain value from paying the attention towards the possibility to find osteoporosis at further lower age groups particularly when it is considered that diagnosis of osteoporosis is seldom included in the admission or discharge reports of patients with fractures of the hip for example.[7] The prevalence of osteopenia/osteoporosis and vitamin D deficiency in rather younger age groups and among males as much as in females could further confirm the concept about the possibility of an existing hidden environmental error which does not exclude an age group or dominates in a particular gender as traditional risk rules usually suggest as regards the challenge of osteoporosis/vitamin D deficiency. This could be furthermore a good answer for a perfect question; has vitamin D deficiency become an epidemic!! or is it real, vitamin D deficiency is pandemic!![46]

As long as some investigators have referred to the correlation between the prevalence of *H. pylori* and the frequency of osteopenia/osteoporosis and vitamin D deficiency, hence the matter is not altogether hidden; those investigators who missed to indicate this relation were looking for gastric *H. pylori* strains employing upper endoscopy but missed to fetch for the colonic strains. Therefore; the truth which is hidden in this subject is the responsibility of the colonic *H. pylori* strains but not the gastric strains on the challenge of osteoporosis/vitamin D deficiency and that the major factor behind the frequency and the dramatic flare up of the phenomena of osteoporosis/vitamin D deficiency during late decades is *H. pylori* not other traditional factors such as lack of sun exposure for example; the influence or impact of traditional risk factors on vitamin D deficiency should be rather similar during latest decades and previous decades. This suggestion is supported by the observational findings in the 5 groups of vitamin D deficiency in spite of sufficient sun exposure constituting the main motive of this study as 60% at least among them were supposed to have good nutrition advantages in addition. Accordingly, what is hidden in the subject is the combined influence of colonic *H. pylori* strains on vitamin D absorption and the onset/progress of osteoporosis. In brief, traditional risk rules remain insufficient to explain the flare up of vitamin D deficiency and osteoporosis during these latest decades on the basis of lack of sun exposure alone which could further indicate that all efforts to control the challenge via employing traditional measures alone would never be adequate or successful without elimination of a newly-existing underlying pathological error.

What is also hidden is the false impression that *H. pylori* existence does not constitute a risk factor for osteoporosis depending on the findings that eradication of *H. pylori* employing antibiotics does not improve the risk of osteoporosis, on the contrary antibiotic eradication might increase it. That is simply because antibiotics are not effective against gastric *H. pylori* strains except forcing them to migrate to the colon; thus antibiotic eradication would increase the possibility for development and progress of osteoporosis.[20,34,43,44]

What is also missed in the subject is the fact that existence of *H. pylori* strains in the stomach is natural existence and gastric *H. pylori* strains even including abnormal behavior within the stomach such as its presence inside the gastric lumen during presence of food would not have distant pathologic sequels beyond the stomach. It is the major existence of *H. pylori* strains in the colon which could influence distant remote adverse effects in the body or it is the co-existence of gastric and colonic strains which is the commonest situation; colonic stains are the pathogens while the gastric are mostly not, investigators are searching for the gastric strains only and get mixed up about the undesirable sequels of *H. pylori* existence in general.[21,42]

What is also hidden and commonly missed in this subject is a common un-realized therapeutic nutritional mistake in recommending low-fat milk products for the purpose of improving dyslipidemia.[28] It has been demonstrated that the reason behind the conflict of dyslipidemia during late decades is mostly colonic due to major existence of *H. pylori* strains in the colon but not the traditional dietary reasons of eating full-fat products. It has been further reported and confirmed that food or specifically fat of the food is innocent as concerns the sequels of dyslipidemia namely the increased serum level of cholesterol and triglycerides; the pathogenesis of dyslipidemia is essentially metabolic not dietary due to intake of full-cream food products.[47-50] Milk products include two components which are having biological correlation with each other which are the fat content and lactic acid content. The fat contains the fat-soluble vitamins

(A, D, E and K) while lactic acid is a healthy stuff. Lactic acid is digestive and works to behave the abnormal behavior of gastric *H. pylori* strains as much as the vinegar does; it was found that bio-organic acids such as lactic, formic and acetic inhibit bacterial growth on solid culture media with the lactic acid demonstrating the maximum inhibition.[51] It was also reported that addition of pyruvate inhibits *H. pylori* growth on culture media and this inhibition was attributed to accumulation of acetate, lactate and formate.[52] The reason for this biological inhibition is the fact that the pyruvate dehdrogenase complex is controlled by the rules of feedback regulation and product inhibition,[36,37] hence these bio-organic acids could interfere with the energy metabolism of bacteria. As lactate is identified among the main metabolic products of glucose utilization,[53] therefore; inclusion of lactic acid in food would interfere with ability of the human body to gain energy from carbohydrates and the body becomes obliged to gain the energy from lipids. Furthermore, as much as vinegar mixed in salad could be used for slimming purposes through forcing the body for consumption of fat,[28] lactic acid content of milk products forces the body to consume the milk fat content and hence getting benefit of the vitamins dissolved in its fat. Therefore; lowering the fat content of milk products reduces the digestive, biological and vitamin supplement values without much benefit on dyslipidemia while in the meantime adding further insult towards vitamin D deficiency due to the poor vitamin D content of low-fat milk products.

The striking association of colonic *H. pylori* strains with osteoporosis and vitamin D deficiency confirm that the existence of these strains in the colon could have a significant influence on the challenge of osteoporosis/vitamin D deficiency during latest decades. It has been furthermore previously confirmed that the existence of *H. pylori* in the colon could compromise the fat-soluble vitamin D absorption via interference with lipid metabolism.[28] Therefore; these findings conform with the results of the current study to support the concept that colonic *H. pylori* strains could constitute a hidden reason behind the flare up of osteoporosis and vitamin D deficiency during late decades. The dilemma of *H. pylori* is essentially a sanitary conflict before it is a medical challenge,[20] sanitary problems are treated with sanitary measures and antiseptics but not antibiotics. The antibiotics violence towards *H. pylori* could lead to major migration of *H. pylori* to the colon and flare up of abnormal-existence/behavior of *H. pylori* strains. Existence of *H. pylori* in the colon is life-long unless eradicated,[20,54] these abnormal-behavior *H. pylori* strains could travel from stomach to stomach via meals and even navigate between countries predisposing to spread of many reasons of chronic and major illness;[20,21,55] that could exactly constitute a grave environmental healthcare error. Therefore; eradication of *H. pylori* strains from the colon via natural measures could be an ideal effective and definitive measure to control the challenge of osteoporosis/vitamin D deficiency; improving vitamin D serum level and stopping progress of osteoporosis even without further vitamin D supplement therapy.

Could osteoporosis be prevented!! The goal of treatment of osteoporosis is prevention of bone fractures by reducing bone loss or preferably by increasing bone density and strength. Although early detection and timely treatment of osteoporosis can substantially decrease the risk of future fractures, none of the available treatments for osteoporosis are complete cure. In other words, it is difficult to completely rebuild bone that has been weakened by osteoporosis. Therefore; prevention of osteoporosis is rather more important than treatment.[7,8]

Osteoporosis prevention: A dream, difficult to access!! But why not? Adequate screening might reveal that the majority of the increased frequency of osteoporosis developing in recent decades could be related to major existence of colonic *H. pylori* strains, these strains could be easily screened and eradicated employing natural measures; complications associated with these strains could be thercforc avoided.

A National Healthcare Program of Screening and Prevention could be suggested; mass screening of colonic *H. pylori* strains for population at risk of developing osteoporosis is in-expensive and possible or empirical colon clear upon developing frank colonic upsets or *H. pylori* dyspeptic symptoms is also easy, safe and healthy. Accordingly; existence of colonic *H. pylori* strains could be therefore raised as a new healthcare predictor for developing osteoporosis among population at risk.

Prevention of osteoporosis is a challenge, treatment of osteoporosis is also a challenge and complications of treatments are further challenge; therefore, implementation of the concept of this study could give good promises for many patients at risk of osteoporosis. If further accurate re-determination is required for the wide practical application of the concept of this study, it should be done without much delay as it could save a lot of osteoporosis misery for so many people, impaired quality of life for many patients with fractures and save an adequate healthcare budget.

Conclusion: A hidden truth in the challenge of osteoporosis/vitamin D deficiency could lie in the prevalence and major existence of ***H. pylori*** strains in the colon that could lead to a significant double influence on the development of both osteoporosis and vitamin D deficiency accounting for the main world's burden of this challenge during latest decades not lack of sun exposure. Whereas gastric ***H. pylori*** strains even including abnormal behavior within the stomach seem rather innocent as regards the conflict of osteoporosis/vitamin D deficiency. Eradication of ***H. pylori*** strains from the colon via natural measures could be therefore an effective and definitive measure for the control of the challenge of osteoporosis and vitamin D deficiency worldwide; improving serum vitamin D level and protecting from an onset of osteopenia or stopping further progress of osteoporosis even without an additional vitamin D supplement therapy.

Conflict of Interest: There is no conflict of interest existing.

REFERENCES:

1. **Wang H, Gong C, Liu X, et al.** Genetic interaction of purinergic P2X7 receptor and ER-☒ polymorphisms in susceptibility to osteoporosis in Chinese postmenopausal women. *J Bone Miner Metab 2017 Sep 7. doi: 10.1007/s00774-017-0862-3. [Epub ahead of print]*

2. **Antika LD, Lee EJ, Kim YH, etal. Dietary phlorizin enhances osteoblastogenic bone formation through enhancing ☒-catenin activity via GSK-3☒ inhibition in a model of senile osteoporosis.** *J Nutr Biochem 2017 Jul 28; 49: 42-52.*

3. **Zhao XL, Chen JJ, Zhang GN, et al. Small molecule T63 suppresses osteoporosis by modulating osteoblast differentiation via BMP and WNT signaling pathways.** *Sci Rep 2017 Sep 4; 7 (1): 10397. doi: 10.1038/s41598-017-10929-3.*

4. **Chen X, Zhi X, Cao L, et al. Matrine derivate MASM uncovers a novel function for ribosomal protein S5 in osteoclastogenesis and postmenopausal osteoporosis.** *Cell Death Dis 2017 Sep 7; 8 (9): e3037. doi: 10.1038/cddis.2017.394.*

5. **Löfdahl E, Rådegran G. Osteoporosis following heart transplantation and immunosuppressive therapy.** *Transplant Rev (Orlando) 2017 Aug 12. pii: S0955-470X(17)30039-3. doi: 10.1016/j.trre.2017.08.002. [Epub ahead of print]*

6. **Kemp JP, Morris JA, Medina-Gomez C, et al. Identification of 153 new loci associated with heel bone mineral density and functional involvement of GPC6 in osteoporosis.** *Nat Genet 2017 Sep 4. doi: 10.1038/ng.3949. [Epub ahead of print]*

7. **Meier C, Uebelhart B, Aubry-Rozier B, et al. Osteoporosis drug treatment: duration and management after discontinuation. A position statement from the SVGO/ASCO.** *Swiss Med Wkly 2017 Sep 5; 147: w14484. doi: smw.2017.14484. eCollection 2017 Sep 5*

8. **Holick MF. Vitamin D deficiency.** *N Engl J Med 2007 Jul 19; 357 (3): 266-81.*

9. **Kizilgul M, Kan S, Ozcelik O, et al. Vitamin D replacement improves tear osmolarity in patients with vitamin D deficiency.** *Semin Ophthalmol 2017 Sep 6: 1-6. doi: 10.1080/08820538.2017.1358752. [Epub ahead of print]*

10. Pilecka I, Sandin S, Reichenberg A, et al. Sun exposure and psychotic experiences. *Front Psychiatry 2017 Jun 19; 8: 107. doi: 10.3389/fpsyt.2017.00107. eCollection 2017.*

11. Rolvien T, Krause M, Jeschke A, et al. Vitamin D regulates osteocyte survival and perilacunar remodeling in human and murine bone. *Bone 2017 Jun 27; 103: 78-87.*

12. Iqbal AM, Dahl AR, Lteif A, et al. Vitamin D deficiency: A potential modifiable risk factor for cardiovascular disease in children with severe obesity. *Children (Basel) 2017 Aug 28; 4 (9). pii: E80. doi: 10.3390/children4090080.*

13. Chen LW, Chien CY, Hsieh CW, et al. The associations between Helicobacter pylori infection, serum vitamin D, and metabolic syndrome: A Community-Based Study. *Medicine (Baltimore) 2016 May; 95 (18): e3616. doi: 10.1097/MD.0000000000003616.*

14. Shih HM, Hsu TY, Chen CY, et al. Analysis of patients with Helicobacter pylori infection and the subsequent risk of developing osteoporosis after eradication therapy: A nationwide population-based cohort study. *PLoS One 2016 Sep 14; 11 (9): e0162645*. doi: *10.1371/journal.pone.0162645. eCollection 2016.*

15. Chung YH, Gwak JS, Hong SW, et al. Helicobacter pylori: A possible risk factor for bone health. *Korean J Fam Med 2015 Sep; 36 (5): 239-44.*

16. Fotouk-Kiai M, Hoseini SR, Meftah N, et al. Relationship between Helicobacter pylori infection (HP) and bone mineral density (BMD) in elderly people. *Caspian J Intern Med 2015 spring; 6 (2): 62-6.*

17. Asaoka D, Nagahara A, Shimada Y, et al. Risk factors for osteoporosis in Japan: is it associated with Helicobacter pylori? *Ther Clin Risk Manag 2015 Mar 6; 11: 381-91.*

18. Al Shaikh AM, Abaalkhail B, Soliman A, et al. Prevalence of vitamin D deficiency and calcium homeostasis in Saudi children. *J Clin Res Pediatr Endocrinol 2016; 8 (4): 461-467.*

19. Kaddam IM, Al-Shaikh AM, Abaalkhail BA, et al. Prevalence of vitamin D deficiency and its associated factors in three regions of Saudi Arabia. *Saudi Med J 2017; 38 (4): 381-390.*

20. Farinha P, Gascoyne RD. Helicobacter pylori and MALT Lymphoma. *Gastroenterology 2005 May; 128 (6): 1579-605.*

21. Nasrat AM, Nasrat SAM, Nasrat RM, et al. Misconception and misbehavior towards Helicobacter pylori is leading to major spread of illness. *Gen Med 2015; S1: 002.* [Open Access]

22. Mizuno S, Matsui D, Watanabe I, et al. Serologically determined gastric mucosal condition is a predictive factor for osteoporosis in Japanese men. *Dig Dis Sci 2015 Jul; 60 (7): 2063-9.*

23. Lin SC, Koo M, Tsai KW. Association between Helicobacter pylori Infection and Risk of Osteoporosis in Elderly Taiwanese Women with Upper Gastrointestinal Diseases: A Retrospective Patient Record Review. *Gastroenterol Res Pract 2014; 2014: 814756. doi: 10.1155/2014/814756. Epub 2014 May 13.*

24. Xu ZH, Zhang J, Yang D, et al. Progress of research between Helicobacter pylori infection and osteoporosis. *Zhongguo Gu Shang 2011 Nov; 24 (11): 966-8.*

25. Suzuki H, Matsuzaki J, Hibi T. Lifestyle-related diseases and H. pylori. *Nihon Rinsho 2009 Dec; 67 (12): 2366-71.*

26. Nasrat SAM, Nasrat RM, Nasrat MN, et al. The dramatic spread of diabetes mellitus worldwide and influence of Helicobacter pylori. *General Med. 2015; 3 (1): 159-62.*

27. Bulut Y, Agacayak A, Karlidag D, et al. Association of CagA+ Helicobacter pylori with adenotonsillar hypertrophy. *Tohoku J Exp Med. 2006 Jul; 209 (3): 229-33.*

28. Nasrat AM, Nasrat RM, Nasrat MM. A pathologic etiology for the rising world challenge of obesity and dyslipidemia during latest three decades. *Am J Med Med Sci 2017; 7 (8): 318-322.*

29. Chen Z, Xu C, Luo L, et al. Helicobacter pylori infection and gastric mucosa change and blood-lipid in people undergoing the physical examination in Changsha. *Zhong Nan Da Xue Xue Bao Yi Xue Ban 2014 Mar; 39 (3): 265-9.*

30. Vijayvergiya R, Vadivelu R. Role of Helicobacter pylori infection in pathogenesis of atherosclerosis. *World J Cardiol 2015 Mar 26; 7 (3): 134-43.*

31. Buzás GM. Metabolic consequences of Helicobacter pylori infection and eradication. *World J Gastroenterol 2014 May 14; 20 (18): 5226-34.*

32. Sharma V, Aggarwal A. Helicobacter pylori: Does it add to risk of coronary artery disease. *World J Cardiol 2015 Jan 26; 7 (1): 19-25.*

33. Nasrat AM, Nasrat SAM, Nasrat RM, et al. The definitive eradication of Helicobacter pylori from the colon. *Gen Med 2015; S1: 1.* [Open Access]

34. Nasrat RM, Nasrat MM, Nasrat AM, et al. Improvement of idiopathic cardiomyopathy after colon clear. J Cardiol Res *2015 Apr; 6 (2): 249-254.* [Open Access]

35. Nasrat AM, Nasrat RM, Nasrat MM. Frequency of leukemia during late decades may indicate that the anti-Helicobacter pylori antibiotic strategy was a therapeutic mistake. *Am J Med Med Sci 2017; 7 (3): 103-107.* [Open Access]

36. Hughes NJ, Clayton CL, Chalk PA, et al. Helicobacter pylori porCDAB oorDABC genes encode distinct pyruvate: flavodoxin and 2-oxoglutarate: acceptor oxidoreductases which mediate electron transport to NADP. *J Bacteriol 1998 Mar; 180 (5): 1119-28.*

37. Berg JM, Tymoczko JL, Stryer L. Biochemistry. *WH Freeman and Company. 2002; 5th Ed: 480.*

38. Mendz GL, Hazell SL. Fumarate catabolism in Helicobacter pylori. *Biochem Mol Biol Int. 1993 Oct; 31 (2): 325-32.*

39. Mendz GL, Hazell SL, van Gorkom L. Pyruvate metabolism in Helicobacter pylori. *Arch Microbiol. 1994; 162(3):187-92.*

40. Nasrat AM. The dramatic spread of diabetes mellitus and influence of Helicobacter pylori. *J Clinic and Appl Res and Educ 2012; 9 (4): 53.*

41. Bulut Y, Agacayak A, Karlidag D, et al. Association of CagA+ Helicobacter pylori with adenotonsillar hypertrophy. *Tohoku J Exp Med. 2006 Jul; 209 (3): 229-33.*

42. Nasrat AM. Biological benefits of Helicobacter pylori and the intelligence of juxta-mucosal ammonia. *Am J Med Med Sci 2017; 7 (7): 281-286.* [Open Access]

43. Kubo N, Kochi S, Ariyama I, et al. Pseudomembranous colitis after Helicobacter pylori eradication therapy. *Kansenshogaku Zasshi 2006 Jan; 80 (1): 51-5.*

44. Schweigart U, Franck H, Schepp W, et al. Toxic megacolon after Helicobacter pylori eradication therapy. *Internist (Berl) 1997 Apr; 38 (4):352-4.*

45. Grünberger B, Wöhrer S, Streubel B, et al. Antibiotic treatment is not effective in patients infected with Helicobacter pylori suffering from extragastric MALT lymphoma. *J Clin Oncol 2006 Mar 20; 24 (9):1370-5.*

46. Shah D, Gupta P. Vitamin D deficiency: Is the pandemic for real? *Indian J Community Med 2015 Oct-Dec; 40 (4): 215-217.*

47. Rosch PJ. Cholesterol does not cause coronary heart disease in contrast to stress. *Scand Cardiovasc J 2008 Aug; 42 (4): 244-9.*

48. Rosch PJ. Saturated fat and cholesterol do not cause coronary heart disease. *The Annual Conference of the Saudi Heart Association, Hofuf, Saudi Arabia, Oct 2008.* Available from URL, *www.sha.org.sa*

49. Ravnskov U. The fallacies of the lipid hypothesis. *Scand Cardiovasc J 2008 Aug; 42 (4): 236-9.*

50. Scherstén T, Rosch PJ, Arfors KE, et al. The cholesterol hypothesis: time for the obituary? *Scand Cardiovasc J 20011 Dec; 45 (6): 322-3.*

51. Midolo PD, Lambert JR, Hull R, et al. In vitro inhibition of Helicobacter pylori NCTC 11637 by organic acids and lactic acid bacteria. *J Appl Bacteriol. 1995 Oct; 79 (4); 475-9.*

52. Mendz GL, Ball GE, Meek DJ, Pyruvate metabolism in Campylobacter spp. *Biochim Biophys Acta 1997 Mar 15; 1334 (2-3): 291-302.*

53. Mendz GL, Hazell SL, Burns BP. Glucose utilization and lactate production by Helicobacter pylori. *J Gen Microbiol 1993 Dec; 139 (Pt 12): 3023-8.*

54. Asaka M. Epidemiology of Helicobacter pylori infection in Japan. *Nippon Rinsho 2003 Jan; 61 (1): 19.*

55. Nasrat AM. The world misconception and misbehavior towards Helicobacter pylori is leading to major spread of illness. *The 7th Anti-Aging Medicine World Congress, Monte-Carlo, Monaco, 2009 Mar.* Available from URL, *www.euromedicom.com*

A SIMPLE SUSTAINED SOLUTION FOR DISSOLUTION OF THE CELLULITE

Introduction: Cellulite refers to a dimpled skin pathology that changes the skin surface appearance into an orange peel morphology. It is multi-factorial in its etiology caused by subcutaneous fat bulging into the dermis leading to cosmetic disfigurement which could be sometimes typically described as cottage cheese-like. Despite its high prevalence affecting a vast majority of **post**-pubertal women (85-98%), it remains a major cosmetic concern for women as it constitutes one of the most intolerable aesthetic imperfections.[1-4]

Although it is of no danger on general health, cellulite is psycho-socially debilitating. Cellulite is manifested by tissue edema and lipodystrophy while its etiology includes multiple factors. Cellulite and lipodystrophy are often found together especially in the areas of the buttocks and thighs. Edema that accompanies cellulite causes disorders of blood flow; therefore, different preparations and procedures that enhance circulation and improve blood perfusion, peripheral lymphedema and metabolism of subcutaneous fat were introduced to support treatment of cellulite. Cellulite in menopause has raised the attention towards female sex hormones, estrogen and progesterone, as the skin is the target of female sex hormones; the texture and appearance of the skin in women are most significantly affected by female sex hormones. Low estrogen during menopause, being responsible for the increased vascular permeability and decreased vascular tone, would lead to impairment of micro-circulation which is an important factor predisposing to the development of cellulite. Accordingly, preparations containing ingredients which help improving the metabolism of subcutaneous fat and enhance blood and lymphatic circulation in cosmetic styles have been reviewed and recommended in menopause for cellulite treatment.[5-9]

An effective and long-term treatment of cellulite has not been well established; it is still difficult to indicate an exclusive and effective single treatment for this condition. Topical treatments, noninvasive energy-based devices and recently developed minimally invasive interventions that may finally provide a solution have been implemented. However, no systematic review has been performed so far in order to evaluate the efficacy of the available treatment options for cellulite.[4,5,10]

Slimming creams have been tested for adequate treatment of cellulite without serious adverse effects, however additional large clinical trials are required to confirm their efficacy. Precise effective delivery of laser energy to the dermal adipose tissue as well as the deep adipose lipodystrophy is feasible as a safe measure for simultaneous treatment of cellulite and lipodystrophy in the buttocks and thighs. Intermittent negative pressure devices were initially developed to enhance circulation, improve blood perfusion and combat lymphedema. Focused ultrasonic lipolysis has been reported effective method for reduction of abdominal cellulite with some amount of circumference reduction reversal occurring in long term follow-up. There is growing evidence that extra-corporeal shock wave therapy is able to improve the degree of cellulite. The safety, efficacy and subject satisfaction with vacuum-assisted precise tissue release in the treatment of cellulite among adult women with moderate to severe degree of cellulite had been further reported. Treatment of abdominal cellulite and circumference reduction of abdomen with radiofrequency and dynamic muscle activation demonstrated that radiofrequency provided beneficial effects as regards reduction of abdominal circumference and cellulite appearance while the benefit of muscle activation needed further accurate determination. Radiofrequency had been always recommended as painless, safe and effective noninvasive skin tightening measure for body contouring and cellulite reduction. Cryolysis has been introduced as a safe effective noninvasive procedure for body contouring and nonsurgical fat reduction. Clinical evaluations demonstrated consistent improvement in skin texture, laxity and cellulite after cryolipolysis as independently assessed by patients and investigators.[2,3,6,8,11-15]

REFERENCES:

1. **Janda K, Tomikowska A.** Cellulite - causes, prevention, treatment. *Ann Acad Med Stetin 2014; 60 (1): 29-38.*

2. **Kaminer MS, Coleman WP 3rd, Weiss RA, et al. Multicenter pivotal study of vacuum-assisted precise tissue release for the treatment of cellulite.** *Dermatol Surg 2015 Mar; 41 (3): 336-47.*

3. **Byun SY, Kwon SH, Heo SH, et al. Efficacy of Slimming Cream Containing 3.5% Water-Soluble Caffeine and Xanthenes for the Treatment of Cellulite: Clinical Study and Literature Review.** *Ann Dermatol 2015 Jun; 27 (3): 243-9.*

4. **Luebberding S, Krueger N, Sadick NS. Cellulite: an evidence-based review.** *Am J Clin Dermatol 2015 Aug; 16 (4): 243-56.*

5. **Green JB, Cohen JL, Kaufman J, et al. Therapeutic approaches to cellulite.** *Semin Cutan Med Surg 2015 Sep; 34 (3): 140-3.*

6. **Petti C, Stoneburner J, McLaughlin L. Laser cellulite treatment and laser-assisted lipoplasty of the thighs and buttocks: Combined modalities for single stage contouring of the lower body.** *Lasers Surg Med 2016 Jan; 48 (1): 14-22.*

7. **Wilczyński S, Koprowski R, Deda A, et al. Thermographic mapping of the skin surface in biometric evaluation of cellulite treatment effectiveness.** *Skin Res Technol 2016 Jun 5. doi: 10.1111/srt.12301. [Epub ahead of print]*

8. **Campisi CC, Ryn M, Campisi CS, et al. Intermittent negative pressure therapy in the combined treatment of peripheral   lymphedema.** *Lymphology 2015 Dec; 48 (4): 197-204.*

9. **Leszko M. Cellulite in menopause.** *Prz Menopauzalny 2014 Oct; 13 (5): 298-304.*

10. **Zerini I, Sisti A, Cuomo R, et al. Cellulite treatment: a comprehensive literature review.** *J Cosmet Dermatol. 2015 Sep; 14 (3):   224-40.*

11. **Moravvej H, Akbari Z, Mohammadian S, et al. Focused ultrasound lipolysis in the treatment of abdominal cellulite: An open-label study.** *J Lasers Med Sci 2015 summer; 6 (3): 102-5.*

12. **Knobloch K, Kraemer R. Extracorporeal shock wave therapy (ESWT) for the treatment of cellulite--A current metaanalysis.** *Int J Surg 2015 Dec; 24 (Pt B): 210-7.*

13. **Wanitphakdeedecha R, Iamphonrat T, Thanomkitti K, et al. Treatment of abdominal cellulite and circumference reduction with radiofrequency and dynamic muscle activation.** *J Cosmet Laser Ther 2015; 17 (5): 246-51.*

14. **Harth Y. Painless, safe, and efficacious noninvasive skin tightening, body contouring, and cellulite reduction using multisource 3DEEP radiofrequency.** *J Cosmet Dermatol 2015 Mar; 14 (1): 70-5.*

15. **Carruthers J, Stevens WG, Carruthers A. Cryolipolysis and skin tightening.** *Dermatol Surg 2014 Dec; 40 Suppl 12: S184-9.*

SCIENTIFIC EVIDENCES ON THE SIMPLE SUSTAINED SOLUTION FOR DISSOLUTION OF THE CELLULITE

A*Simple Sustained Solution for Dissolution of the Cellulite:* Published in the American Journal of Medicine and Medical Sciences; 2017; 7 (9):331-337. Nasrat et al. A simple sustained solution for dissolution of the cellulite. *Am J Med Med Sci 2017; 7 (9):331-337. [doi: 10.5923/j.ajmms.20170709.02]*

Background: Cellulite refers to a dimpled skin pathology that changes the skin surface appearance into an orange peel morphology. It remains a major cosmetic concern for women as it affects the vast majority of women. Cellulite is manifested by tissue edema and lipodystrophy whereas its etiology includes multiple factors. Cellulite is a frequent skin condition for which treatment remains a challenge, a wide variety of treatments are available but an effective and long-term treatment of cellulite has not been well established, it is still difficult to indicate an effective exclusive single treatment for this condition.[1-4]

Although it is of no danger on general health, cellulite is psycho-socially debilitating. Cellulite is manifested by tissue edema and lipodystrophy while its etiology includes multiple factors. Preparations containing ingredients which help improving the metabolism of subcutaneous fat and enhance blood and lymphatic circulation in cosmetic styles have been recommended in menopause for cellulite treatment.[5-10]

From slimming creams to laser energy, ultrasound lipolysis, radiofrequency and cryolysis; many advanced technical measures have been employed but clinical results and women satisfaction are still controversial.[2,3,6,8,11-15]

Objective: Demonstration of the frequency of existence of colonic strains of ***Helicobacter pylori*** among a sample of women with cellulite and illustration of the role of these colonic ***H. pylori*** strains in the pathogenesis of cellulite.

Design& Setting: A prospective clinical study done in Jeddah/Saudi Arabia between October 2013 and May 2017.

Patients& Methods: A group of 30 women with moderate to severe cellulite, variable body weight/ body mass index (BMI) and an age range of 34-49 years were included in the study and investigated for the existence of colonic ***H. pylori*** strains employing ***H. pylori*** fecal antigen test.[16] The women who were found positive for colonic ***H. pylori*** strains followed a natural measure for eradication of ***H. pylori*** from the colon which consisted of the senna leaves extract purge colon clear and vinegar therapy. The senna purge was employed every month for three successive times to ensure eradication of the colonic ***H. pylori*** strains while vinegar therapy was used to protect from recurrence of the abnormal-existence/behavior colonic ***H. pylori*** strains via buffering the bacterium ingested with any query meal. Vinegar therapy consisted of a vinegar-mixed salad with principal meals, once or twice daily/five days a week for six months.[17] They had also received suction cupping therapy massage three times every week for one month then twice per week for one month and once a week for one further month.[18] The follow-up of women continued for three years as assessed independently by the women themselves and investigators based on longevity of follow up and observation of the body weight/BMI, subcutaneous fat reduction, skin texture/laxity and improvement of cellulite.[15] Women were not following any particular diet regimen, slimming measures or procedures for cellulite treatment. They were allowed to follow their own style of life except extreme restriction of outside-home meals to avoid recurrence of the colonic *H. pylori* strains. Women were advised to watch their colonic condition and repeat the senna purge and vinegar therapy whenever they develop colonic strains of *H. pylori* or frank colonic upsets.

Results: All women with cellulite were found positive for colonic *H. pylori* strains, their weight was ranging between 109-117 KG with BMI ≥25. All women became negative for colonic *H. pylori* strains after the senna purge as confirmed by the *H. pylori* fecal antigen test. Marked significant slimming was demonstrated in 27 women (90%) within 3-5 months and improvement of their BMI with a range of body weight of 81-92 KG. Slimming was frankly characterized by stretched skin without any redundancy or wrinkles as the loss of weight occurred just gradual.[19] Cellulite markedly improved in 24 women (80%) within three months as independently assessed by the women and investigators based on appearance, laxity and texture of the skin together with disappearance of lumps and dimples. Another three women (10%) showed the same good improvement in cellulite after further two months. Three women (10%) did not complete the study due to travelling from the area while 6 women (20%) gained weight within 18-20 months due to overeating but they did not develop any recurrence of cellulite.

Ethical Considerations: An informed signed consent was taken from all women, they were made aware about safety of the natural vinegar therapy and senna extract purge, they were free to quit the study whenever they like. The research proposal was approved and the study followed the rules of the Research Ethics Committee.

Discussion: Cellulite, those lumps and bumps constituting the modern woman's dilemma, seems to be growing in an epidemic way during the latest thirty years. In the past few years the interest of scientists in this problem has clearly increased. Several theories on the patho-physiology of cellulite have been produced. A number of different therapeutic regimens have been developed using modern technology. However, despite the many treatment options for cellulite, patient satisfaction is extremely the most important question as regards this noisy skin condition.[1]

Cellulite is a frequent skin condition for which treatment remains a challenge; a wide variety of treatments are available but most procedures offer sub-optimal clinical effect and/or delayed therapeutic outcome. Only few therapeutic options have proven effective in the treatment of cellulite. Despite the growing popularity of noninvasive ultrasonic lipolysis procedures, there is lack of evidence about the efficacy of this method. Long-term follow-up results beyond one year are lacking as well as details on potential combination therapies in cellulite such as with low level laser therapy, cryolipolysis and other procedures.[11-13]

An obscure etiology with indefinite cure results for a challenging frequent problem of a recent growing history should direct the clinical attention towards an underlying environmental error. The shortest access to identify an underlying error is to search out for a common reason which is directly related to other medical challenges spreading during the same period.

The latest reports in literature demonstrate a definite flare up of many medical challenges in rather a dramatic way through different reasons. Some reports consider disease spread a consequence of progress and lifestyle change.[16,19-24] In spite of that, traditional risk rules do not appear fully sufficient to explain the rising figures of chronic illness spread in the world. Prevalence of the phenomena of obesity constituting an actual growing challenge worldwide has been emphasized during the latest few decades.[25-28] The latest three decades confirm the prevalence of abnormal-existence/behavior colonic *H. pylori* strains with flare up of a lot of medical challenges related to these strains through immune, inflammatory, toxic or different unknown reasons.[16,17] The pathologic influence of these abnormal-existence colonic *H. pylori* strains has been demonstrated as concerns the challenge of obesity during the latest three decades;[19] therefore, the influence of these strains in cellulite could be strongly considered.

H. pylori colonized the stomach since an immemorial time as if both the stomach wall and the bacterium used to live together in peace harmless to each other. *H. pylori* could migrate or get forced to migrate to the colon under the influence of antibiotic violence to become a foreign structure to the tissues beyond the stomach as the bacterium is recognized only to the gastric wall tissues. *H. pylori* outside the stomach is rendered a poison itself by inducing auto-immunity and a source of poison by leading to inflammatory reactions and local tissue pathology. Colonic *H. pylori* strains will continue producing ammonia for a reason or no reason, un-opposed or buffered by any acidity, leading to accumulation of profuse toxic amounts of ammonia that could cause different adverse toxic sequels in the body.[16,17] Different reports in literature have confirmed the association of cytotoxin-associated gene A (cagA) with colonic *H. pylori* strains and emphasized that cagA of *H. pylori* encodes a highly immunogenic and virulence-associated protein; the presence of this virulent gene in the body could affect the clinical outcome in many patients.[29,30]

Cellulite skin has got characteristic manifestations induced by lipodystrophy and tissue edema leading to the orange peel appearance of the skin with lumps and dimples;[1,6-9] that is exactly the possible influence of colonic *H. pylori* strains on the skin of cellulite. It has been reported that colonic *H. pylori* strains interfere with fat turnover, lipid metabolism, lipid-lipoprotein metabolism and glucose metabolism in the body through increasing insulin resistance, these sequels could be sufficient reasons for development of lipodystrophy in the skin of cellulite.[19,31,32] Ammonia is a smooth muscle tonic, accumulation of excess amounts of ammonia in the colon could be smooth muscle spastic leading to multiple colonic spasms and a high rectal spasm causing a colonic re-absorptive error with consequent retention of fluids in the body. These fluids, being colonic contents, are expected to include salts and toxins that could induce inflammatory and undesirable pathologic effects.[17,28,33,34] These re-absorbed fluids from the colon are expected to become directed mostly towards the subcutaneous compartment in the lax areas of the body like the buttocks, thighs and abdomen as evidenced by the observational finding that pitting edema over the shaft of the leg among those people appears and increases with colonic troubles while it improves or disappears with improvement of these colonic troubles. This matter could match with the answer of the question; why cellulite selects some areas like the thighs, abdomen and buttocks and spares other areas!! It selects the lax areas where the inflammatory fluids can accumulate; these are at the mean time the same areas of fat deposition which in the presence of the inflammatory fluids could easily go into dystrophy. Accumulation of toxic inflammatory fluids within the subcutaneous tissues is simply sufficient to account for abnormal skin features such as in cellulite. The resulting tissue edema would be responsible for the orange peel appearance of the skin "peau d'orange" with dimpled skin morphology as the skin is normally attached to the dermis by subcutaneous fibrous septa which in presence of edema cause dimples on the surface.[2] The principle of employing the senna extract purge in the current study is to eradicate and ensure eradication of the colonic *H. pylori* strains which are the suggested pathogenic reason for development of cellulite. Eradication of *H. pylori* from the colon could also help slimming and reduce body fat which is in favor of cellulite improvement.[19] The senna leaves extract purge was demonstrated as the typical natural measure for definitive eradication of *H. pylori* from the colon. Three-times dilution of the standard senna leaves extract was found directly lethal to *H. pylori* strains on culture media.[34-36] Whereas employment of the vinegar therapy was meant to protect from recurrence of any abnormal-behavior *H. pylori* strains via buffering any query food intake. The complex nutritional requirements of *H. pylori* are achieved via its unique energy metabolism as the major routes of generation of energy for *H. pylori* are acquired via pyruvate while the activity of the pyruvate dehydrogenase complex is controlled by the rules of product inhibition and feedback regulation.[37,38] As acetate is demonstrated as an end product among the metabolic pathway of *H. pylori*;[39,40] therefore, addition of acetic acid (dietary white vinegar 6%) to the atmosphere around *H. pylori* could compromise the energy metabolism of *H. pylori* or interfere with the organism's respiratory chain metabolism. So long the matter includes interference with the energy metabolism and respiratory chain metabolism of **H. pylori**, an immediate dramatic lethal effect on the bacterium could be considered. Twenty times-dilution of dietary white vinegar 6% was found directly lethal to **H. pylori** strains upon brief immersion or on different culture media.[33,34] Accordingly and in the same mechanism, vinegar could interfere with ability of the human body to gain energy from carbohydrates forcing it to consume lipids for gaining energy; therefore, vinegar in this study could participate in slimming purposes also to improve the general state of the skin and cellulite.

The principle of employing the cupping suction massage in this study is enhancement of the circulation, treating tissue edema via encouraging lymphatic drainage and improving the micro-circulation;[18] tissue edema, lack of proper circulation and inadequate micro-circulation are known underlying pathologic elements in leading to cellulite.[7-9] Further previous studies have used the intermittent negative pressure therapy and the vacuum-assisted precise tissue release to improve peripheral lymphedema, enhance circulation and assist blood perfusion for the treatment of cellulite.[2,8] Cupping suction improves the micro-circulation because of the endothelial-derived nitric oxide liberation via a shear stress effect caused by the action of repeated suction.[18] The wonderful effect of cupping massage in eliminating inflammatory edema together with the intelligence of nitric oxide in enhancing the micro-circulation are sufficient, after eradication of the pathologic etiology, to clear out the miserable skin features of cellulite.

Fundamental definitive cure is treatment of the cause with elimination or withdrawal of pathology not just treatment of the symptoms. This study is concerned essentially with eradication of the colonic **H. pylori** strains which are the hypothesized pathogenic reason of cellulite together with preventing recurrence of the pathologic etiology via vinegar therapy and cure of symptoms by means of suction cupping therapy massage. The possible reason that previous efforts in treatment of cellulite did not achieve definitive or exclusive results is focusing their work on cure of symptoms but not the causative pathology. In brief, this study was working on three main elements which are withdrawal of pathology via the natural senna purge, avoiding recurrence of pathology by employing the vinegar therapy and curing the symptoms via improving tissue edema, encouraging blood and lymphatic circulation and enhancing the micro-circulation by means of the suction cupping therapy massage.[16-18]

Revision of literature studies for comparative reasons with rather similar sample size of subjects revealed that treatment of cellulite features without eradication of the underlying pathology brought inadequate results and the resulting improvement was not satisfactory or persistent. In a multi-center study of side-firing laser therapy for cellulite treatment among 57 individuals using clinical photographs for evaluation of the results of therapy, it was found that the average improvement score at 6 months was 1.7 for dimples and 1.1 for contour irregularities while at 12 months the average improvement score was 1.4 for dimples and 1.0 for contour irregularities on a 5-point scale;[41] it means that improvement declined in short time. In a further study of laser cellulite treatment combined with laser-assisted lipoplasty of buttocks and thighs among 16 subjects using Nurnberger-Muller scale and global aesthetic improvement scale for evaluation of therapy, similar results were also achieved.[6] In a study of the effect of noninvasive ultrasonic lipolysis for treatment of abdominal cellulite among 28 subjects where evaluation of results was based on contour measurement, a significant average of 1.89 cm decrease of circumference was observed in each ultrasonic lipolysis therapy session whereas the mean pre-treatment to post-treatment circumference reduction was 8.21 cm that declined to 7 cm at the three-month follow-up visit;[11] which is also a short time. Radiofrequency employed for 25 females receiving six-weekly treatments for abdominal cellulite has given suboptimal clinical or delayed therapeutic effect of 25-49% after 1-4 weeks follow-up as evaluated by the standard photographs and the measurement of abdominal circumference, improvement was also not sustained as it was less in the fourth week follow-up visit.[13] Based on independent assessments by the subjects and investigators, cryolipolysis has shown consistent but mild to moderate improvement on skin texture/laxity and the cellulite.[15] A further study in favor of cryolipolysis in fat reduction in the flanks among 19 subjects reported reduction of fat as measured by ultrasound in 79% of subjects but a variety of side-effects such as paradoxical adipose hyperplasia or adipose hypertrophy following cryolipolysis were also encountered.[42-44] Efficacy of slimming creams was tested on 15 females for circumference reduction employing a standard visual scale score, thigh and upper-arm circumferences decreased by 0.7 cm and 0.8 cm respectively after 6 weeks but itching and flushing were commonly reported.[3] Single treatment of vacuum-assisted precise tissue release for the treatment of cellulite was done for 55 women with moderate to severe cellulite employing the blinded assessments of subject photographs, a validated Cellulite Severity Scale and the Global Aesthetic Improvement Scale. The mean baseline score of 3.4 decreased to 1.3 at 3 months and 1.4 at one year.[2] Intermittent negative pressure therapy was studied on 50 patients with lymphedema and it was found that it caused 7% improvement in the volume of edma; therefore, it was recommended to be included in the treatment of cellulite.[8] Throughout this comparison, the vacuum assisted precise tissue release and intermittent negative pressure therapy seem most promising, safe and satisfactory.

Procedure	Subjects No	Results	Decline of Effect	Side-Effects
Laser Therapy	57, 16	Mild-Moderate	+	Minimal
Ultrasonic Lipolysis	28	Mild-Moderate	+	-
Radiofrequency	25	Mild-Moderate	+	-
Cryolipolysis	19	Mild-Moderate	+	++
Slimming Creams	15	Mild	++	+
Vacuum-Assisted Tissue Release	55	Good	+	-
Intermittent Negative Pressure Therapy	50	Good	+	-
Combined Colon Clear& Cupping Suction Massage	30	V. Good	-	-

The table illustrates a comparison between different procedures of cellulite treatment as concerns the effect, sustain/decline of the effect of therapy and possibility of side-effects.

Cellulite is a complicated compromise; a woman with cellulite has to lose weight, reduce subcutaneous fat, get rid of tissue fluid retention, improve local and general circulation and enhance micro-circulation of the affected areas. All these criteria or most of them constitute challenges to patients and physicians which explains to a great extent why investigators did not approach maintained satisfactory results in treatment of cellulite. The combined senna purge, vinegar therapy and suction cupping therapy massage via withdrawal of the most possible etiologic pathology which is the colonic *H. pylori* strains could help to reduce weight and body fat, push out tissue edema and encourage general and micro-circulation.[16-19,33]

Several measures has been planned to guide assessment of therapy in cellulite such as biometric thermo-graphic images mapping of the skin, the modified Nurnberger-Muller scale, the global aesthetic improvement scale, the validated Cellulite Severity Scale, the ultrasound-measured subcutaneous tissue thickness, the standard visual scale score and the standardized clinical photographs with measurements of body weight and abdominal circumference.[2,3,6,7,13]

Clinical evaluation of the results of therapy among women of the current study demonstrated consistent improvement in the skin texture, skin laxity, body weight, BMI, reduction of fat and improvement of cellulite as independently assessed by the women themselves and the investigators. Independent assessment was followed in this study as individual satisfaction was considered an adequate judge for clinical improvement. A further study has employed the independent assessment of the results of therapy in cellulite based on individual's satisfaction and investigators evaluation, it was found that this way of assessment is satisfactory and practical.[15] Independent assessment by individuals and investigators could be just adequate so long the improvement is frank and obvious as the individual satisfaction is the main target of therapy. Previous records of the research team of this study denoted that patient satisfaction in skin problems could be a reliable monitor for clinical improvement as the skin appearance is the important target and patient satisfaction with his skin would be therefore an adequate mirror image for improvement of the clinical condition.

Conclusion: Clinical evidences seem supporting the finding that the abnormal existence of colonic ***H. pylori*** might be a hidden reason behind the recent medical challenge for most women known as the "***cellulite***"; therefore, eradication of these colonic ***H. pylori*** strains via natural measures could be an effective scientific approach to control the spread of cellulite worldwide. Combined senna purge and vinegar therapy together with suction cupping therapy massage could be promising simple, safe and effective measure for sustained treatment of cellulite among people with positive colonic ***H. pylori*** strains.

Conflict of Interest: There is no conflict of interest existin

REFERENCES:

1. Janda K, Tomikowska A. Cellulite - causes, prevention, treatment. *Ann Acad Med Stetin 2014; 60 (1): 29-38.*

2. **Kaminer MS, Coleman WP 3rd, Weiss RA, et al. Multicenter pivotal study of vacuum-assisted precise tissue release for the treatment of cellulite.** *Dermatol Surg 2015 Mar; 41 (3): 336-47.*

3. **Byun SY, Kwon SH, Heo SH, et al. Efficacy of Slimming Cream Containing 3.5% Water-Soluble Caffeine and Xanthenes for the Treatment of Cellulite: Clinical Study and Literature Review.** *Ann Dermatol 2015 Jun; 27 (3): 243-9.*

4. **Luebberding S, Krueger N, Sadick NS. Cellulite: an evidence-based review.** *Am J Clin Dermatol 2015 Aug; 16 (4): 243-56.*

5. **Green JB, Cohen JL, Kaufman J, et al. Therapeutic approaches to cellulite.** *Semin Cutan Med Surg 2015 Sep; 34 (3): 140-3.*

6. **Petti C, Stoneburner J, McLaughlin L. Laser cellulite treatment and laser-assisted lipoplasty of the thighs and buttocks: Combined modalities for single stage contouring of the lower body.** *Lasers Surg Med 2016 Jan; 48 (1): 14-22.*

7. **Wilczyński S, Koprowski R, Deda A, et al. Thermographic mapping of the skin surface in biometric evaluation of cellulite treatment effectiveness.** *Skin Res Technol 2016 Jun 5. doi: 10.1111/srt.12301. [Epub ahead of print]*

8. **Campisi CC, Ryn M, Campisi CS, et al. Intermittent negative pressure therapy in the combined treatment of peripheral lymphedema.** *Lymphology 2015 Dec; 48 (4): 197-204.*

9. **Leszko M. Cellulite in menopause.** *Prz Menopauzalny 2014 Oct; 13 (5): 298-304.*

10. **Zerini I, Sisti A, Cuomo R, et al. Cellulite treatment: a comprehensive literature review.** *J Cosmet Dermatol. 2015 Sep; 14 (3): 224-40.*

11. **Moravvej H, Akbari Z, Mohammadian S, et al. Focused ultrasound lipolysis in the treatment of abdominal cellulite: An open-label study.** *J Lasers Med Sci 2015 summer; 6 (3): 102-5.*

12. **Knobloch K, Kraemer R. Extracorporeal shock wave therapy (ESWT) for the treatment of cellulite--A current metaanalysis.** *Int J Surg 2015 Dec; 24 (Pt B): 210-7.*

13. **Wanitphakdeedecha R, Iamphonrat T, Thanomkitti K, et al. Treatment of abdominal cellulite and circumference reduction with radiofrequency and dynamic muscle activation.** *J Cosmet Laser Ther 2015; 17 (5): 246-51.*

14. **Harth Y. Painless, safe, and efficacious noninvasive skin tightening, body contouring,**

and cellulite reduction using multisource 3DEEP radiofrequency. *J Cosmet Dermatol 2015 Mar; 14 (1): 70-5.*

15. Carruthers J, Stevens WG, Carruthers A. Cryolipolysis and skin tightening. *Dermatol Surg 2014 Dec; 40 Suppl 12: S184-9.*

16. Farinha P, Gascoyne RD. Helicobacter pylori and MALT Lymphoma. *Gastroenterology 2005 May; 128 (6): 1579-605.*

17. Nasrat AM, Nasrat SAM, Nasrat RM, et al. Misconception and misbehavior towards Helicobacter pylori is leading to major spread of illness. *Gen Med 2015; S1: 002.* [Open Access]

18. Nasrat AM, Nasrat MM. The scientific theory in cupping therapy; the highly selective pooling of the whole circulation within a localized sector of the capillary bed over a limited interval. *Am J Med Med Sci 2017; 7 (7): 302-307.* [Open Access]

19. Nasrat AM, Nasrat RM, Nasrat MM. A pathologic etiology for the rising world challenge of obesity and dyslipidemia during latest three decades. *Am J Med Med Sci 2017; 7 (8): 318-322.* [Open Access]

20. Katulanda P, Sheriff MH, Matthews DR. The diabetes epidemic in Sri Lanka-a growing problem. *Ceylon Med J 2006 Mar; 51(1): 26-8.*

21. Wissow LS. Diabetes, poverty and Latin America. *Patient Educ Couns 2006 May; 61 (2): 169-70. Epub 2006 Apr 18.*

22. Einecke D. Like a tsunami: diabetes wave floods the whole world. *MMC 2006 Apr 6; 148 (14): 4-6.*

23. Yach D, Stuckler D, Brownell KD. Epidemiologic and economic consequences of the global epidemics of obesity and diabetes. *N Med 2006 Jan; 12 (1): 62-6.*

24. Reddy KS, Naik N, Prabhakaran D. Hypertension in developing world: a consequence of progress. *Curr Cardiol Rep 2006; 8 (6): 399-404.*

25. Parikh Y, Mason M, Williams K. Researchers' perspectives pediatric obesity research participant recruitment. *Clin Transl Med 2016 Dec; 5 (1): 20. Epub 2016 Jun 23.*

26. Xiao C, Dash S, Morgantini C, et al. Pharmacological Targeting of the Atherogenic Dyslipidemia Complex: The Next Frontier in CVD Prevention Beyond Lowering LDL Cholesterol. *Diabetes 2016 Jul; 65 (7): 1767-78.*

27. Grammer T, Kleber M, Silbernagel G, et al. Residual risk: The roles of triglycerides and high density lipoproteins. *Dutsch Med Wochenschr 2016 Jun; 141 (12): 870-7.*

28. Hossain P, Kawar B, El Nahas M. Obesity and diabetes in developing world-a growing challenge. *N Engl J Med 2007 Jan18; 356 (3): 213-5.*

29. Nasrat SAM, Nasrat RM, Nasrat MN, et al. The dramatic spread of diabetes mellitus worldwide and influence of Helicobacter pylori. *General Med. 2015; 3 (1): 159-62.*

30. Bulut Y, Agacayak A, Karlidag D, et al. Association of CagA+ Helicobacter pylori with adenotonsillar hypertrophy. *Tohoku J Exp Med. 2006 Jul; 209 (3): 229-33.*

31. **Buzás GM. Metabolic consequences of Helicobacter pylori infection and eradication.** *World J Gastroenterol 2014 May 14; 20 (18): 5226-34.*

32. **Moretti E, Gonnelli S, Campagna M, et al. Influence of Helicobacter pylori infection on metabolic parameters and body composition of dyslipidemic patients.** *Intern Emerg Med 2014 Oct; 9 (7): 767-72.*

33. **Nasrat AM, Nasrat SAM, Nasrat RM, et al. An alternate natural remedy for symptomatic relief of Helicobacter pylori dyspepsia. Gen Med 2015**; *3 (4).* **[Open Access]**

34. **Nasrat RM, Nasrat MM, Nasrat AM, et al. Improvement of idiopathic cardiomyopathy after colon clear. J Cardiol Res** *2015 Apr; 6 (2): 249-254.* **[Open Access]**

35. **Nasrat AM, Nasrat SAM, Nasrat RM, et al. The definitive eradication of Helicobacter pylori from the colon. Gen Med 2015**; *S1: 1.* **[Open Access]**

36. **Nasrat AM, Nasrat RM, Nasrat MM. Frequency of leukemia during late decades may indicate that the anti-Helicobacter pylori antibiotic strategy was a therapeutic mistake.** *Am J Med Med Sci 2017; 7 (3): 103-107.* **[Open Access]**

37. **Hughes NJ, Clayton CL, Chalk PA, et al. Helicobacter pylori porCDAB oorDABC genes encode distinct pyruvate: flavodoxin and 2-oxoglutarate: acceptor oxidoreductases which mediate electron transport to NADP.** *J Bacteriol 1998 Mar; 180 (5): 1119-28.*

38. **Berg JM, Tymoczko JL, Stryer L. Biochemistry.** *WH Freeman and Company. 2002; 5ᵗʰ Ed: 480.*

39. **Mendz GL, Hazell SL. Fumarate catabolism in Helicobacter pylori.** *Biochem Mol Biol Int. 1993 Oct; 31 (2): 325-32.*

40. **Mendz GL, Hazell SL, van Gorkom L. Pyruvate metabolism in Helicobacter pylori.** *Arch Microbiol. 1994; 162 (3):187-92.*

41. **DiBernardo BE, Sasaki GH, Katz BE, et al. A multicenter study for cellulite treatment using a 1440-nm Nd: YAG wavelength laser with side-firing fiber.** *Aesthet Surg J 2016 Mar; 36 (3): 335-43.*

42. **Kilmer SL. Prototype CoolCup cryolipolysis applicator with over 40% reduced treatment time demonstrates equivalent safety and efficacy with greater patient preference.** *Lasers Surg Med 2016 Jun 21. doi: 10.1002/lsm.22550. [Epub ahead of print]*

43. **Kelly E, Rodriguez-Feliz J, Kelly ME. Paradoxical adipose hyperplasia after cryolipolysis: A report on incidence and common factors identified in 510 patients.** *Plast Reconstr Surg 2016 Mar; 137 (3): 639e-640e.*

44. **Stefani WA. Adipose hypertrophy following cryolipolysis.** *Aesthet Surg J 2015 Sep; 35 (7): NP218-20.*

CHARACTERISTICS OF HELCOBACTER PYLORI-RELATED DYSPEPSIA

The published related article; *Characteristics of Helicobacter Pylori-Related Dysglycemia:* Published in Journal of General Medicine 2015; S1: 4. (Open Access). Nasrat et al. Characteristics of Helicobacter pylori-related dysglycemia. *General Med 2015; S1: 4. [doi: 10.4172/2327-5146.1000S1-004]*

Characteristic manifestations of *Helicobacter pylori* dyspepsia:

1. In addition to heart burn, burping, distension and constipation; passage of small hard pieces of dried stool indicates existence of multiple colonic spasms due to the smooth muscle spastic effect of excess ammonia produced by *H. pylori* in the colon.

2. Loss of the main colonic function of formation of the bowel contents manifested in passage of soft unformed motions due to presence of high rectal and high sigmoid spasms with consequent dilatation of the colon in order to accommodate its contents is also a frequent observation.

3. Sometimes, patients with H. pylori-induced diabetes do not feel hungry but they feel they like to eat because of feeling some colic in the centre of abdomen falsely believing it as hunger pains, hence they do not feel satiety after intake of food as colic does not stop; the solution in this situation is having vinegar-mixed food after a small snack and this could help relief of colonic spasms via inhibition of ammonia production by H. pylori.

4. Recurrent breathing discomfort on minor effort or even upon turning on either side while lying in bed may also happen due to pressure on the diaphragm by the distended or multiply-spastic colon with consequent embarrassment of the lung's vital capacity.

5. Recurrent faint focal stinging potash-like taste sensation related to some teeth felt by tip of the tongue occurs due to production of ammonia by dental H. pylori colonization; these dental strains are famous of causing gastric recurrence, the solution is mouth wash with diluted vinegar; twice per week are sufficient.

6. Constitutional symptoms such as burning sensation in sole of feet, heaviness and swelling in extremities and pitting edema of lower limbs particularly the left or the frequently dependant side during sleep are constant features most of the time and are related to salt and fluid retention in the body from the colonic contents; the treatment is definitely colon care and colon clear.

7. Motion symptoms like false sensations to pass motion or passing flatus instead, difficulty in passing motion and passage of hard pieces of dry stool are due to colonic spasms, while passing soft unformed motion or frequent need to pass small amounts of soft motion after every food intake are due to the continuously loaded colon.

8. A normal individual does not need urgently passing motion whenever he is having a heavy meal unless he is constipated or not visiting the toilet for few days as the colon forms and accommodates the colonic contents to pass the motion once or twice per day or even once every 2-3 days on habitual convenient times; while in H. pylori dyspeptic person and due to the condition of the loaded colon, a person may sometimes run to pass only a scanty amount of soft motion whenever he is having any size of a meal.

9. The smaller the size of pieces of stool and its situation of dryness are related to the severity and amount of colonic spasms which are related in turn to heaviness of the existing colonic H. pylori strains and the amount of colonic ammonia.

10. The thickness of the mucus surrounding the pieces of stool is also related to heaviness of the existing colonic H. pylori strains; whenever H. pylori exists in heavy percentage, the more viscous and thick is the mucus around the stool.

11. Involuntary incontinence to an abundant amount of soft stool is very unusual event; if happens, it is due to a loaded colon or a loaded rectum inducing a local recto-colic mass reflex; it is simply like a retention with overflow event. The treatment of this matter is colon clear by the natural senna purge.

12. Passage of continent watery motions or just mucoid secretions, single or repeated times, not associated with fever or colic is also a very unusual event; it is due to severely resistant high rectal or high sigmoid spasm or both as demonstrated by sigmoidoscopy and colonoscopy; leading in turn to severe multiple colonic spasms attempting to reduce the size of the colonic contents, the squeezed colonic contents leaves its watery component to pass out as watery motion. Diffuse minute abdominal colics audible on auscultation and a contracted rectum on P/R examination associated with this condition of watery motion are usually due to the ammonia contained in the colon, rectum and sigmoid. This condition usually follows heavy set-up of colonic H. pylori colonization after a query meal. The treatment of this watery motion is immediate colon clear by the potent senna purge but never by any constipating or anti-diarrhea mixture.

13. Prolapsed piles is a common association with H. pylori-relateded dypepsia because of constipation and straining as straining is useless effectiveless with the presence of high sigmoid and/or high rectal spasm; therefore, patients should not sit too long for passing motion, they should avoid un-necessary straining and better learn how to do two-finger anal dilatation (gentle straining and gradual finger anal dilatation) while passing motion to remove small rectal contents in order to protect from prolapse of piles in addition to avoiding any increase of the colonic re-absorptive error pump with straining.

14. If patients can not help to remove some high small rectal contents by finger evacuation, they should not insist long time for that and they better leave it to pass it out later when a proper motion reflex is initiated or the patient can have a vinegar-mixed food after a small snack; this could help passing a motion and clearing the rectum as the vinegar could relieve colonic spasms via inhibition of ammonia production.

15. Constipation associated with H. pylori dyspepsia is sometimes so severe being induced by the spastic effect of excess ammonia in the colon, it does not respond to adequate antispasmodic and laxative measures; it can not be overcome except with vinegar-mixed food as it inhibits ammonia production by H. pylori. Colonic contents should be cleared by the senna purge as it is the best measure to readily clear the colon in such situation.

16. Constipation related to H. pylori dyspepsia even so severe and associated with abdominal distension can not be confused with intestinal obstruction because it is not absolute constipation as there is frequent passage of winds due to liberation of ammonia in the lower colon; P/R examination in many instances reveals an empty contracted rectum due to the effect of ammonia or a rectum contracted over small pieces of stool. However, containment or entrapment of excess ammonia within a closed simple loop or multiple loops could hurt integrity of the gut tissues leading very rarely to severe critical sequels simulating intestinal obstruction.

17. Frequency of micturition is not necessary all the time to be due to uncontrolled blood sugar, it is in many times due to a local axon reflex because of urethral irritation caused by accumulation of ammonia in the pelvic colon or local irritation caused by small dried pieces of stool in the rectum; the frequent urine in such situations is not ample and diluted, on the contrary it is in many times scanty and concentrated.

18. Slipping of small pieces or piece of dried stool into the rectum can not be prevented by the sigmoid as being small sized, these small dried pieces of stool do not usually initiate a motion desire or a motion reflex because of their small size but would continue to cause bladder irritation and urgency for passing urine even of small amounts because of the continuously produced ammonia by H. pylori contained in these small pieces of stool; finger evacuation of these small pieces of stool could be a good solution.

19. Incontinence of few drops of urine or occasional loss of control of the whole urine could also very infrequently happen due to the same reason of local irritation by the local axon reflex; however this matter is self-limited and is improving spontaneously even without using any therapeutic measures due to adaptation of the bladder to the underlying local irritation. Until this adaptation develops, a person while outside home should try to evacuate the bladder whenever possible in order not to face an embarrassing situation. While at convenient situations where there is easy reach of a bathroom, a person may try to practice ignoring the desire to pass urine as possible so as to develop adaption towards that local urethral irritation.

20. It is quite apparent that urgency of micturition in H. pylori-related dyspepsia is mainly rather a sort of stress condition due to local irritation via a local reflex caused by ammonia in the pelvic colon leading to urethral irritating sensation to urgently pass the urine or leading to reduced or contracted bladder capacity as in many times of these urgency situations the person finds the voided urine scanty not abundant or concentrated or both.

21. A normal individual usually does not leave the bed for urgency of urine as the urinary bladder accommodates the urine until the person gets up from sleep. In the same way, in normal situations a subject does not leave the bed for urgency to pass motion as the colon forms and accommodates the colonic contents to pass the motion in convenient times, once or twice per day or more than one day. An H. pylori dyspeptic person may need to leave the bed in order to clear the rectum from small contents causing frequent urgency sensation for urination due to urethral or bladder irritation via a local reflex.

22. In situations of resistant epigastric discomfort that does not respond to symptomatic measures, P/R examination reveals many times a contracted rectum over impacted small pieces of stool; finger evacuation of the rectum relieves a reflex spasm of the cardio-esophageal sphincter with subsequent relief of the epigastric discomfort.

23. Unexplained spacing between two teeth or more was attributed to gingivitis or gingival hyperplasia caused by the dental H. pylori colonization.

24. Blood sugar level could be frankly affected by the colonic upsets or the indigestive condition; in many times, blood sugar level is difficult to control in spite of extreme carefulness in diet; this could be due to the toxic effect of excess colonic ammonia on the pancreas.

25. Asthmatic discomfort due to embarrassment of the chest by the loaded or spastic colon, morning or daytime throat secretions with unexplained cough or bronchial spasm and nasal sinuses symptoms could be also associated features in patients with H. pylori dyspepsia

On conclusion, the ideal strategy in dealing with the challenge of *H. pylori*-related dysglycemia is natural eradication of colonic *H. pylori* strains via employing the senna leaves extract purge, maintenance of colon care by vinegar therapy, guard against gastric recurrence form dental colonization by mouth wash with diluted vinegar twice/week, control of fecal-oral re-infection by disinfecting hands with white vinegar after washing with soap and water and protection from re-set up of abnormal-behavior gastric colonization via oral intake by having a vinegar-mixed food after any query meal.

It is necessary to pay the attention that this chapter *"characteristics of Helicobacter pylori-induced dysglycemia"* includes no references as it is an observational subject of patient's symptoms studied by the authors over more than 10 years. The authors are the pioneers to observe, describe, record, interpret, deal with and manage these symptoms; therefore, a previous experience to describe these symptoms is not available or reported, accordingly references do not have place in this chapter. This chapter is an attempt to precisely describe the individual symptoms associated with *H. pylori* dyspepsia that interferes with quality of life as experienced and expressed by the patients themselves and explain how to deal with these symptoms in order to help improving the lost patient's quality of life due to their dyspeptic troubles.

COLON CARE AND VINEGAR THERAPY

The published related article; *An Alternate Natural Remedy for Symptomatic Relief of Helicobacter pylori Dyspepsia:* Published in Journal of General Medicine 2015; 3 (4): 1000200. (Open Access). Nasrat et al. An alternate natural remedy for symptomatic relief of Helicobacter pylori dyspepsia. *General Med 2015; 3 (4): 1000200. [doi: 10.4172/2327-5146.1000200]*

Vinegar is a food that includes health or healthy values and is not a medicine to drink or to be diluted in warm water and taken on empty stomach as advised by alternate medicine therapists otherwise it would be very drastic to the natural bacteria worse than any antibiotic.[1] Normal behavior of natural bacteria of the gut does include its existence inside the lumen during presence of food, therefore; vinegar mixed with food would not harm except the bacteria which have deviated from its nature. Accordingly, vinegar-mixed food works to behave and kill the abnormal behavior gastric ***Helicobacter pylori*** strains; thus protecting from their spontaneous migration to the colon, that's what is meant by colon care. On the other way, vinegar on empty stomach terrifies the natural bacteria and would definitely force many sound-behavior ***H. pylori*** strains to migrate to the colon.[1-3] These facts explain the development of lower esophagitis in women who followed intake of vinegar in warm water advised by natural therapists for slimming purposes instead of having it mixed with food. Observational studies have proposed a protective role of ***H. pylori*** infection against the development of gastro-esophageal reflux disease, and suggested that ***H. pylori*** eradication treatment may increase the incidence of reflux symptoms.[4]

The fact that vinegar has got an antibacterial activity that can induce immediate in vitro inhibition of growth of pathogenic bacteria allowing its use in different practical applications, has been reported in literature.[5,6] It has been also reported that bacterial growth on fish fillets media was highly inhibited by relatively small concentrations of acetate (less than 0.3%).[7]

In vitro inhibition of ***H. pylori*** growth was demonstrated due to the effect of pH of bio-organic acids, lactic and acetic, with the lactic acid demonstrating the greatest inhibition.[5] The complex nutritional requirements of ***H. pylori*** are achieved via its unique energy metabolism, which exhibits characteristic dislocation sites. These sites can be considered as targets that should attract any attempts to fight the organism.[8,9] As acetate is demonstrated as an end product among the metabolic pathway of ***H. pylori***;[10,11] therefore, addition of acetic acid to the atmosphere around ***H. pylori*** could compromise the energy metabolism of ***H. pylori*** or interfere with the organism's respiratory chain metabolism. This suggestion is supported by the fact that the major routes of generation of energy of ***H. pylori*** are via pyruvate and the activity of the pyruvate dehydrogenase complex is controlled by the rules of product inhibition and feedback regulation.[12,13] For the same reason, addition of pyruvate to different solid culture media was found to inhibit bacterial growth, and this inhibition was attributed to accumulation of acetate and formate;[14] Accordingly, vinegar interferes with ability of the body to gain energy from carbohydrates forcing it to consume lipids for gaining energy; therefore, vinegar could be used for slimming purposes and treating dyslipidemia.

<u>Method of employing Vinegar-mixed food therapy</u>: 1-2 table spoonful of dietary white vinegar and 1-2 table spoonful of pure corn oil mixed with a cup of plain yoghurt, a salad or fruits could be also added, and to be taken once or twice daily with lunch and/or dinner, 3-5 days per week. Colon care means getting rid of the abnormal gastric **H. pylori** strains before reaching the colon.[3]

Vinegar can be added to warm drinks such as green tea after principal meals for slimming purposes in addition to behaving or getting rid of the abnormal behavior gastric **H. pylori** strains, but it should be strictly and directly after food but not on empty stomach, particularly after the meal that contains excess calories. Vinegar could be also added to a soup dish instead of lemon for the same slimming purpose and it should be preceded by few bites of food or a snack.[1,3]

Vinegar is a food that includes health and cure but is not a medicine that can be mixed with water and drunk on empty stomach while corn oil is also a food staff that could be of laxative or lubricant value to the bowel motion, therefore; the amount of vinegar and corn oil in vinegar therapy is not a fixed dose but can be changed as desired and could be dealt with exactly such as the amount of salt in food which is added according to what is palatable by the person. Palatable taste of vinegar-mixed food is important for avoiding noise to normal gastric **H. pylori** strains in order to avoid pushing them to migrate to the colon or escape from the stomach to anywhere else.[3]

REFERENCES:

1. **Farinha P, Gascoyne RD.** Helicobacter pylori and MALT Lymphoma. *Gastroenterology 2005 May; 128 (6): 1579-605.*

2. **Nasrat AM. The world misconception and misbehavior towards Helicobacter pylori is leading to major spread of illness.** *The 7th Anti-Aging Medicine World Congress, Monte-Carlo, Monaco, 2009 Mar.* **Available from URL,** *www.euromedicom.com*

3. **Baron S. Baron's medical microbiology.** *Churchill Livingstone. 2000; 4th Ed: 346.*

4. **Labenz J, Blum AL, Bayerdorffer E, et al. Curing Helicobacter pylori infection in patients with duodenal ulcer may provoke reflux esophagitis.** *Gastroenterology 1997; 112: 1442-47.*

5. **Midolo PD, Lambert JR, Hull R, et al. In vitro inhibition of Helicobacter pylori NCTC 11637 by organic acids and lactic acid bacteria.** *J Appl Bacteriol. 1995 Oct; 79 (4): 475-9.*

6. **Makino SI, Cheun HI, Tabuchi H, et al. Antibacterial activity of chaff vinegar and its practical application.** *J Vet Med Sci. 2000 Aug; 62 (8): 893-5.*

7. **Debevere J, Devlieghere F, van Sprundel P, et al. Influence of acetate and CO2 on the TMAO – reduction reaction by Shewanella baltica.** *Int J Food Microbiol 2001 Aug 15; 68 (1-2):115-23.*

8. **Ge Z. Potential of fumarate reductase as a novel therapeutic target in Helicobacter pylori infection.** *Expert Opin Ther Targets 2002 Apr; 6 (2): 135-46.*

9. **endz GL, Hazell SL, Burns BP. Glucose utilization and lactate production by Helicobacter pylori.** *J Gen Microbiol 1993 Dec; 139 (Pt 12): 3023-8.*

10. **Mendz GL, Hazell SL. Fumarate catabolism in Helicobacter pylori.** *Biochem Mol Biol Int. 1993 Oct; 31 (2): 325-32.*

11. **Mendz GL, Hazell SL, van Gorkom L. Pyruvate metabolism in Helicobacter pylori.** *Arch Microbiol. 1994; 162 (3):187-92.*

12. <u>Hughes NJ, Clayton CL, Chalk PA, et al. Helicobacter pylori porCDAB oorDABC genes encode distinct pyruvate: flavodoxin and 2-oxoglutarate: acceptor oxidoreductases which mediate electron transport to NADP.</u> *J Bacteriol 1998 Mar; 180 (5): 1119-28.*

13. <u>Berg JM, Tymoczko JL, Stryer L. Biochemistry.</u> *WH Freeman and Company. 2002; 5th Ed: 480.*

14. <u>Mendz GL, Ball GE, Meek DJ, Pyruvate metabolism in Campylobacter spp.</u> *Biochim Biophys Acta 1997 Mar 15; 1334 (2-3) : 291-302.*

COLON CLEAR AND THE SENNA LEAVES EXTRACT PURGE

The published related article; *The Definitive Eradication of Helicobacter pylori from the Colon:* Published in Journal of General Medicine 2015; S1: 5. (Open Access). Nasrat et al. The definitive eradication of Helicobacter pylori from the colon. *General Med 2015; S1: 5. [doi: 10.4172/2327-5146.1000S1-005]*

The senna is an herb, the leaves and the fruit (seeds or pods) of this plant are used in medicinal preparations. The senna is an FDA-approved non-prescription laxative used to treat constipation. It contains senna glycosides called sennosides which are a group of organic compounds commonly found in plants. The effect of the senna is processed via a chain of fatty acids that promote its digestion and fermentation until finally conversion of these glycosides into a potent purgative. The senna seeds are gentler than the leaves and are used as mild laxative while the senna leaves (sennoside folium) are used as a potent purgative to treat severe forms of constipation, to help weight loss or clearing the bowel contents before diagnostic procedures such as colonoscopy.[1-3]

Data from observational findings did not report any side effects or hepato-toxic influence due to employment of the traditional doses of the senna leaves extract purge. The senna is a wild plant which is found in many countries, it has been used in India for thousands of years as a laxative. The senna leaves could be obtained from herbal or health food stores.[2,4,5]

It has been reported that the senna has got an antidiabetic, antibacterial, anti- inflammatory or antiseptic, antiviral and antihelminthic effects.[3,6-10] In further studies by the authors, it was found that addition of three times dilutions of the senna leaves extract is directly lethal to **Helicobacter pylori** culture media.[1,11,12]

As the senna leaves extract purge exists in many countries at least for many decades as a traditional remedy, therefore; the authors did their best to collect the mostly accepted method of its employment as approved by adequate sources in order to provide the best ideal way of using it. It was observed that the senna leaves purge differs from many medicinal or pharmaceutical preparations as with intake of ample amounts of warm drinks, it is very specific for clearing the colonic contents where diarrhea ceases spontaneously once the colonic contents are completely cleared out even the individual continues oral fluid intake; the fluids taken after clear of colonic contents will not be lost. The senna as a purgative respects the medical rules in causing no colic so long the user keeps drinking adequate amounts of warm drinks before and during the diarrhea; although many medicinal and pharmaceutical laxative preparations fall in this mistake leading in turn to habituation and intolerance. The senna purge restores and maintains the colonic function as it can be repeated only every one month (4 weeks, no less than 3 weeks) and the user has to reduce the dose gradually until reaching a minimal maintenance dose that causes watery diarrhea once or twice, this minimal dose (1/3-1/4 of a glass) could be repeated every 4-8 weeks for the purpose of keeping the colon clear. This means that the colon is depending upon itself in performing its integral function; that is unlike many medicinal and pharmaceutical laxatives where the patient has to increase the dose in order to achieve the same effect until intolerance could not be avoided. In addition to colon contents clear, the senna was found to kill and expel all the bacteria in the colon as checked and proved by **H. pylori** fecal antigen and culture sensitivity tests. Tamarind which is an herbal food staff is included in the constituents of the classic senna purge tradition, it helps to adsorb and fix the toxins in the colon, eliminating them out.[1]

The classic tradition of employing the senna leaves extract purge:

It is a soak method as the rule in herbs is to soak the leaves, boil the roots while seeds could be soaked for 5-10 minutes or boiled for 1-2 minutes.

1 cup (paper cup) of the senna leaves is used and should be cleaned from branches, seeds and impurities, wash in a pot, add 1 table spoon of Shamar (fennel) seeds, add 50 grams of dry Tamarind, add 1-3 spoons of sugar as required, honey, plant sugar or add artificial sweetener after it is prepared as concerns diabetic persons, soak altogether in 2 glasses/cups of boiled water late at night (3-4 hours only) until it is room temperature, filter and drink one cup (200 ml) only in the morning on empty stomach, then have only warm drinks and no food until diarrhea starts and stops, diarrhea starts within 3-4 hours, lasts for 3-4 times diarrhea within 1-2 hours almost. Drinks should be warm but never cold (like tea, tea with milk, green tea, soaked mint drink, soaked Shamar (fennel) seeds drink and clear soups), room temperature drinks such as water or juices could be permissible in few sips. After diarrhea stops, light soft diet but no meat such as boiled rice, macaroni and vegetables, also cheese and bread, can be taken until end of the day.

The next day: regular diet plus yoghurt with vinegar to complete disinfection of the gut.

The following 3-4 days: it is expected to have no bowel motions, it is not constipation or rebound effect to the purge but the colon is just clean and contents are insufficient to move the bowel. Therefore; bowel movement is encouraged by regular diet in addition to yoghurt mixed with white vinegar and corn oil twice daily with lunch and dinner until motion habit becomes regular, then it can be once or twice daily not necessary twice, 3-5 days a week not necessary every day.

The senna purge is recommended every month while a minimal maintenance dose (150 ml) could be repeated every 4-8 weeks as far as possible. The initial dose of the senna is meant to completely clear the colonic contents while the minimal dose is required to maintain the colon clear. The initial dose of the senna leaves purge is once monthly for three times while the maintenance senna could be every 4-8 weeks or even 4-12 weeks as a lifestyle.[1]

REFERENCES:

1. **Nasrat AM.** The world misconception and misbehavior towards Helicobacter pylori is leading to major spread of illness. *The 7th Anti-Aging Medicine World Congress, Monte-Carlo, Monaco, 2009 Mar.* Available from URL, *www.euromedicom.com*

2. **Rosenthal I, Wolfram E, Meier B. An HPLC method to determine sennoside A and sennosde B in Sennae frctus and Sennae folium.** *Pharmeur Bio Sci Notes 2014; 2014: 92-102.*

3. **Thilagam E, Parimaladevi B, Kumarappan C, et al. ⊠-Glucosidase and ⊠-amylase inhibitory activity of Senna surattensis.** *J Acupunct Meridian Stud 2013 Feb; 6 (1): 24-30.*

4. **Vitalone A, Di Giacomo S, Di Sotto A, et al. Cassia angustifolia extract is not hepatotoxic in an in vitro and in vivo study.** *Pharmacology 2011; 88 (5-6): 252-9.*

5. **Slva MG, Aragao TP, Vasconcelos CF, et al. Acute and subacute toxicity of Cassia occidentalis L. stem and leaf in Wistar rats.** *J Ethnopharmacol 2011 Jun 22; 136 (2): 341-6.*

6. **Varghese GK, Bose LV, Mabtemariam S. Antidiabetic components of Cassia alata leaves: identification through ⊠-glucosidase inhibition studies.** *Pharm Biol 2013 Mar; 51(3): 245-9.*

7. Keskin D, Toroglu S. **Studies on antimicrobial activities of solvent extracts of different species.** *J Environ Biol 2011 Mar; 32 (2): 251-6.*

8. Guarizel L, Costa JC, Dutra LB, et al. **Anti-inflammatory, laxative and intestinal motility effects of Senna macranthera leaves.** *Nat Prod Res 2012; 26 (4): 331-43.*

9. Quintero A, Fabbro R, Maillo M, et al. **inhibition of hepatitis B virus and human immunodeficiency virus (HIV-1) replication by Waescewiczia coccinea (Vahl) KI. (Rubiaceae) ethanol extract.** *Nat Prod Res 2011 Sep; 25 (16): 1565-9.*

10. Eguale T, Tadesse D, Giday M. **In vitro anthelmintic activity of crude extracts of five medicinal plants against egg-hatching and larval development of haemonchus contortus.** *J Ethnopharmacol 2011 Sep 1; 137 (1): 108-13.*

11. Nsarat SAM, Nasrat AM. **An alternative approach for the rising challenge of hypertensive illness via Helicobacter pylori eradication.** *J Cardiol Res 2015 Apr; 6 (1): 221-225.*

12. Nsarat RM, Nasrat MM, Nasrat AM, et al. **Improvement of idiopathic cardiomyopathy after colon clear.** *J Cardiol Res 2015 Apr; 6 (2): 249-254.*

THE ADVANTAGE OF FOLLOWING THE STRATEGIC INSTRUCTIONS OF THE "NEW CONCEPTS IN CONTROL OF DISEASE SPREAD"

Last but not least, what is the advantage of following the rules and instructions included in the "*New Concepts in Control of Disease Spread*"!!

For example, many patients with newly discovered diabetes could readily recover the diabetic condition and with simple carefulness towards out-side home meals can lead normal life. Other patients who do not recover the diabetic condition can adapt with time the biological stress condition caused by accumulation of toxins in the colon and can reach optimal control of their diabetes relying only on diet control without any need to use pills. Patients with established diabetes at least will enjoy good control of blood sugar upon their own medications; they might even be able to reduce these medications, therefore; they could maintain/ensure protection from diabetes complications in the foot and heart that result mainly from longstanding uncontrolled diabetes. A world with complications-free diabetes is not just a dream of the "*New Concepts in Medicine*" but it can be also a possible and an accessible target. Concerning childhood diabetes, the matter is most favorite as children are given insulin as earliest which gives the pancreas physiological rest avoiding over stress of the pancreas caused by the oral pills.

Again, most hypertensive patients could quit medications and maintain normal blood pressure values after colon clear. As regards cardiomyopathy, most cases of cardiomyopathy during latest decades are not due to viral myocarditis but toxic myocarditis, therefore; they could revert back to their normal achieving complete cure after elimination of potential toxins through colon clear employing natural measures. Similar promises could be also achieved with many other diseases.

It has got no sense to find and diagnose acid reflux in children without defining an underlying real pathologic etiology. Moreover, a person with spastic colonic symptoms would suddenly astonish and realize after following the natural measures in this book for colon care/colon clear that spastic colitis is a big scientific lie and that it was just illogic to swallow such amount of chemical pills for a long life.

Gout is not a disease of youg adults with perfeft kidney function unless there is an underlying missed pathology, definition of the real etiology is adequate to correct the condition. Also, endometriosis and ovarian cystic disease are being treated without decision of definite reasons, discovery and dealing with the real reasons could prevent these conditions and stop progress of any established illness at least.

If autism is not a disease of definitive cure when established but so long it could be a typical disease of definite prevention, hence the problem could have solution via following the natural measures of this book same as hopeless conditions such as poliomyelitis and small pox that have vanished after routine vaccination. Through following the proper natural measures of this book, Alzheimer disease also could be readily delayed until end of life of a person.

People can manage their obesity and dyslipidemia even enjoying their food and discover that dyslipidemia was the fake of last century; Paul Rosch has said that food is innocent towards dyslipidemia particularly animal source fat, he related dyslipidemia to a metabolic error but not the food itself while the most accepted pathologic etiology was precisely decided in the "*New Concepts in Disease Spread& Control of Disease Spread*" The scientific published articles of Paul Rosch have been mentioned within references of the related chapter of this book.

The strategic instructions of the "*New Concepts in Disease Spread& Control of Disease Spread*" could safely confirm that leukemia can never constitute an influenzea among youg adults and that vitamin D deficiency or osteoporosis can never run among people such as common or uncommon cold.

As it was mentioned that the two main hidden reasons behind major, chronic illness and cancer are the accumulation of toxic inflammatory mediators in the circulation and accumulation of potential toxins in the colon which together constitute around 90% of the reasons of curable diseases; the scientific references of these facts were included with the related articles of the book. Hence; three fundamental elements of the "*New Concepts of Control of Disease Spread*" which are the senna purge, vinegar therapy and cupping therapy are quite legable to achieve withdrawal and dealing with pathology of most current diseases. Accordingly and according to this scientific base-evidenced concept; which has got better advantage and benefit in therapy, to have more than one line of treatment of the modern medicine for every disease which are all neither successful or completely decisive or to have three fundamental therapies only for most diseases which are usually adequate and successful as concerns definitive cure!! Here lies a true valuable advantage of the "*New Concepts in Disease Spread& Control of Disease Spread*".

The "*New Concepts in Disease Spread& Control of Disease Spread*" is wishing that the current world's challenging burden of "*Disease Spread*" gets reverted back to its traditional figures and most patients could find solution for their condtions in this book in addition to the many people who could get protected from chronic and major illness.

Remarks: Colon clear means clear of colonic contents employing the senna leaves extract purge, while colon care with watching the colonic condition means getting rid of the abnormal-behavior gastric Helicobacter pylori strains before reaching the colon via intake of vinegar therapy-mixed food, avoiding foods known to the person to cause colonic upsets and carefulness towards outside-home meals.

The future Part II of the "New Concepts in Disease Spread& Control of Disease Spread"' is expected to include also new definitive strategic concepts for the control of spread of further many diseases. Until then, people can consult for any query concerning a current illness on the phone or e-mail as shown at end of the following chapter of questionnaires and queries.

HOW SHOULD THE WORLD MANAGE THE CHALLENGE OF HELICOBACTER PYLORI!!

The published related articles: *1. Misconception and Misbehavior towards Helicobacter pylori is leading to Major Spread of Illness:* Published in the Journal of General Medicine 2015; S1: 002. (Open Access). Nasrat et al. Misconception and misbehavior towards Helicobacter pylori is leading to major spread of illness. *General Med 2015; S 1: 002. [doi: 10.4172/2327-5146.1000S1-002]*

2. Biological benefits of Helicobacter pylori and the intelligence of juxta-mucosal ammonia: Published in the American Journal of Medicine and Medical Sciences; 2017; 7 (7): 281-286. Nasrat et al. Biological benefits of Helicobacter pylori and the intelligence of juxta-mucosal ammonia. *Am J Med Med Sci 2017; 7 (7): 281-286. [doi: 10.5923/j.ajmms.20170707.01]*

Now, should we fight and kill or save *Helicobacter pylori*!! We should save *H. pylori* for its huge biological benefits and the grave risk caused by forcing it to change behavior or shelter.[1,2] This hot exciting topic will be discussed in full details with all its published articles in the future volume III of "*New Concepts in Medicine*" which is "*New Concepts in Helicobacter pylori*".

The last three decades have shown prevalence of abnormal-behavior *H. pylori* strains and rising figures of many medical challenges related to these abnormal strains. It means that the last three decades demonstrated the rediscovery of *H. pylori*, the antibiotic aggression towards it, the prevalence of its abnormal-behavior strains instead of getting rid of it and the flare up of a lot of medical challenges related to these abnormal *H. pylori* strains.[1-3] A medical study which does not correlate between these obvious findings is definitely not employing a clinical sense.

H. pylori colonized the stomach since an immemorial time;[1] as if both the stomach wall and the bacterium used to live together in peace harmless to each other. *H. pylori* in the stomach leads a physiological behavior identical with that of natural bacteria; namely its existence since an immemorial time, having mostly-harmless long history inside the stomach before being attacked by antibiotics, its huge biological talents of survival inside the stomach and the fact of its unavoidable gastric recurrence. In addition to that, *H. pylori* is protective against reflux disease and the development of low acidity-related carcinoma of the cardia of stomach.[1,2]

Although eradications regimens seem to efficiently eradicate *H. pylori* from the stomach; the emergence of antibiotic-resistant *H. pylori* strains and the severe side effects are major drawbacks of these treatments.[1] Apparently *H. pylori* is not eradicated from the stomach but forced to migrate elsewhere, major complications therethen start as evidenced by the re-appearance of *H. pylori* in unusual existence exceeding limits of the stomach together with the development of new unusual symptoms and complications.[1,2] More efficient, economic and friendly drugs should be developed.

H. pylori could migrate or get forced to migrate to the colon under the influence of antibiotics where it will continue to produce ammonia for a reason or no reason leading to accumulation of profuse amounts of ammonia un-opposed or buffered by any acidity. Accumulation of profuse amounts of ammonia is toxic and constitutes a biological stress to the body that could lead to different adverse effects.[1-3]

Colon clear with the senna leaves extract purge and vinegar-mixed food therapy have been recently demonstrated effective towards the challenge of *H. pylori* including eradication of colonic and abnormal-behavior gastric *H. pylori* strains in addition to prevention of further gastric recurrence of abnormal *H. pylori* strains via query meals.[2,3]

H. pylori, being a natural bacterium,[1,2] could travel from stomach to stomach via meals. As long as rich people tour in poor countries and poor people travel to work in rich countries; therefore, bad *H. pylori* strains would in this way promote disease navigation from country to country all over the world.

Therefore; countries and health organizations should follow a strategic health policy towards *H. pylori*:

Peace should be started with the stomach bacterium *H. pylori* unless it is abnormal behavior or abnormal existence strains that cause frank dyspeptic symptoms and would lead to development of complications.

Cease all the fire and the antibiotic fight against *H. pylori* except natural measures so long it is nomal behavior/existence strains; normal strains do not cause bad symptoms, also undetectable by specific laborstory measures and they are always associated with good digestive and bowel functions.[2-4]

Allow all suitable climate for its stay and function inside the stomach by avoiding bad food habits and antibiotics unless strictly indicated; thanks for antibiotics but against *H. pylori*, no thanks. All regards to antibiotics in many fields and indications but against *H. pylori*, no thank you very much.

No medicine that attacks or annoys the stomach bacterium should be employed; proton pump inhibitors and gastric sedatives entailing anti-urease activity that destroys the main talent of *H. pylori* for survival in the stomach should be subjected to severe discussion and accurate re- determination.

Patients and family education as concerns misbehavior in food habits and antibiotic use as bad food habits pushes it to change behavior while inside the stomach while antibiotic abuse forces it to change shelter.

Orientation programs in primary health care units as concerns the natural manures towards *H. pylori*-related dyspepsia.

Stop searching and researching after *H. pylori* and redirect these research funds for raising life standards and sanitary water supply standards in poor and developing countries as rich people tour in poor countries and poor people travel to work in in rich countries; bad *H. pylori* strains in such way travel from stomach to stomach and from country to country promoting disease navigation all over the world.

Food handlers should strictly and frequently disinfect hands with vinegar and travelers should make vinegar a friend with their meals while touring.

REFERENCES:

1. **Farinha P, Gascoyne RD.** Helicobacter pylori and MALT Lymphoma. *Gastroenterology 2005 May; 128 (6): 1579-605.*

2. **Nasrat AM. The world misconception and misbehavior towards Helicobacter pylori is leading to major spread of illness.** *The 7th Anti-Aging Medicine World Congress, Monte-Carlo, Monaco, 2009 Mar.* **Available from URL,** *www.euromedicom.com*

3. **Nasrat SAM, Nasrat RM, Nasrat MM, et al. The dramatic spread of diabetes mellitus worldwide and influence of Helicobacter pylori.** *General Med J 2015; 3 (1): 159-62*

4. **Nasrat AM, Nasrat SAM, Nasrat RM, et al. Misconception and misbehavior towards Helicobacter pylori is leading to major spread of illness.** *Gen Med 2015; S1: 002.* **[Open Access]**

COMMON PATIENT'S AND PRACTITIONER'S QUESTIONNAIRES OR QUERIES:

How does this book depend upon vinegar therapy and the senna purge only for controlling all these diseases!! *The advanced knowledge of the modern medicine itself confirms that the abnormal strains of the bacterium Helicobacter pylori is behind a lot of chronic and major illness; the definitive control of the challenge of the abnormal strains of H. pylori is the natural therapy which is vinegar and the senna. In addition, it is a definite scientific fact that accumulation of potential toxins in the colon is the second main hidden reason behind major and chronic illness; the first reason being the accumulation of undesired elements and inflammatory mediators in circulation, colon care and colon clear via employing vinegar therapy and the senna purge are the most ideal, effective and simple way to deal with colonic toxins.*

If this book gives fundamental solutions for all these medical dilemmas, deos it mean that the knowledge included in this book deserve the Nobel Prize!! *The question should be reversed, does Nobel Prize deserve this book!! As Nobel Prize has been rewarded in 2005 for two Australian scientists who claimed the discovery/re-discovery of a stomach bug, we got it a bacterium surviving in the hell of the stomach acid, it should be the reason behind gastric ulcer and cancer and they suggested the antibiotic violence against it that was the start of human misery of chronic illness. The knowledge of this book corrects the mistake of the blind Nobel Justice towards an innocent bacterium and the world's health, hence it justifies the unfair medical battle against a tiny bacterium and towards humanity; accordingly, which deserves which!!*

How could the author or investigator of this book hold one medical speciality which is general surgery and is dealing with all these medical problems that still constitute challenges to specialts and scientists in their own field!! *That is the favor of having the background of Natural Fundamental Therapy Elements which is the reputation culture of the author.*

Can vinegar be diluted in water and taken in the morning on empty stomach!! *Vinegar is a food that includes health but not a medicine to be diluted diluted in water and taken on empty stomach; vinegar should be mixed wth salad and taken among the meal.*

Why it is white vinegar not apple cider vinegar!! *All vinegar is vinegar; acetic acid 5 or 6% but the whit vinegar especially the artificial or industrial is preferable because of low chance of faulty preparation during fermentation process as it happens to find famous brands of apple cider vinegar that smell alcohol and taste alcohol.*

Why it is corn oil not olive oil!! *The idea of the oil in vinegar therapy is to lubricate the bowel. Olive oil has got high nutritional value, so it is all absorbed and does not reach the colon to help as contact laxative unless it is old and oxidized where it not absorbed and causes loose stool. Corn oil is healthy, cholesterol free and of low fat contet but it is not of high nutritional value, therefore; good amount reaches the colon to work as laxative.*

Is vinegar harmful to throat or esophagus or can cause lower esophagitis!!: *Vinegar is not harmful to the mucosa; esophagitis that develops after drinking vinegar on empty stomach as advised by alternative therapists is due to forcing gastric H. pylori strains to migrate from stomach with loss of their protective value and consequent gastric acid reflux which is the reason of lower esophagitis in such situations.*

Could repeated monthly use of the senna leaves extract purge be of any harm to the colon!!: *Repeated employment of the senna purge on monthly basis has demonstrated no harm to colonic wall, even weekly use includes no harm to the colonic wall but it is against the principle of the senna purge therapy because of leaving no chance for the colon to practice its function; the monthly basis of the senna is indicated so that the colon can restore and perform its function.*

Why the senna is used every month not every week!! *The monthly basis of the senna is indicated so as to give the chance to restore and maintain the colonic function.*

How can vinegar therapy be supplied to children!! *Vinegar therapy (yoghurt/vinegar/oil) can be blended with honey and fruits such as orange with banana or apricot with strawberry.*

What is the dose of vinegar and oil in vinegar therapy!!: *Vinegar is a food but not a medicine and corn oil is a food staff; therefore, the amount of vinegar and corn oil in vinegar therapy is not a fixed dose but can be adjusted as desired and could be dealt with exactly as the amount of salt in food which is added according to what is palatable by the person; It is approximately one or two table spoonful of each of them on a salad dish or small cup of yoghurt.*

What are the purposes of using vinegar for children!!: *Vinegar therapy is healthy to children helping digestion and bowel motion in addition to management of medical problems related to the abnormal-behavior strains of Helicobacter pylori.*

What is against the apple vinegar in your view!! *All types of vinegar are acetic acid 5-6%, the main healthy value of vinegar is due to the acetic acid and not the contents of the apple juice, vinegar of apple cider has got the disadvantage of being commercial, acceleration of fermentation for commercial reasons would leave residual alcohol traces, therefore; best vinegar is white vinegar even industrial as it never include alcoholic smell or taste.*

What yoghurt to use, full-cream, low-fat or skimmed!!: *Full cream yoghurt because of its adequate content of the healthy lactic acid that also assists the antibacterial effect of vinegar. There should be no worry from the yoghurt fat as it is animal fat, the human body consumes the required energy to the body and the fat soluble vitamins (A, D, E& k) while the rest is lost in the colon helping to lubricate motion.*

How to choose between different brands of yoghurt!!: *Choose the brand which when left sealed outside freege for 1-3 days leaves a liquid on top which is the lactic acid of yoghurt and the yoghurt itself gets more sour meaning that preservatives are less and fermentation goes on producing healthy probiotics.*

How to get a pure corn oil!!: *The content of oil in corn is not commercial; therefore, ideal or pure corn oil is supplemented with medicinal, artificial or mineral oils like parafin oil which are cholesterol/fat free and even non-absorbable, it does not withstand frying as it gets dried, more important it does not cause upsets when mixed with salad. If corn oil is mixed with hydrogenated oils like palm or sunflower oil which are made for frying not eating, hence it could withstand frying and it causes stomach upsets when taken with salad or food.*

Questions and queries could be answered via the e-mails:
abdullahmnasrat@gmail.com
abdullahalnasrat@hotmail.com
Phone: +966 (0) 5651 37361
Future Publications
"New Concepts in Helicobacter pylori"
"New Concepts in Blood-Let out Cupping Therapy"
"New Concepts in Fundamental Therapy& Definitive Cure"
"New Concepts in Natural Nutritional Drug-Free Therapy"
"New Concepts in Physio-Benefits of Human Body Balance"

Scientific Research Activity of the Author Published with Digital Object Identification (doi) in International medical journals; mostly American and Canadian

1. The Dramatic spread of diabetes mellitus worldwide and influence of Helicobacter pylori. *Published in General Med 2015; 3 (1): 159. [doi: 10.4172/2327-5146.1000159]*

2. An alternative approach for the rising challenge of hypertensive illness via Helicobacter pylori eradication. *Published in J Cardiol Res 2015; 6 (1): 221-225. [doi: 10.14740/cr382e]* Epub 2015 Feb 9. PubMed PMID: 28197229; PubMed Central PMCID: PMC5295557.

3. Improvement of idiopathic cardiomyopathy after colon clear. *Published in J Cardiol Res 2015 Apr; 6 (2): 249-254. [doi: 10.14740/cr398e]* Epub 2015 Apr 6. PubMed PMID: 28197234; PubMed Central PMCID: PMC5295537.

4. Functional Dyspepsia. *Published in General Med 2015; 3 (3): 192. [doi: 10.4172/2327-5146.1000192]*

5. Role of blood-let out cupping therapy in angina and angina risk management. *Published in General Med 2015; 3(3): 191. [doi: 10.4172/2327-5146.1000191]*

6. Role of blood-let out cupping therapy in taming the wild hepatitis B virus. *Published in Intern J Recent Sci Res Jul 2015; 6 (7): 5049-5051. [Open Access]:* Available at International Journal of Recent Scientific Research (www.recentscientific.com)

7. An influence of Helicobacter pylori in thrombocytopenia in children. *Published in Intern J Recent Sci Res Jul 2015; 6 (7): 5052-5054. [Open Access]:* Available at International Journal of Recent Scientific Research (www.recentscientific.com)

8. An alternate natural remedy for symptomatic relief of Helicobacter pylori dyspepsia. *Published in General Med 2015; 3 (4): 1000200. [doi: 10.4172/2327-5146.1000200]*

9. The challenge of childhood diabetes. *Published in General Med 2015; 3 (4): 193. [doi: 10.4172/2327-5146.1000193]*

10. Diabetic leg critical ischemia; early clinical detection and therapeutic cupping prophylaxis. *Published in General Med 2015; 3 (4): 1000201. [doi: 10.4172/2327-5146.1000201]*

11. Characteristics of Helicobacter pylori-related dysglycemia. *Published in General Med 2015; S1: 4. [doi: 10.4172/2327-5146.1000S1-004]*

12. Are tonsils and adenoids secondary reservoirs for Helicobacter pylori in children? Why it matters!! *Published in General Med 2015; S1: 6. [doi: 10.4172/2327-5146.1000S1-005]*

13. The definitive eradication of Helicobacter pylori from the colon. *Published in General Med 2015; S1: 5. [doi: 10.4172/2327-5146.1000S1-005]*

14. Therapeutic effect of combined colon clear and cupping therapy on idiopathic skin pathology. *Published in General Med 2015; 3 (5): 209. [doi: 10.4172/2327-5146.1000209]*

15. Why do physicians diagnose gout in young adults with perfect kidney function!!. *Published in General Med 2015; 3 (5): 208. [doi: 10.4172/2327-5146.1000208]*

16. Role of blood-let out cupping therapy in female pelvic congestion syndrome. *Published in General Med 2015; S1: 3. [doi: 10.4172/2327-5146.1000S1-003]*

17. A comparative study of natural eradication of Helicobacter pylori Vs antibiotics. *Published in General Med 2015; S1: 1. [doi: 10.4172/2327-5146.1000S1-001]*

18. Misconception and misbehavior towards Helicobacter pylori is leading to major spread of illness. *Published in General Med 2015; S1: 2. [doi: 10.4172/2327-5146.1000S1-002]*

19. The biology of combined colon clear and blood-let out cupping therapy in female health. *Published in General Med 2015; 3 (4): 203. [doi: 10.4172/2327-5146.1000203]*

20. The real fact in irritable bowel syndrome. *Published in General Med 2015; 3(6): 213. [doi: 10.4172/2327-5146.1000213]*

21. New approach for hidden reasons behind cervical disc pathology during late decades. *Published in General Med 2015; 3 (6): 214. [doi: 10.4172/2327-5146.1000214]*

22. Endometriosis and ovarian cystic disease; why so linked as if born simultaneous!! *Published in General Med 2016; 4 (1): 1000221. [doi:10.4172/2327-5146.1000221]*

23. Male pelvic congestion; obscure reasons for an obvious phenomenon among the young. *Published in General Med 2016; 4 (2): 1000236. [doi: 10.4172/2327-5146.1000236]*

24. Hematologic challenges of Helicobacter pylori in children. *Published in General Med 2015; 3 (6): 1000212. [doi: 10.4172/2327-5146.1000212]*

25. A therapeutic answer for the controversy of insulin cardio-protection among dysglycemic patients. *Published in General Med 2015; 3 (6): 1000216. [doi: 10.4172/2327-5146.1000216]*

26. Hepatitis C virus; its eradication from the circulation is just possible. *Published in General Med 2016; 4 (3): 1000249. [doi: 10.4172/2327-5146.1000249]*

27. How should the world manage the challenge of diabetes mellitus!! *Published in General Med 2016; 4 (1): 1000223. [doi: 10.4172/2327-5146.1000223]*

28. Frequency of leukemia during late decades may indicate that the anti-Helicobacter pylori antibiotic strategy was a therapeutic mistake. *Published in Am J Med Med Sci 2017; 7 (3): 103-107. [doi: 10.5923/j.ajmms.20170703.03]*

29. A biologic influence on the integrity of the natural desire, sense of libido and sexual drive. *Published in Intl J Health Sci Res 2017; 7 (3): 250-255. [Open Access]:* Available at International Journal of Health Sciences & Research (www.ijhsr.org)

30. Stop fighting the stomach bacterium Helicobacter pylori; esophageal reflux was not as such before the anti-H. pylori antibiotics. *Published in Am J Med Med Sci 2017; 7 (4): 196-201. [doi: 10.5923/j.ajmms.20170704.07]*

31. Autism; an approach for definite etiology and definitive etiologic management. *Published in Am J Med Med Sci 2017; 7 (5): 108-118. [doi: 10.5923/j.ajmms.20170703.04]*

32. Alzheimer and Helicobacter pylori; should we fight and kill or save H. pylori!! We should save H. pylori. *Published in Am J Med Med Sci 2017; 7 (5): 221-228. [doi: 10.5923/j.ajmms.20170705.03]*

33. Autism and Alzheimer; the etio-pathologic twins. *Published in Am J Med Med Sci 2017; 7 (6): 277-280. [doi: 10.5923/j.ajmms.20170706.07]*

34. The secret of the silence of the silent maxillary sinus syndrome. *Published in Am J Med Med Sci 2017; 7 (6): 242-247. [doi: 10.5923/j.ajmms.20170706.03]*

35. Biological benefits of Helicobacter pylori and the intelligence of juxta-mucosal ammonia. *Published in Am J Med Med Sci 2017; 7 (7): 281-286. [doi: 10.5923/j.ajmms.20170707.01]*

36. The scientific theory in cupping therapy. *Published in Am J Med Med Sci 2017; 7 (7): 302-307. [doi: 10.5923/j.ajmms.20170707.03]*

37. A pathologic etiology for the rising world challenge of obesity and dyslipidemia during latest three decades. *Am J Med Med Sci 2017; 7 (8): 318-322. [doi: 10.5923/j.ajmms.20170708.03]*

38. A simple sustained solution for dissolution of the cellulite. *Am J Med Med Sci 2017; 7 (9):331-337. [doi: 10.5923/j.ajmms.20170709.02]*

39. The hidden truth behind osteoporosis and vitamin D deficiency. *Am J Med Med Sci 2017; 7 (11):369-377. [doi: 10.5923/j.ajmms.20170711.02].*

CPSIA information can be obtained
at www.ICGtesting.com
Printed in the USA
LVHW070402250520
656347LV00007B/309